Hutchison's Clinical Methods

Seventeenth Edition

STUART MASON MD, FRCP
Consultant Physician to The London Hospital

MICHAEL SWASH MD, MRCP
Consultant Physician to The London Hospital

D0543474

BAILLIÈRE TINDALL · LONDON

A BAILLIÈRE TINDALL book published by
Cassell Ltd.,
35 Red Lion Square, London WC1R 4SG

and at Sydney, Auckland, Toronto, Johannesburg

an affiliate of
Macmillan Publishing Co. Inc.
New York

First published 1897
Sixteenth edition 1975
  Reprinted 1976, 1978
Seventeenth edition 1980

ISBN 0 7020 0801 X

Educational Low-priced Book Series Edition 1980
Spanish edition (Salvat Editores, Barcelona) 1972

Set by D. P. Media Limited, Hitchin, Hertfordshire and printed in
Great Britain by Hazell Watson and Viney Ltd, Aylesbury, Bucks

British Library Cataloguing in Publication Data

Hutchison, *Sir* Robert, *bart*
  Hutchison's clinical methods. – 17th ed.
  1. Diagnosis
  I. Mason, Stuart   II. Swash, Michael
  616.07′5   RC71

  ISBN 0-7020-0801-X

Contents

List of Plates

Preface

In 1897, Robert Hutchison began his preface: 'The title *Clinical Methods* probably describes the scope of this book better than any other. It is not intended as a treatise upon medical diagnosis. On that subject there is already a sufficiency of good works in existence. It aims rather at describing those methods of clinical investigation by the proper application of which a correct diagnosis can alone be arrived at. To every student when he first begins work in a medical ward the question presents itself: How shall I investigate this case? To that question the present work is intended to provide an answer. The first chapter deals, therefore, with the methods of case-taking in general, and includes a general scheme for the investigation of medical cases. The rest of the book is really an expansion of that scheme, each system being taken up separately, and the methods of investigating it described in detail.'

Six years have elapsed since the 16th edition of *Hutchison's Clinical Methods*. Once again the book has undergone a thorough revision and on this occasion we have taken the opportunity to replace some of the older illustrations. This seventeenth edition contains several new chapters. In particular those on haematology and the abdomen are entirely new and we have added a chapter on the examination of the unconscious patient. Despite these changes, the aim of the book is unchanged. We cannot express this more clearly than in the words of Robert Hutchison's preface to his first edition of 1897.

Richard Bomford has now retired from editorship, but his wise influence can be seen still. Donald Hunter, that great teacher, died in 1978. We are greatly indebted to all our colleagues, who are listed in the acknowledgements for their contributions to this edition but responsibility for any errors or omissions is ours.

January 1980

STUART MASON
MICHAEL SWASH

Acknowledgements

We wish to thank the following for their help:

F. P. Marsh, MB, FRCP	The Urine
H. O. F. Currey, MMed, FRCP	Examination of Joints
A. D. M. Jackson, MD, FRCS, DCH	Examination of Children
D. T. D. Hughes, MB, FRCP	The Respiratory System
G. G. Jenkins, MD, FRCP	Haematology
B. T. Colvin, MB, MRCP	Haematology
D. Maclean, MB, FRCS	The Abdomen
A. MacDonald, MB, FRCP	The Cardiovascular System
A. W. Morrison, MB, FRCS, DLO	The Ear
P. Mckelvie, MD, ChM, FRCS, DLO	The Nose and Throat
A. Mushin, MB, FRCS, DO	The Eye
J. Pegum, MD, FRCP	The Skin

S.M.
M.S.

1

Case taking

It is easy to talk of the principles of medicine but difficult to provide accurate succinct definitions. One statement that gets near to the truth is that 'diagnosis should precede treatment whenever possible'. There are two steps in making a diagnosis. The first is observation by history taking, physical examination and ancillary investigations. The second is interpretation of the information obtained in terms of a disorder of function and structure, then in terms of pathology. This book is about observation rather than interpretation; pathology, the study of disease, is largely outside its scope. However, information and interpretation go hand in hand. The nature of further observation is determined by interpretation of information already obtained. In practice, of course, patients do not present with a diagnosis; they come with problems. The wise doctor does not think of himself as a diagnostician but rather as someone who elucidates human problems.

THE HISTORY

The aim is to get from the person concerned an accurate account of his complaint and to see this against the background of his life as a whole. The findings should be recorded under the following headings:

1. Presenting complaint
2. History of present illness
3. Previous history of illness
4. Menstrual history
5. Treatment history
6. Family history
7. Social and occupational history

Some doctors prefer to record the patient's social and occupational history and the past and family histories before the history of the presenting complaint, since the patient's presenting illness is then viewed more clearly in the context of what has happened before. Further, it is often wise to find out about the patient's life, at least to some degree, before tackling the presenting illness itself. However, in taking the history it is neither possible nor desirable to tie a patient down to any particular sequence. He must be allowed to tell his story in his own way. Further, a good doctor begins the examination of a patient as the latter walks into the room—his general appearance, the way he walks, the way he answers questions and so on—and only finishes taking the history when the consultation is over. Occasionally a vital piece of information may come out just when the patient is leaving.

The list of headings may appear formidable and it does take some experience to know in a given case which part of the history is particularly worth pursuing. If, for instance, the patient's complaint is undue bleeding, a careful *family history* may virtually make the diagnosis. If he has chest symptoms, the fact that he worked with asbestos even twenty years earlier (*occupational history*) may be the vital clue. If his complaints are those of a severe anaemia, the fact that he has been treated with chloramphenicol (*treatment history*) may be all-important. If he has a fever, the fact that his plane put down in West Africa (*social history*) may be the clue. These are rare examples; more commonly it may be his *social circumstances*—his relations with his wife or his employer—that are at fault. When students start case taking they are wise to make at least some enquiry under all the headings listed. When they have had more experience, they may know on which they should concentrate; but in a difficult case even the most experienced doctor would be unwise to neglect any of the headings listed.

In a simple case—provided one can be sure that the case in point is simple—a few direct questions may obtain all the necessary information. In a difficult one it is best just to let the patient talk, even if the process seems time-consuming. One should 'listen to the patient telling one the diagnosis': the woman complaining of an itching skin rash may end her story with a remark that her husband irritates her.

History taking is a *special form of the art of communication*. It is necessarily a two-way business. At an intellectual level it is important that doctors and students, as well as patients, should confine themselves to words the meaning of which cannot easily be misunderstood. At a deeper level there is no doubt that some doctors inspire confidence in patients and some do not. A better understanding of what is referred to as the doctor–patient relationship can be developed by active participation in sensitivity groups of the kind pioneered for doctors in this country by the late Dr Michael Balint. Members of such groups hope to gain insight into their own personalities and so to acquire greater skill in interpersonal relationships in general and in the doctor–patient relationship in particular.

Doctors often tend to overlook the importance of *non-verbal forms of communication*, which play a big part in their relationships with their patients. The eyes sometimes convey more information than words; the clenched fist may demonstrate latent tension, and touch may be equally important.

There is a taboo in our culture against the touching of other humans, though this does not extend to horses and dogs. If you are one of those with inhibitions about touch, then on the next occasion that you visit a frightened old lady in hospital try holding her hand. You may well find that when you want to withdraw it, she will grip so that release is difficult; and next time you visit, the hand will be there waiting to be held. For the old lady finds the touch of your hand much more comforting than all your carefully phrased verbal reassurance.

When it comes to physical examination, does the patient feel the doctor's touch as an attack or a caress? There is nothing new in such a suggestion: a distinguished surgeon wrote that abdominal palpitation, to be successful, must be like a caress. Patients often derive great satisfaction from being examined, albeit just the taking of the pulse or blood pressure. It may well be that non-verbal means of communication of this sort go a long way to explaining why some doctors inspire more confidence than others.

It is important to realize that *apparent evasiveness* on the part of the patient is almost never deliberate. It can occasionally be due to sub-normal intelligence, but is much more often due to nervousness or actual fright. One must realize that a visit to the doctor or by a doctor is a real ordeal for some patients, quite as bad as a *viva voce* for some students; for the doctor, like the examiner, may be felt at the margins of consciousness to be an all-powerful figure. Thus on approaching a patient who does not know you, tell him who you are and why you have come to see him. Greet him by his own name whenever possible. It is often wise to open the interview with some entirely non-committal chat in the hope that a friendly relationship and some confidence may be established. The discovery of a common county of origin or a common interest in bowls may work wonders. Make clear that the patient has your whole attention. Invite confidence. Your stance and facial expression should assure the patient that you will not be shocked or angered by what he says. Inattention or the continuous writing of notes will put off the patient as he tells his story.

There is another and more subtle reason for apparent evasiveness. Sometimes the symptoms are psychological ones and the patient has difficulty in describing them precisely. Moreover, physical illness is respectable but many people and some doctors consider that psychological symptoms are not. There is therefore a tendency to present the doctor with a physical symptom, though the complaints are really psychological, and the patient comes to the doctor with a rather vague physical discomfort. Only later may he be able to say that everything is flat and hopeless, and that life is not worth living, or in other words that he is depressed. An anxious patient may present with discomfort in any system or organ in the body, but only later may he be able to voice his ever-present feeling that something awful is going to happen. Indeed this feeling has become so much a part of him that he is almost unaware of it. Evasiveness is, of course, particularly common when the real problem is a sexual one. It is important that the doctor recognizes the reason for the apparent evasiveness of his patients and does not get angry with them. Unfortunately doctors vary greatly in their ability to tolerate patients with psychological problems. If a patient does in fact make one angry, it is useless simply to try and suppress the feeling. It is much better to say, 'I am afraid I find what you are saying difficult to follow. Let's start again.'

In spite of a huge proliferation of ancillary aids, *history taking and physical examination remain essential skills for the doctor*, if only for two simple reasons. Those who work in large modern hospitals are apt to forget that most of the world's population have to be treated either where there are no ancillary aids or where these are very restricted. Even where these aids are freely available, they are in varying degrees costly and are not without discomfort or risk to the patient. It was the original author of this book who wrote: 'From making the cure of the disease more grievous than the endurance thereof, good Lord deliver us.'

Special investigations should therefore be used with discretion; that is, they should be used selectively, when simpler clinical methods have indicated what further investigations are likely to be profitable. It is our view too that no doctor should request any special investigation unless he knows what information relevant to the problem it is likely to provide, and has some idea of its cost and of its possible dangers to the patient.

Thus case taking—the taking of histories and the performance of physical examinations under supervision during the period of medical clerking—remains an essential part of medical education. In this first chapter we deal with history taking and physical examination in general terms. In later chapters we shall elaborate by considering different systems individually and the book ends with a short section about cooperation with the laboratory.

There is no one method of history taking applicable to all patients in all situations. The method will vary according to whether the history is being taken in the wards, the out-patient clinic, the surgery or the home, and according to the state of the patient and the time available. It is wise to open a non-urgent consultation with some general question such as 'What can I do for you?' This gives the patient an opportunity to say what he wants from the consultation. To know this at the outset may be valuable and may indeed save time. Here we attempt to describe the methods that we think should be used by students undertaking medical clerking in hospital. We shall consider these for convenience under the headings mentioned above, but must emphasize once more that patients cannot be tied down to an orderly sequence. They must be allowed as far as possible to tell their story in their own words and in their own way. Only when they have done this should they be asked to enlarge on what appear to be the more important aspects of the story and only after that should specific questions be asked. Personal history taking must never become a stereotyped routine of asking standard questions and recording the answers, though questionnaires may be useful for special purposes.

The presenting complaint

Try to define the main complaint and its duration. The presenting complaint is simply the complaint which made the patient come to the doctor. The remarks above about apparent evasiveness may apply here, but most patients with physical disease have no difficulty. They have pain in the belly or headache or shortness of breath. In writing up the history students should avoid the temptation to include a mini-history under the presenting complaint. In most cases there is one symptom which made the patient come to the doctor and ideally this is all that should be included under this heading. One must admit, however, that some patients have more than one main complaint and a few have so many that it is impossible to identify a presenting complaint.

The question of duration may be difficult. First, many people, particularly the elderly, cannot remember the duration of their symptoms. One could indeed regard this as the normal state of affairs and suspect the patient who can remember every detail of his illness of being unduly introspective and hypochondriacal.

Most patients with long-standing symptoms tend to date them by events rather than by years, even though there is no causal relationship. The symptoms started 'after my husband died' or 'at the time of the last General Election'. With patience it is possible to get at the likely duration. After that it is wise to ask some such question as 'Did you ever have anything wrong before that?' or even 'When were you last perfectly well?' In this way earlier symptoms, which the patient regards as unimportant, may be revealed. One should remember too that patients often use the word 'chronic' to mean 'severe', rather than of prolonged duration.

The history of the present illness

Ask the patient to tell you the story of his illness from the beginning. Ideally you should allow him to do this without interruption, but this may be a counsel of perfection. It may require some tactful encouragement to make a dour or nervous patient tell you his story at all, while some talkative ones cannot keep anywhere near the point. A particular difficulty is the patient who will use pseudo-medical terms or terms of which he does not know the medical meaning. Patients who insist on talking about rheumatism, migraine, acidity, catarrh or disc should be gently discouraged and asked to describe what they actually feel to be wrong. Others will insist on talking about 'what my other doctors said'.

When the patient has told you all that he will spontaneously, ask him to enlarge on any points that you may think to be important. Also try to clear up any doubt about the time of onset and the duration of the main symptoms. Some patients have symptoms which come and go, and it is important to try to find out whether the relapses and remissions are related in any way to times, seasons or events in the patient's life.

When you think that you have the patient's story clearly, you should take each main symptom in turn and examine it in detail. The first step is to try to make sure that you and the patient are talking about the same thing. A patient may, for instance, complain of wind or flatulence. Since flatus is considered in our culture to be an indelicate subject, it may be assumed that he means bringing up wind, whereas he may well mean passing wind by the bowel; or he may mean that he has a feeling that he wants to get rid of wind but is unable to do so. One must therefore enquire directly: 'Do you mean that you bring the wind up or that you pass it down or that you feel that you want to get rid of it but can't?' It should be unnecessary to point out that one should avoid leading questions, which themselves suggest the answer expected, as far as possible, but some questions, such as 'Have you ever spat blood?' may be essential.

Perhaps the commonest complaint which brings a patient to a doctor is a *pain* of some sort and this will serve to illustrate one way in which this nature of a symptom can be further explored.

Ask about the following points:

Site.   Where is it? Note whether the patient points to one spot or spreads his hands over a wide area.

Radiation.   Does it stay in one place or does it move or spread?

Severity.   Does it interfere with his activities and does it ever keep him awake at night? If it never interferes in any way with his activities and never keeps him awake at night, he is probably talking about what should properly be called discomfort. Patients who use such exaggerated terms as continual agony are usually seeking sympathy and one should try to discover the real reason for their distress, which is often social or psychological.

Timing.   When did it start? When does it come and when does it go?

Character.   What is it like? Most descriptions of the character of a pain, e.g. stabbing, burning, pricking or gnawing, are unhelpful. A distinguished professor of medicine pointed out that to describe a pain as gnawing really conveys no information unless the listener has had the experience of being gnawed. Yet, said the professor, some patients will not only describe a pain as gnawing but will 'specify the species of rodent concerned'. On the other hand the distinction between a colic, which waxes and wanes and may cause a patient to roll about, and a steady pain like that of peritonitis, which causes the patient to try to avoid all movement, may be very important.

The following points are often particularly helpful in deducing what disturbance of normal function is responsible for the pain:

Occurrence or aggravation. What brings it on? And what makes it worse? A pain in the centre of the chest which always comes on after a certain amount of exertion, or is made worse by exertion, is almost certainly due to ischaemia of the heart. A very similar pain which comes on a short time after eating is probably oesophageal.

Relief. What makes it better? Pains may be relieved by simple measures. Pain arising in the musculoskeletal system for instance, may be relieved by a change of position. Upper gastrointestinal pains, e.g. duodenal ulcer, are usually promptly relieved by eating. Lower gastrointestinal pains are relieved by defaecation or the passage of wind. Many cardiac pains, brought on by exertion, are relieved by rest. Any definite relief by simple things of this sort may be a valuable clue to the disturbance of function or structure involved.

The effect of drugs may also be of diagnostic value. Ischaemic cardiac pain is usually promptly relieved by trinitrites. Musculo-skeletal pains are usually relieved by simple analgesics like aspirin, while discomforts associated with stress and tension are not. Most physical back pains are therefore relieved to some extent by aspirin, while tension pains usually are not so relieved. In the rare event of a back pain made worse by aspirin, one would have to think of an abdominal cause, e.g. a peptic ulcer adherent to the posterior abdominal wall.

Pain is a symptom which can usually only be further explored in clinical terms. It may, however, be possible to explore other symp-toms, thirst for example, in more precise physiological terms.

Thirst must first be distinguished from the dry mouth of oral infections or of defective salivary secretion; occasional patients with neurosis or compulsive water drinking may complain of thirst. But it is most commonly the prime symptom of loss of body water (with or without loss of salt). The principal causes of loss of body water are diminished intake, vomiting, diarrhoea, increased sweating, increased output of urine and severe haemorrhage. Observation or simple questions will therefore uncover the immediate disorder of function or functions that are responsible for the symptom, but further questions and investigations may be necessary to explain it in terms of pathology.

If, for instance, the thirst appears to be due to loss of body water due to increased urinary output, one must recall that the huge output of urine of low specific gravity of diabetes insipidus and the similar output of urine of high specific gravity (due to glucose) of diabetes mellitus can both cause severe thirst. The passage of large amounts of urine with a specific gravity of 1010 (isotonic with plasma) in renal failure may be sufficient to cause thirst. Hypercalcaemia, by diminishing the action of antidiuretic hormone and so increasing water loss, may produce thirst and finally the administration of diuretics (or even excessive tea or coffee drinking) may promote salt and water loss with increased urine volume and so thirst.

These two examples—pain and thirst—will serve to illustrate different ways in which all important symptoms should be explored, with the object of identifying, if possible, the disturbance of function and/or structure responsible for them.

While concerning oneself with the details of a patients' symptoms it is important not to lose sight of what may be called the shape of the illness. Is it something that began insidiously and has gradually got worse up to the present time? Or something intermittent? Or something which began acutely and is slowly getting better, but has not yet gone? Sometimes this shape of the illness may be more significant than individual symptoms.

Another valuable question in patients with long-standing symptoms (particularly psychological ones) is: '*What made you decide to come and see me at this particular time?*' The answer is sometimes illuminating. It may well be: 'I wouldn't have dreamt of coming, but my wife made me', or it may be because an acquaintance has recently died with what appeared to the patient to be rather similar symptoms.

On pages 14–24 there is a scheme, arranged under systems, of the kind of questions that doctors usually ask when taking a history. Such a scheme is of limited value. When the patient has told his story and the stage of examining individual symptoms is reached, the doctor should be asking himself first, 'Are we both talking about the same thing?' and then, 'What does this thing (i.e. symptom) mean in terms of disturbance of function and/or structure?' and should be framing his questions accordingly, rather than be repeating a list of standard questions. It is usual, however, to conclude the history of the present illness with a brief review of the other systems which do not appear to be implicated.

Previous history of illness

The previous history should include all important illnesses from infancy onwards. Beware of accepting ready-made diagnoses, particularly, as explained above, in the case of such terms as influenza, arthritis, rheumatism and so on. Even if more precise diagnostic terms are used, it is wise to ask a few questions about the nature of the illness to check whether the diagnosis seems likely. Questions about common infections should usually include a tactful enquiry about venereal disease and its treatment.

In some cases it may be necessary to communicate with doctors or hospitals that have treated the patient in the past to obtain information necessary for correct treatment. The name and, if possible, the address of the doctor or hospital concerned with the treatment of a previous illness should therefore be recorded, together with the name and address of the patient at the time of the previous illness, if this has changed in the interval, and in the case of a married woman her name before marriage.

The menstrual history

Women should be asked about menstruation. In the majority of cases menstruation occurs every 28 days, but the intervals may be longer or shorter according to the patient's habit. Ask at what age menstruation began and if menstruation has ceased, ask how long it has been absent. The menopause usually occurs about the forty-fifth year or later. Enquire also whether the patient is losing more or less blood than usual. The menstrual flow is to be regarded as abnormal if it lasts for fewer than 2 or more than 8 days. Ask about premenstrual tension and about the presence or absence of pain at the periods; and ask whether the patient is or has been taking oral contraceptives.

The treatment history

The treatment history should include details of drugs taken, including psychotropic drugs, surgery, radiotherapy and psychotherapy. Adverse reactions to drugs, including hypersensitivities (especially to penicillin) are most important. A major difficulty is that patients may not be able to remember, nor may any record exist, about past treatments. Many of his remedies may in any case have been bought across the counter. In this case, and probably always, it helps to ask about remedies taken for particular complaints, e.g. 'What do you take when you have a headache?'; 'What do you take for the bowels?' Patients' memories can be aided by asking them to bring up the whole contents of their medicine store. It is often extensive and outdated. Relatives often remember more than the patient if he is very old, very young or mentally sick. It is important to discover not only whether someone was given a drug to take, but whether he took it and for the appropriate time. If the drugs were not taken as prescribed, the reasons for them not being taken must be discovered. Patients frequently do not comply with instructions. Vocabulary matters: medicines often mean something liquid or something sold in a pharmacy; drugs may mean doctors' prescriptions or illicit narcotics to a patient; and tablets may not be distinguished from capsules. It is often better to ask a patient what remedies he took for particular complaints and whether these ever disagreed with him, than to use technical terms. Drug manufacturers can usually help with the names of unusual drugs imported from overseas. Much difficulty would be avoided if all doctors used official rather than proprietary names.

The family history

Note the patient's position in the family and the ages of the children if any. Usually it is only necessary to record the state of health, the important illnesses and the cause of death of immediate relatives. If, however, there is any question of an hereditary disorder one should enquire about all known relations and attempt to contruct a family tree showing those affected and those not affected.

The social and occupational history

Enquire about what may be grouped together as the patient's physical and emotional environment, his surroundings both at home and work, his habits and his own mental attitude to life and to his work. Try to visualize his life, sharing his emotions and viewing step by step his home, family, daily habits, diet and work. It may help to ask him to give an account of a typical day. Ask about:

1. The *exact nature of his occupation* (not just the name of his trade but what precisely his work involves) and whether it exposes him to injurious influences. Former occupations should also be noted. One should ask about his attitude to his work, his employers and his workmates. Sometimes one should enquire into a patient's business affairs and the possibility of financial worries.

2. His *domestic and marital relationships*, his feelings about other members of his family, his interests, hobbies, hopes, fears, the holidays he gets and whether he enjoys them, the amount of exercise he takes, the games he plays, and, in general, the sort of life he leads and the sort of person he is.

3. His *home surroundings*, their sanitary condition and the possible existence of overcrowding or of loneliness. What pets does he keep? Where did they come from and were they recently imported?

4. His *diet* and his *use of alcohol and tobacco*. It is important to ask about past habits in these respects. A man who says that he neither drinks nor smokes may have been a heavy drinker or smoker in the past. Remember too that many alcoholics will convincingly deny their dependence. Distinguish between cigarette smoking and pipe or cigar smoking.

5. *Whether or not he has lived abroad* and if so whether he was ill there. Recent travel may be important; a patient may for instance suffer from malaria in the U.K. if he has recently travelled from or even through a malarious area.

The psychiatric history

Patients coming to a general physician may resent psychiatric case taking. It is important therefore to introduce it in an acceptable form. Most patients find it reasonable if the doctor says that pains (or headaches, breathlessness, dizziness—whatever has been complained of) may sometimes be made worse by worry: 'Have you any special worries?' If 'yes' follow up the reply with appropriate supplementary questions. If 'no' ask tactfully worded leading questions about *work, social and sexual relationships*. These are the three main areas of human concern. Other common psychoneurotic symptoms may be asked about directly such as anxiety, specific fears (phobias), obsessive thoughts and compulsive acts and depression. A useful leading question if severe mental disturbance is suspected is: 'Have you had any unusual experiences recently?' which may stimulate the patient to talk about false beliefs (delusions) or false sensations or perceptions (hallucinations). A question about getting on with people may disclose paranoid ideas (of persecution). Much of a psychiatric history is covered by the headings used in taking a medical history: complaint, history of present illness, previous history of illness, family history, etc. The main exception is the personal history. More detail is gathered about early family life, schools, further education, jobs, marriage and children. In the case particularly of children and old persons, information from relatives or neighbours may be important.

There are two more points about history taking which should be mentioned. *First* it is sometimes as important to record that a symptom was not present as to record that it was present. Under each system therefore the absence of the most important symptoms, e.g. breathlessness and cough in the case of the respiratory system, breathlessness on exertion or cardiac pain in the case of the cardiovascular system, and paralysis, headache or fits in the case of the nervous system, should be recorded.

Secondly the history does not end when the patient is first seen. Continuation notes should record the disappearance of symptoms of the appearance of new ones, or any other relevant fact which becomes apparent while the patient is under observation.

There follows a scheme of the kind of questions which most doctors ask in taking a history.

ROUTINE QUESTIONS

General

Weight. Is it increasing, decreasing or stationary?

Sleep. Has the sleeping pattern changed? Is there difficulty in getting to sleep or unusually early waking? Is the patient sleepy during the day?

Energy. Tiredness is a universal complaint. Is it loss of energy or boredom? Is it part of general malaise?

Gastrointestinal system, abdomen and pelvis

1. Symptoms point to an affection of the *upper alimentary tract*. Inquire about:

Pain. What is its severity and site? Is it localized or diffuse? Does it radiate in any particular direction? For how long has the patient had it? Does he have intervals of freedom? If so, for how long? What is its relation to meals (if any)? Does it wake him at night? What things aggravate it? What affords relief (e.g. food, antacid powders, vomiting)? Distinguish especially between 'pain' and 'sense of discomfort' or 'fullness'.

Appetite. Is it increased or reduced? If reduced, is his appetite really bad, or is the patient afraid to eat on account of pain?

Vomiting. Frequency. Its relation to pain; does it relieve pain or not? Distinguish between vomiting (contraction of abdominal muscles and diaphragm) and regurgitation (contraction of stomach muscles against closed pylorus).

General characteristics of vomited matter. Its amount and colour. Does it ever contain blood? Does it ever look like 'coffee-grounds'? Is it ever sour and frothy? Does it contain residues of food taken the day before?

Flatulence. Does the wind tend to escape downwards or upwards? Does either form relieve the symptoms?

Water brash. Does the patient ever experience excessive secretion of saliva into the mouth, with regurgitation of mouthfuls of clear, tasteless fluid?

Heartburn. Does the patient suffer from pain behind the sternum? Does it come on especially when he is lying down?

Dysphagia. Is there any difficulty in swallowing? If so, where does the food appear to 'stick'? Is it worse with liquids or with solids? Is swallowing painful?

2. Symptoms point to an affection of the *lower alimentary tract*. Inquire about:

Diarrhoea.   Number and time of occurrence of motions during the day; their relation to meals or to special articles of food. Colour of the motions; are they formed, unformed, porridge-like, frothy, or frankly watery? Do they float in the lavatory pan or are they difficult to flush away? Has he ever passed any blood or slime? Is there pain during defaecation? Does the patient use purgatives or does he take anything else, e.g. beer, likely to produce loose motions?

Constipation.   What is the patient's usual bowel habit? Has there been any recent change in habit? If so, can this be explained by change in diet, medicines, etc.? Does the constipation alternate with diarrhoea? If so, can this be explained by the taking of purgatives? Has he any colicky pain? Has he passed blood? Has he had any vomiting? Does he take codeine in any form?

Pain.   Site, radiation and character? Persistent or intermittent? Where is it felt worst? Is it relieved by defaecation or by the passage of flatus?

3. Symptoms point to an affection of the *liver* or *gallbladder*, e.g. patient is jaundiced or has pain in the region of the liver. Inquire about:

Jaundice.   Has the patient noticed any change of colour of the urine or faeces? Does the skin itch? Have there been any other cases of jaundice among his family, friends or workmates? Has he had any kind of injection in the last three or four months?

Pain.   Its site. Has the patient ever had attacks of very severe pain, coming on suddenly and lasting for a few hours? If so did the pain radiate and in what direction? Was he yellow after it subsided? Has he ever had pain in the tip of the shoulder or in the middle of his back?

Inquire also regarding his digestion on the lines already laid down.

4. Symptoms point to an affection of the *genital system*:
Patients will usually talk spontaneously about structural things,

such as a urethral discharge, swelling of the testicles or ulceration of the penis or scrotum in the male; and gynaecological abnormalities in the case of the female. (See specialized textbooks.)

Often, however, their real complaint is of a disorder of function which is to them intensively personal and embarrassing. Tact and sympathetic listening may enable such patients to discuss disorders of coital function, such as impotence, premature ejaculation or frigidity, problems of infertility and possible anxieties about masturbation or homosexuality.

Cardiovascular system

If the symptoms point to an affection of the *circulatory system* inquire about:

Rheumatic fever or chorea. A history of rheumatic fever or chorea is significant. If the patient is a child, also ask about sore throats and 'growing pains'.

Dyspnoea. How short of breath is the patient? When does it come on? Is it present at rest or only on exertion? What degree of exertion is necessary to produce it? Does he have attacks of breathlessness at night (paroxysmal nocturnal dyspnoea)? Does he have to sit up or can he sleep lying down?

Pain or distress. What is its exact site and character? Does it radiate to the left arm, neck, shoulder or interscapular region? If so, in what direction? What precipitates it, and what, if anything, relieves it?

Palpitation. What brings on palpitation and how long does it last? Does the heart give an occasional thump now and then? Has the patient ever felt his own pulse during an attack? Enquire also about cough, sputum and haemoptysis, as under respiratory system.

Do the feet swell?

Does he ever have pain in the calves when walking? Or is there undue coldness, redness or blueness of the extremities?

The blood

If the symptoms and appearances point to a blood disorder, inquire about:

Family history of bleeding. Has the patient had any loss of blood? Has he noticed any red spots in the skin? Does he bruise easily? Do his gums bleed? Has he been taking aspirin in any form? Are the stools ever black? Has he bleeding piles? (If a woman, is menstruation excessive or diminished?) What kind of a diet does he eat? What drugs has he been taking and to what chemical substances is he exposed in his work or home?

Such subjective sensations as breathlessness on exertion, headache, giddiness or palpitation.

Do the feet swell?

The respiratory system

If the symptoms point to an affection of the *respiratory system*, ask about:

Family history of tuberculosis or allergies; occupation (including past occupations) and possible exposure to animal, mineral or vegetable dusts. Ask particularly about smoking habits, past and present.

Cough. Whether dry or productive. Worst at which time of day? Worsened by any particular conditions, such as cold, dust or pollen? Painful or not?

Sputum. Quantity. Most produced at what time of day? Consistency, colour, and odour. Purulent or not? Ever blood-stained, and if so whether with streaks or clots, and on how many occasions?

Breathing. Is the patient dyspnoeic? Does dyspnoea occur at rest, or after varying degrees of exertion? Various 'grades' of dyspnoea have been described, but for the student it is best to inquire from the patient what sort of activity (e.g. walking upstairs, running for a bus, etc.) produced dyspnoea. Patients with severe pulmonary disease may be dyspnoeic at rest.

Wheeze. Wheezing may be associated with dyspnoea. The student should inquire when wheezing occurs. Is it constant or intermittent? Does anything provoke it? Is it worse at any particular time of day or night?

Chest pain. Where is it? Is it aggravated by deep breathing or coughing? Was it associated with increase in cough, sputum or dyspnoea? Was the onset sudden, as in spontaneous pneumothorax?

The urinary system

If the symptoms point to an affection of the *kidneys*, e.g. oedema, or *urinary system*, e.g. pain on micturition, ask about:

History of tonsillitis or previous renal disease. Family history of renal disease or high blood pressure. What analgesics has the patient taken?

Has he any pain in the lumbar region or any attacks of acute pain shooting down into the groin or testicles?

The following remote symptoms: headache, vomiting, drowsiness, fits, dimness of vision, dyspnoea.

Does the face ever look puffy in the morning? Are the ankles swollen?

What is the state of the bowels?

Inquire regarding micturition, as follows:

Urine.   Is the urine altered in amount? Does the patient have to get up at night to pass it?

Is it altered in colour? Is it clear or turbid when passed? Any blood in it? If so, at what period of micturition is it present? Is the urine frothy?

Is there any increased frequency of micturition? Is the increase by day or by night? Is there an increase in volume passed? Is frequency associated with undue thirst? Distinguish between *polyuria* as in diabetes and chronic renal failure and *frequency* as in cystitis.

Is there any pain during micturition? Is it before, during or after the act? What is its character, and where is it felt?

Skin diseases

Inquire carefully into the patient's personal habits as regards diet, clothing and washing. What is his occupation? Does he handle chemical substances or other irritants? Ask if he has been taking any drugs recently. It may be necessary to inquire carefully regarding syphilis. Does the eruption itch? If so, when is the itching worst? Did the eruption appear all at once or in crops? Does he suffer from asthma, hay fever or any other allergic conditions? What are his hobbies? Is he in contact with animals, with insects, with plants? What has he applied to his skin on his own initiative, or on the instructions of his doctor? What cosmetics does she use? Is there a *family* history of skin disease, asthma, hay fever, urticaria? Is there a family history of loss of hair or of excessive hair?

The nervous system

If symptoms point to an affection of the nervous system, ask about:

A family history of mental illness, paralysis, or fits. The nature of the patient's work; is he exposed to any poisons, e.g. lead, mercury, manganese, carbon disulphide or other volatile substances? Syphilis and alcohol should be inquired about. Has he been exposed to tropical infestations?

It is always important to inquire about discharge from the ear and about recent or remote head injury.

Should the patient complain of *fits* or *blackouts* the following questions should be asked in order to clarify the nature of the attacks:

Age at first attack? Describe the first attack. When did the second occur? What has been shortest and longest interval be tween attacks? Do they occur in sleep or not? Has he any premonition or *aura*? What is its character? Does the patient go rigid? Does he lose consciousness? Is the onset sudden or gradual? Are convulsions present? Are they general or local? Where do they begin and end? Does he fall? Has he ever hurt himself? Does he bite his tongue, micturate or defaecate during the fit? Are there any after-symptoms, such as sleep, headache, automatism or paralysis? Is there any subsequent mental disturbance? Because these patients are seldom clear as to the exact nature of their fits, it is essential to interview separately a reliable person who has seen the patient in a fit. The word 'fit' is often undesirable and 'attack' or 'seizure' is preferable.

If he complains of *paralysis* or *stroke* inquire regarding:

Symptoms of heart disease, hypertension, or diabetes (see Circulatory and Urinary Systems). Had he any premonitory symptoms before the onset? How did the paralysis come on? Suddenly or gradually? Has he any headache or vomiting? Where is the headache situated? (Other subjective symptoms of nervous disease are considered in Chapter 8.)

The locomotor system

If the symptoms point to an affection of the bones or joints:

Inquire for previous manifestations of rheumatoid arthritis, rheumatic fever or gout. Ask about possible associated conditions in the skin (e.g. dermatomyositis, psoriasis, disseminated lupus erythematosus, scleroderma and erythema nodosum), the bowels (ulcerative colitis) and the eyes (e.g. conjunctivitis, uveitis and Sjøgren's disease). Ask about the presence of a urethral discharge in the male or of vaginal discharge in the female. Has the patient been exposed to rubella? Tuberculosis and syphilis may occasionally be important. Is there a family history of gout or other rheumatic disorder?

If there is pain referred to a bone, ask whether it is worse in the day or in the night. Bone pains are often described as being deep and boring.

If the pain is in a joint, ask whether it is present constantly or only when the joint is moved. Has the joint been visibly swollen? Does the pain move from one joint to another, as is characteristic of acute or subacute rheumatism?

Children

If the patient is a young child, the following special questions should be put to the mother or other responsible person:

How many other children are there in the family? What are their sexes and ages? Have there been any miscarriages or stillbirths? If so, when? Is there a history of illness in the parents or siblings, or in the parents' near relatives?

Was the mother well during pregnancy and did she take any drugs? Was this a full-term infant? What was the birth weight? Was the child born at home or in hospital, and was the labour normal? Were there any unusual symptoms, such as jaundice, cyanosis or fits, in the newborn period?

Was the baby breast-fed, and for how long? If bottle-fed, what type of milk was used? Were vitamin supplements given? When was mixed feeding introduced? Was there a satisfactory weight-gain in infancy? What immunizations were given, and when?

It is particularly important to inquire about the 'milestones of development' (p. 423). When did the baby first smile, sit up, walk and talk? When did he acquire control of bowels and bladder?

What are the child's present habits with regard to eating, sleeping, bowels and micturition? What is his general behaviour like in comparison with his siblings or other children of the same age? If the child is of school age, does he attend school regularly, does he get on well with his lessons, and does he like school?

Has the child ever been separated from his mother? If so, when and for how long? What is the social background? Are the living conditions satisfactory? Does the mother go out to work? If she does, who looks after the child while she is away? Is this an immigrant family? If so, where do they come from, and how long have they been in this country?

Finally, inquire about previous illnesses, their nature and severity, and the ages at which they occurred—infectious diseases, fits, bowel disturbances, upper respiratory infections, discharging ears. If there is a history of cough, was it spasmodic, associated with vomiting, particularly bad at night? And was there a whoop? What drugs has the child received? Has the child ever been in hospital? Have there ever been any accidents involving physical injury, burns or poisoning?

In taking the history try to discover what is really worrying the parents. It may be something deeper than is suggested by the child's symptoms, for example leukaemia or some other serious disease which affected another child in the family.

The occupational history

In clinical practice the occupational history is often valuable, and there are few surer and quicker means of gaining a patient's confidence than the display of an intelligent knowledge of his or her job. It is a wise rule to take the occupational history from the time the patient left school. Record the dates and items of all subsequent jobs. He may be exposed to a noxious substance responsible for his ill-health in his present occupation, but this should not be assumed. A man describing himself as an ice-cream vendor may have cancer of the skin of the hand due to work in the pitch-beds of a gasworks 20 years before, or a mesothelioma due to exposure to asbestos many years before. Cancer of the genito-urinary tract may be the result of exposure in the past to certain aromatic amines used as intermediates in the dye-stuffs industry, as an anti-oxidant in rubber and cable-making and in the laboratory handling of such substances as benzidine, once used for occult blood tests, but no longer available. Ask the patient the name of his trade, the processes employed, the tools used and the substances handled. The name of an occupation may be misleading, for different names are used for the same process in different places.

It often happens that workmen and foremen refer to chemical substances by their popular names and not by their chemical names. Examples of such names are lunar caustic for silver nitrate, chrome yellow for lead chromate, wood spirit for methyl alcohol, and oil of mirbane for nitrobenzene. The man may be ignorant of the nature of a substance he uses and know it only by a trade name. In such cases it is best to communicate with his works manager and ask what is the nature of the substance in question.

Question him as to the general conditions at his place of work. If necessary ask him to sketch on paper a plan of his workshop and of the apparatus he uses. Is the job dusty, and if so what tools make the dust? Are there fumes or vapours, and if so what are the chemical substances involved? Most of the toxic substances encountered in the dangerous trades enter the body by inhalation. Ask whether a hood is installed over his bench, and whether it is connected to a suction system. Ask about the provision of protective clothing at his place of work. Does he wear a special suit, gloves or goggles, and why? Finally ask whether any similar illness has befallen a fellow workman.

Whenever serious doubts and difficulties arise, it is advisable to visit the factory in order to ascertain the conditions of work on the spot. In difficult cases the practitioner should enlist the help and advice of HM Factory Inspectorate, through the Chief Medical Adviser, Baynards House, Chepstow Place, London W2 (01 229 3456).

Other aspects of the history are no less important. A particular illness may render a man temporarily or permanently unfit to do his work. The doctor should know that conditions peculiar to certain trades may cause disease which predisposes to infection. Thus, silicosis leads to an excessive mortality from pulmonary tuberculosis and also from pneumonia. Diseases other than infections may be involved. For example, a heavy mortality from cirrhosis of the liver as well as from tuberculosis exists among publicans, barmen, brewers' draymen and others who have ready access to alcohol.

The doctor should have regard for his patient's work, even when he is suffering from a disease which is non-occupational; one must know whether a man does a job which makes him a danger to others. A dairyman with open tuberculosis can contaminate milk with tubercle bacilli by coughing into it, and those who handle food can initiate outbreaks of typhoid fever, dysentery and *Salmonella* infection by acting as carriers. Those who drive heavy goods or public transport vehicles come under stringent medical regulations. The possible effect of any drug on the patient's occupation must always be considered.

THE PHYSICAL EXAMINATION

The examination of the general state of the patient and of the different systems is described in Chapters 2 to 14. Though the findings should be recorded under systems, patients in medical wards are usually examined from above downwards, by the methods of inspection, palpation, percussion and auscultation, as may be appropriate to the different parts of the body. One should therefore develop a routine of physical examination which combines speed with thoroughness, but disturbs the patient no more than necessary. With practice a routine examination of the kind outlined here can be performed in 15 minutes or less. It need hardly be said that the examination must be carried out as gently as possible, without tiring or exposing the patient more than necessary. In the case of severely ill patients it may be necessary to postpone a routine examination and to perform only the minimum necessary for a provisional diagnosis and treatment. Ill patients must obviously be treated with special care and consideration.

Different doctors have different routines for examining patients in different circumstances, and for writing up their case notes.

The following is the kind of routine examination which students are expected to carry out on patients in medical wards in hospital. Such a routine may have to be modified according to the needs of the patient (e.g. minimum necessary examination in an acutely ill patient; complete examination of the nervous system in a patient with neurological symptoms; see Chapter 8) or according to the circumstances (e.g. in the doctor's surgery or in the patient's home).

During the taking of the history and the performance of the examination the following should be observed:

General

General appearance of illness (does the patient look healthy, unwell or ill)
Intelligence (see p. 267)
Mental state (see p. 264)
Expression
Build
State of nutrition, obesity, oedema
Skin colour, cyanosis, anaemia, jaundice, pigmentation
Skin eruptions, petechiae, spider naevi (see Chapter 3)
Body hair
Deformities, swellings
Temperature, pulse, respiration rate

Hair

Area of scalp covered
Texture

Eyes

Simple tests of visual acuity
Exophthalmos or enophthalmos
Ptosis
Oedema of the lids
Conjunctivae: anaemia, jaundice or inflammation
Pupils: size, equality, regularity, reaction to light, accommodation
Eye movements, nystagmus, strabismus
Ophthalmoscopic examination of the fundi

Face

Facies
Function of motor part of fifth nerve
Function of seventh nerve

Mouth and pharynx (a torch and tongue depressor should be used)

Breath odours
Lips: colour and eruptions
Tongue: protrusion and appearance
Teeth and gums (if patient has dentures, notice whether they fit and ask whether they are worn for meals or only for adornment)
Buccal mucous membrane: colour and pigmentation
Pharynx
Movement of soft palate
State of tonsils

Neck

Movements
Veins
Lymphatic glands
Thyroid
Carotid pulses

Upper limbs

General examination of arms and hands
Fingernails: clubbing or koilonychia
Pulse rate, rhythm, volume and character
State of arterial wall of radials and brachials
Axillae, lymphatic glands
Blood pressure
Test for power, tone, reflexes, coordination and sensation
Joints

Thorax

Anteriorly and laterally
  Type of chest, asymmetry if any, breasts

Rate, depth and character of respiration
Pulsations
Dilated vessels
Position of trachea by palpation
Look for and palpate apex beat
Palpate over praecordium for thrills
Palpate respiratory movements
Estimate tactile vocal fremitus
Percuss the lungs
Auscultate the heart sounds
Auscultate the breath sounds
Estimate vocal resonance
Posteriorly (patient sitting)
Inspect and palpate respiratory movement
Estimate tactile vocal fremitus
Percuss the lung resonance
Auscultate the breath sounds
Estimate vocal resonance
Note movements and deformities of the spine
Palpate from behind, cervical glands, thyroid
Look for sacral oedema

Abdomen

Inspection: size, distension, symmetry
Abdominal wall: movement, scars, dilated vessels
Visible peristalsis or pulsation
Pubic hair
Hernial orifices
Palpation: tenderness, rigidity, hyperaesthesia, splashing, masses, liver, gallbladder, spleen, kidneys, bladder
Percussion: masses, liver, spleen, bladder
Auscultation: bowel sounds, murmurs
Impulse on coughing at hernial orifices
Inguinal glands
Genitalia: penis, scrotum, spermatic cord
Abdominal reflexes
Rectal examination when indicated
Gynaecological examination when indicated

Lower limbs

General examination of legs and feet
Oedema
Varicose veins
Test for power, tone, reflexes (including plantar response),
   coordination and sensation
Joints
Peripheral pulses
Temperature of feet

Examination of excreta

Urine, sputum, stools, vomit: examine by naked eye and
   measure or estimate amount.
Test urine for specific gravity, sugar, protein and blood

WRITING OUT THE HISTORY AND EXAMINATION

Different doctors record the history and examination in different
ways. The aim is to write a complete yet concise record of a
patient's illness. For easy reference this is best done in note form,
with important facts starred or underlined.

The physical examination, although performed from above
downwards, should be written out under systems. A short statement of the findings under each system should be included, for the
absence of signs, as well as of symptoms, can be as important as
their presence. The minimum statement about a patient's cardiovascular system might for example read as follows:

pulse 76 regular
neck veins not distended
BP 130/80
apex beat not displaced
heart sounds I and II heard in all areas
no murmurs

Simple line drawings can often convey more information than
much writing. It is usual for a student to conclude his writing-up of
a case with a list of tentative diagnoses and a list of investigations

required, followed by continuation notes. This part of the medical record in particular has been much criticized. A formal scheme of recording with the self-explanatory title, 'Problem-orientated medical records' or POMR, has been adopted by some institutions, and was well described in the *British Journal of Hospital Medicine* (1972) **7**, 603. However the decision to adopt POMR is really one for the department or unit rather than for the individual student, although tentative diagnoses, if not the records, can be problem-orientated with advantage.

PRESENTING A CASE

The value of a student's or doctor's notes on a case is much diminished if he is unable to communicate them in concise form to other students or doctors. Students should therefore practise making a short summary of their findings, emphasizing both important positive findings and relevant negative ones. The summary should always begin with the name, age, sex and occupation of the patient, and can with advantage end with a brief statement of the problems to which the findings have given rise.

INTERPRETATION

The object of history taking, physical examination and ancillary investigations is the *making of a diagnosis*. In the past this has often been taken simply to mean the detection of a disease process, e.g. 'This patient has Hodgkin's disease'. If no disease process was detected the complaints were described as functional. This was illogical since all disease involves some disorder of function. The majority of patients consult a doctor about bodily disorders that express mental distress. The detection and alleviation of these problems are as important as the diagnosis of an organic disease process. Furthermore, the patient's own concept of his disease and his reaction to it has to be assessed alongside the doctor's diagnosis. Ultimately, it is the patient's symptoms that must be relieved.

One should begin the process of making a diagnosis by asking oneself some such broad questions as 'What is this person's problem?' and 'Has he a disability?' If one decides that he has a disability, one should ask:

1. *How far* can this person's disability be explained by his environment, i.e. in geographical, socio-economic and cultural terms?
2. *How far* can this person's disability be explained by his own attitude and mental make-up, i.e. in psychological terms?
3. *How far* can this person's disability be explained by a disease process or processes, i.e. in pathological terms?

Such an approach is clearly more reasonable than to search for a disease process and then to label as functional any disability not so accounted for.

It used also to be axiomatic that one should try to account for all a patient's symptoms by one disease process. But a surprising number of patients have in fact more than one (e.g. coronary artery disease and an hiatus hernia, both of which may produce central chest pain) and still more have a disease process which either does not explain their symptoms at all or does not explain all their symptoms (e.g. weakness and tiredness in a patient with mild angina pectoris or mild anaemia).

In making a diagnosis one should try to account for a person's total disability and should not be dismayed if this involves mentioning more than one item. This the diagnosis in an old lady with multiple symptoms might well be:

1. Loneliness
2. Depression
3. Mild osteoarthrosis

or in a young man with dyspepsia:

1. Impending marriage
2. Anxiety state
3. Duodenal ulcer

A diagnosis of this kind gives a truer picture of the state of affairs than a statement that the patient has osteoarthrosis or duodenal ulcer with functional overlay.

2

General considerations and appearances

The physical state
The mental state

THE PHYSICAL STATE

A good physical examination requires a cooperative patient and a quiet, warm and well-lit room. Daylight is better than artificial light because the latter may mask changes in skin colour, for example the faint yellow tinge of slight jaundice. Although in practice the examination may have to be made under all sorts of circumstances, every attempt should be made to reassure and relax the patient. For a complete examination the patient should be asked to take off all his clothes and should then be covered by a blanket or dressing gown. Patients are often examined while wearing underpants; but it is essential to remember to examine the buttocks and genitalia. Ideally a chaperone should be present when a male doctor is examining a female patient and during rectal and vaginal examinations, both to reassure the patient and to protect the doctor from subsequent accusations of impropriety.

Considering the general appearance, the most important step is to make a rapid assessment of the *degree of 'illness'*. This is not making a diagnosis. One has simply to answer the question: 'Does this patient look well, mildly ill, or severely ill and therefore in need of urgent attention?' Experienced nurses are often highly skilled in this kind of assessment and their opinion should never be ignored. Some severely ill patients complain little; occasionally one meets a patient whose appearance of excellent health belies his protestations of unbearable agony.

It has already been said that a good doctor begins his examination as soon as he meets the patient, and continues taking the history until the consultation ends. The examination of systems may provide information about organs and functions, but in physical examination as well as in history taking it is important to try to view the patient as a whole person and to find his reaction to his illness.

The mental and emotional state

One should therefore make some assessment of the patient's intelligence and of his mental and emotional state. Simple tests of intelligence (p. 267) and mental state (p. 264) may be necessary. Observation, as well as the history, may assist in the assessment of the emotional state. Thus an anxious person may be restless, with wide palpebral fissures and sweating palms. Is the anxiety reasonable in the circumstances or is the patient over-anxious? In rare cases of classical hysteria the patient may have an apparently severe disability, but shows a complete lack of the appropriate anxiety—*la belle indifférence*. The lowered mood, inability to concentrate or make decisions, mental retardation, apathy or even obvious misery of a depressed patient may be clearly evident; but so-called 'masked depression', in which these features are less obvious, is an important cause of physical symptoms.

The attitude

The attitude of a patient may give valuable information. Severely ill patients slip down into the most uncomfortable attitudes and are unable to correct their position for themselves. Patients with congestive heart failure may become dyspnoeic if they lie flat (*orthopnoea*). Patients with abdominal pain due to peritonitis lie still, while patients with colic are restless or even roll about in futile attempts to find relief. Patients with painful joint diseases often have an attitude of helplessness. Various neurological disorders produce characteristic attitudes (Chapter 8). In the severest cases of meningitis the neck may be bent backwards so that the head appears to bore into the pillow (*neck retraction*).

The gait

The gait should be observed in patients able to walk. Important abnormalities of the gait are described in Chapters 8 and 10, but note that simple things like a painful corn, an ill-fitting shoe or a strained muscle may produce a temporary limp.

Physique

A lot can be gained from a general inspection of the patient's physique. Is his appearance consistent with his age? Is he tall, short, fat, thin, muscular or asthenic? Are there any obvious deformities and is the body proportionate? Height should be roughly equal to the finger-tip to finger-tip measurement of outstretched arms and twice the leg length from pubis to heel. Dwarfism with a stocky body and very short legs is characteristic of achondroplasia. Hypopituitarism arising in childhood produces a proportionate, but dwarfed, adult with an unusually youthful appearance.

Table 2.1. IDEAL WEIGHTS FOR MEN AGED 25 AND OVER

| Height | | Small frame | | Medium frame | | Large frame | |
ft	in	cm	lb	kg	lb	kg	lb	kg
5	2	157·5	112–120	50·8–54·4	118–129	53·5–58·5	126–141	57·2–64·0
5	3	160·0	115–123	52·2–55·8	121–133	54·9–60·3	129–144	58·5–65·3
5	4	162·6	118–126	53·5–57·2	124–136	56·2–61·7	132–148	59·9–67·1
5	5	165·1	121–129	54·9–58·5	127–139	57·6–63·0	135–152	61·2–68·9
5	6	167·6	124–133	56·2–60·3	130–143	59·0–64·9	138–156	62·6–70·8
5	7	170·2	128–137	58·1–62·1	134–147	60·8–66·7	142–161	64·4–73·0
5	8	172·7	132–141	59·9–64·0	138–152	62·6–68·9	147–166	66·7–75·3
5	9	175·3	136–145	61·7–65·8	142–156	64·4–70·8	151–170	68·5–77·1
5	10	177·8	140–150	63·5–68·0	146–160	66·2–72·6	155–174	70·3–78·9
5	11	180·3	144–154	65·3–69·9	150–165	68·0–74·8	159–179	72·1–81·2
6	0	182·9	148–158	67·1–71·7	154–170	69·9–77·1	164–184	74·4–83·5
6	1	185·4	152–162	68·9–73·5	158–175	71·7–79·4	168–189	76·2–85·7
6	2	188·0	156–167	70·8–75·7	162–180	73·5–81·6	173–194	78·5–88·0
6	3	190·5	160–171	72·6–77·6	167–185	75·7–83·5	178–199	80·7–90·3
6	4	193·0	164–175	74·4–79·4	172–190	78·1–86·2	182–204	82·7–92·5

Heights are measured wearing ordinary shoes and weights in ordinary indoor clothing.
Notice that tables of this kind make no allowance for 'middle-aged spread'.

Table 2.2. IDEAL WEIGHTS FOR WOMEN AGED 25 AND OVER

Height		Small frame		Medium frame		Large frame	
ft in	cm	lb	kg	lb	kg	lb	kg
4 10	147·3	92– 98	41·7–44·5	96–107	43·5–48·5	104–119	47·2–54·0
4 11	149·9	94–101	42·6–45·8	98–110	44·5–49·9	106–122	48·1–55·3
5 0	152·4	96–104	43·5–47·2	101–113	45·8–51·3	109–125	49·4–56·7
5 1	154·9	99–107	44·9–48·5	104–116	47·2–52·6	112–128	50·8–58·1
5 2	157·5	102–110	46·3–49·9	107–119	48·5–54·0	115–131	52·2–59·4
5 3	160·0	105–113	47·6–51·3	110–122	49·9–55·3	118–134	53·5–60·8
5 4	162·6	108–116	49·0–52·6	113–126	51·3–57·2	121–138	54·9–62·6
5 5	165·1	111–119	50·3–54·0	116–130	52·6–59·0	125–142	56·7–64·4
5 6	167·6	114–123	51·7–55·8	120–135	54·4–61·2	129–146	59·5–66·2
5 7	170·2	118–127	53·5–57·6	124–139	56·2–63·0	133–150	60·3–68·0
5 8	172·7	122–131	55·3–59·4	128–143	58·1–64·9	137–154	62·1–69·9
5 9	175·3	126–135	57·2–61·2	132–147	59·9–66·7	141–158	64·0–71·7
5 10	177·8	130–140	59·0–63·5	136–151	61·7–68·5	145–163	65·8–73·9
5 11	180·3	134–144	60·8–65·3	140–155	63·5–70·3	149–168	67·6–76·2
6 0	182·9	138–148	62·6–67·1	144–159	65·3–72·1	153–173	69·4–78·5

Heights are measured wearing ordinary shoes and weights in ordinary indoor clothing.
Notice that tables of this kind make no allowance for 'middle-aged spread'.

'*Ideal*' *weights*, as used in life insurance assessment, are listed in Tables 2.1 and 2.2. Obesity is a problem of developed countries. In other parts of the world signs of malnutrition such as wasting, apathy, anaemia and skin changes may be encountered; they should also be looked for in neglected elderly patients in the UK. A history of weight gain or loss can be checked by observation, remembering that fluid retention (*oedema*) will increase weight. Obvious weight loss, mainly from loss of adipose tissue, when food intake has increased is seen in thyrotoxicosis and diabetes mellitus. Psychogenic loss of appetite in girls (anorexia nervosa) causes extreme emaciation while physical activity remains unimpaired.

The face

Observe the patient's face. His expression, and particularly his eyes, may indicate his real feelings better than do his words. The characteristic facies of various diseases, e.g. myxoedema, thyrotoxicosis, acromegaly, third and seventh cranial nerve palsies (pp. 283, 297) and paralysis of the cervical sympathetic (Horner's syndrome) (p. 293), must be learnt in practice.

Parotid swellings are obvious on inspection of the face. The temporary tender bilateral parotid swelling of mumps or the unilateral swelling with reddening of the skin from acute parotitis can be contrasted with the non-tender bilateral persistent enlargement, accompanied by dry tearless eyes of Sjøgren's syndrome, or the more irregular unilateral lump of a mixed parotid tumour.

The *cheeks* give some information regarding the patient's health: in anaemia and hypopituitarism they are pale; in the nephrotic syndrome they are pale and puffy; in cases of mitral stenosis there is sometimes a bright circumscribed flush over the malar bones; in many persons who lead an open-air life they are red and high-coloured; in congestive heart failure they may also be high-coloured, but the colour is of a bluish tint which cannot be mistaken for the red cheeks of weather-beaten people. In some cases of disseminated lupus erythematosus there is a red raised eruption on the bridge of the nose extending on to the cheeks in a 'bat's-wing' distribution.

The skin

Look at the skin. The most important abnormalities in a general examination are pallor, yellowness, pigmentation, cyanosis and cutaneous eruptions. Feel its texture. In dehydration the skin is dry and inelastic, it can be pinched up into a ridge. The skin is atrophied by age and exposure to excess glucocorticoids. It is thickened, greasy and loose in acromegaly.

Pallor depends on the thickness and quality of the skin, and the amount and quality of blood in the capillaries. It is thus seen in persons with thick or opaque skins who are always pale; in states where the blood flow in the capillaries is diminished, such as shock, syncope or left heart failure; locally in a limb deprived of its blood supply; or in the fingers or toes when arterial spasm occurs on exposure to cold, as in Raynaud's disease. Generalized pallor may also occur in severe anaemia. Anaemia, however, is to be judged 'by the colour of the blood rather than that of the patient' and the colour of the skin may be most misleading; that of the mucous membranes of the mouth and conjunctivae gives a better indication, and so does the colour of the creases in the palm of the hand. *Yellowness* may be due to haemolytic jaundice, when the tint is pale lemon-yellow, or to obstructive jaundice, when it may be of a dark yellow or orange tint. In obstructive jaundice there may be scratch marks that result from the itching which the bile salts evoke. In rare cases yellowness may be due to carotinaemia. *Pigmentation* is most commonly racial or actinic. Other forms are described in Chapter 3. The pigmentation of Addison's disease affects the buccal mucous membranes as well as the skin of exposed parts and parts subject to friction. *Cyanosis* is a bluish colour of the skin and mucous membranes due to an increase in the amount of reduced haemoglobin in the blood. It may be divided into central and peripheral. Central cyanosis results from imperfect oxygenation of blood, as in heart failure and some lung diseases, or from the mixture of arterial and venous blood in the presence of right-to-left or venous–arterial shunts in the heart. In this case the cyanosis is general and the cyanosed extremities are warm. It characteristically affects the tongue. Peripheral cyanosis is due to excessive reduction of oxyhaemoglobin in the capillaries when the flow of blood is slowed. This may happen on exposure to cold, when there is venous obstruction or in heart failure. The cyanosed extremity or extremities are then cold and the tongue is unaffected. One should note, however, that the cyanosis of heart failure is often of a mixed type, due to both central and peripheral causes. A similar bluish or leaden colour may in rare cases be produced by methaemoglobinaemia or sulphaemoglobinaemia, usually due to the taking of drugs such as phenacetin. This should be considered in any patient who is cyanosed but not breathless. Carbon monoxide poisoning produces a generalized cherry-red discoloration.

Cutaneous eruptions are described in Chapter 3. Purpuric haemorrhages (petechiae), which do not disappear on pressure, are of great importance in blood diseases and in infective endocarditis. Spider naevi (telangiectases), which have typically a red centre and spidery branching tributaries and which do disappear on pressure, are a useful sign of liver disease.

When an excess of fluid is present in the subcutaneous tissue the condition is known as *oedema*. Thus in acute nephritis an early symptom is oedema of the face, which is most marked when the patient rises in the morning. In dependent oedema, however, which is typically present in congestive heart failure, and in conditions associated with a low plasma protein level, the swelling first appears at the ankles and over the dorsum of the foot, and only gradually mounts to the legs, thighs and trunk. In local venous obstruction, the oedema is confined to the parts from which the return of blood is impeded. In this way one finds oedema of an arm when malignant glands constrict the axillary vein or oedema of a leg in thrombosis of the popliteal or femoral vein. Oedema of the whole upper part of the body may result from intrathoracic tumours. Oedema may be recognized by the pallid and glossy appearance of the skin over the swollen part, by its doughy feel, and by the fact that it pits on finger pressure. In recumbent patients oedema often appears first over the sacrum. In eliciting pitting it is important to press firmly and for a sustained period, or slight oedema may be missed.

Localized oedema may be due to local changes in capillary permeability, as in angioneurotic oedema and giant urticaria.

Subcutaneous emphysema is uncommon, but if present can be readily recognized by the crackling sensation which is detected on pinching the part affected.

The hands

The hands of the patient should be examined (Plate I). Notice the strength of grip as he shakes hands; this often indicates improvement or deterioration with considerable accuracy. Their general shape should be noted, along with the state of the joints, the character of the nails, the presence or absence of finger-clubbing and the presence of staining with nicotine. In osteoarthrosis the finger joints are often implicated, and bony nodules, known as *Heberden's nodes*, are formed at the bases of the terminal phalanges. In rheumatoid arthritis there is characteristically a spindle-shaped swelling of the interphalangeal joints and later an ulnar deviation of the fingers. *Trophic changes* in the skin may be present in neurological disease and in disorders of the peripheral circulation (e.g. Raynaud's disease). Characteristic movements or attitudes of the hand may also be seen in athetosis, tetany, and lead palsy. *Tremor* of the hands may occasionally be congenital. In other cases it is due to nervousness, senility, parkinsonism, thyrotoxicosis, alcoholism, disseminated sclerosis, uraemia, hepatic failure or mercurial poisoning. This and other abnormal movements are considered on p. 324. In ulnar paralysis the hand becomes deformed by over-extension of the first phalanges, combined with excessive flexion of the rest, so that a claw-like attitude is produced. This is known as the '*main en griffe*'. Wasting of the small muscles of the hand, due for example to median or ulnar nerve lesions, cervical root (C8) disease or loss of anterior horn cells at the same level, gives the hand a flattened appearance. In *Dupuytren's contracture* there is a thickening of the palmar fascia, which may lead to a flexion contracture of the ring and other fingers. In acromegaly the hands are massive, the fingers spatulate with square tips and the skin thickened. In *clubbing of the fingers* the tissues at the base of the nail are thickened, and the angle between the nail base and the adjacent skin of the finger is obliterated. The nail itself loses its longitudinal ridges and becomes convex from above down as well as from side to side. In extreme cases the terminal segment of the finger is bulbous like the end of a drumstick. The condition may occasionally be congenital. Gross degrees of clubbing are found in association with severe chronic cyanosis, as in congenital heart disease; and in association with chronic suppuration within the chest, as in bronchiectasis and empyema. Lesser degrees may be found in carcinoma of the lung, pulmonary tuberculosis, and chronic abdominal conditions such as polyposis of the colon, Crohn's disease and ulcerative colitis. Clubbing is also an important sign of subacute bacterial endocarditis, when it may be associated with Osler's nodes, tender transient swellings about the size of a pea in the pulp of the fingers and toes, and 'splinter' haemor-rhages beneath the nails. In hypertrophic pulmonary osteo-arthropathy there is, besides clubbing of the fingers, thickening of the periosteum of radius, ulna, tibia and fibula. This gives rise to swelling above the wrist and ankle. *Koilonychia* occurs in iron-deficiency anaemia. The nails are soft, thin and brittle. The nor-mal convexity is lost and replaced by a concavity.

The feet

The feet must not remain obscured under bedclothes or socks. Apart from looking for pitting oedema, the condition of the skin of the feet is of importance, especially in diabetics and the elderly. Peripheral vascular disease will make the skin shiny and hair does not grow on ischaemic legs or feet. The dorsalis pedis and posterior tibial pulses may be reduced or absent. If the toes of an ischaemic foot are compressed their dull purple colour will blanch and only slowly return. Painless trophic lesions, often with deep ulceration, on the soles are seen frequently in diabetic peripheral neuropathy.

The neck

The neck should be inspected and palpated. Swellings in the neck are usually felt best from behind. Note:

The lymphatic and salivary glands.   In infected conditions of the tonsils the glands at the angles of the jaw are enlarged, and those below the jaw in cases of malignant disease in the mouth. Glands draining an inflammatory focus are usually tender. Enlarged tuberculous glands may occur in groups or in long chains beside the sterno-mastoid, and scars may mark the points of past suppuration in severe untreated cases. In Hodgkin's disease and other reticuloses the glands are enlarged and discrete. In lymphatic leukaemia there may be great enlargement of the glands on both sides. In secondary syphilis the glands under the upper part of the trapezius are often palpable. If enlarged glands are found either in the neck or elsewhere, it is important to observe whether they are firm and distinct, or fused together, whether fluctuation can be elicited, and whether they are adherent to adjacent structures. The *submandibular salivary glands* should also be palpated when the neck is being examined from behind. If they are swollen and tender, the opening of their ducts into the mouth should be inspected with the tip of the patient's tongue rolled upwards; a salivary calculus may be seen.

The thyroid gland.   Inspect the neck for any general or local enlargement of the gland, and observe its movement with the larynx as the patient swallows. Patients find this easier if they are given a glass of water. Then stand behind the patient and palpate the gland with one hand on each side of the neck. Determine if any swelling exists, and if so whether it is uniform or nodular, hard or soft. Sometimes such enlargements press on the trachea and occasionally extend into the thorax behind the sternum; at other times, particularly if the disease is malignant, the recurrent laryngeal nerves may become implicated. In cases where there is difficulty in determining whether a tumour is connected with the thyroid, it is helpful to remember that the gland and any tumour connected with it moves up and down on swallowing. Minor degrees of enlargement of the thyroid are often better seen than felt. A bruit on auscultation shows that the gland is hyperactive.

Pulsations.   Pulsations in the vessels must be recorded. Any arterial pulsation is both seen and felt as a distinct thrust, whereas venous pulsation is seen but is not felt as a thrust, if it is felt at all. In aortic incompetence the carotid arteries are seen to pulsate forcibly. In aortic stenosis a systolic thrill is felt. Women patients with hypertension sometimes show kinking of the right common carotid artery which simulates aneurysm. The jugular veins may be distended and pulsatile in congestive heart failure (p. 202). In superior mediastinal obstruction due to retrosternal goitre or malignant neoplasm in the mediastinum, non-pulsatile distended veins may be seen over the neck and upper part of the body; cyanosis and oedema of the upper part of the body may accompany this sign. Distended neck veins may also be seen in large pericardial effusions.

The breasts

The chance of finding a treatable cancer should make a full examination of the breasts a necessary feature of every general examination of a woman. With the patient reclining, arms to the sides, inspect the development and symmetry of breasts and nipples. Look for any reddening of the skin, ulceration or dimpling (*peau d'orange*). Retraction (rather than inversion) of one nipple may signpost the cancer beneath. If there is a discharge from the nipple determine whether it is bloody, serous or milky.

Palpate each breast with the flat of the fingers, working over the whole breast as if it was mapped out in quadrants. Repeat this when the patient has her hands placed behind her head. If a lump is found the qualities to be observed are those that hold good for any lump felt anywhere in the body. Determine the situation, size, shape, surface and edge; feel its consistency and mobility in relation to deep and superficial structures.

Axillae.   Then examine the axillae. It is difficult to feel enlarged lymph glands unless the patient's arm is raised to allow the examining fingers to be pushed high into the axilla. The arm is then lowered and palpation is continued downwards along the chest wall. Any swelling of the male breast is likely to be seen at a glance. The swelling can be distinguished as breast tissue rather than pectoral fat by palpation when the patient's hands are behind his head. At some stage of puberty the majority of normal boys will have a palpable disc of breast tissue beneath the areola.

Temperature

When taking the temperature, the following practical points must be attended to:

1. The thermometer must be accurate and of NPL standard.

2. The thermometer must be kept in position long enough to allow the mercury to reach the body temperature. It is advisable to exceed the period which the instrument professes to require. The ordinary 'half-minute' thermometer should be left in position for one or two minutes. Collapsed, comatose and elderly patients should have the rectal temperature taken with a special 'low-reading' thermometer. Accidental hypothermia is not uncommon in the elderly.

3. In conscious adults the temperature is taken in the mouth or in the axilla. In young children the thermometer should be placed in the fold of the groin, and the thigh flexed on the abdomen; or it may be inserted into the rectum. The temperature of the mouth and rectum is generally at least half a degree higher than that of the

groin or axilla. When the temperature is taken in the mouth, the patient must breathe through the nose and keep the lips firmly closed during the observation.

4. Before inserting the thermometer, make it an invariable rule to wash it in antiseptic or in cold water, and see that the mercury is well shaken down. Wash it again before replacing it in its case. The Centigrade (Celsius) scale is in general use, although in Great Britain many people are still more familiar with the Fahrenheit scale (for comparison of the two scales see p. 476).

Normal	36·6–37·2°C	(98–99°F)
Subnormal	below 36·6°C	(below 98°F)
Febrile	above 37·2°C	(above 99°F)
Hyperpyrexia	above 41·6°C	(above 107°F)
Hypothermia	below 35°C	(below 95°F)

In many conditions, notably acute fevers, there is a disturbance of heat regulation, which may be looked on as the setting of the 'thermostatic' mechanism controlling heat gain and loss at a higher level than normal. While the temperature is rising to this new level, heat is being conserved, the skin vessels are constricted so that the body surface feels cold, and the patient may even shiver violently. This shivering is referred to as a *rigor*. When the higher temperature is reached, heat loss again becomes apparent; the skin vessels dilate and the body surface feels warm. This is the state of affairs present in sustained fever or *pyrexia*.

There are three classical *types of fever*—the continued, the remittent and the intermittent. When fever does not fluctuate more than about 1°C (or 1·5°F) during the twenty-four hours, but at no time touches the normal, it is described as *continued*. When the daily fluctuations exceed 2°C, it is known as *remittent* (Fig. 2.1); and when fever is present only for several hours during the day it is called *intermittent*. When a paroxysm of intermittent fever occurs daily, the type is *quotidian*; when on alternate days, *tertian*; when two days intervene between consecutive attacks, *quartan* (Fig. 2.2). However, with the use of antibiotics and other specific drugs these classical types of fever are not often seen.

Pulse

Count the pulse for a full minute when the patient is at rest and composed. Abnormalities due to cardiovascular causes are

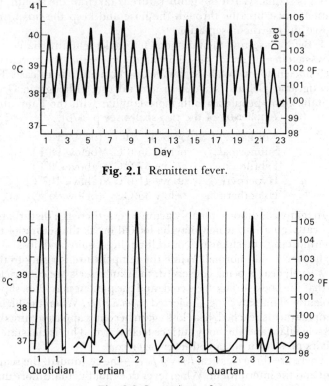

Fig. 2.1 Remittent fever.

Fig. 2.2 Intermittent fever.

described in Chapter 7. The rate in health and under conditions of a medical examination varies from about 60 to 80 beats a minute. The common causes of a rapid pulse are recent exercise, excitement or anxiety, shock (e.g. bleeding), fever and thyrotoxicosis. A slow pulse is characteristic of severe myxoedema and of complete heart block.

Respiration

Count the patient's respirations for a full minute when his attention is distracted from his breathing. It is convenient to do this when he thinks you are still counting his pulse. The normal rate in an adult under the conditions of a medical examination is about 16 to 22 respirations a minute, but wide variations occur in health. The main causes of fast breathing (tachypnoea) are exercise, nervousness and fever; pulmonary, pleuritic and cardiac conditions causing hypoxia; cerebral disturbance, metabolic acidosis and hysterical overbreathing, which later may give rise to alkalosis and attacks of tetany.

Changes in the character of respiration are discussed in Chapter 6, but one should notice that obstruction in different parts of the respiration tract may give rise to recognizable varieties of noisy breathing. Obstruction in the nasal passages may cause sniffing or bubbling sounds. Paralysis of the soft palate causes a snoring noise. Obstruction in the region of the larynx causes inspiratory stridor of which one example is the 'whoop' of whooping cough. Obstruction in the trachea may produce growling or rattling noises, as in the 'death rattle', when the lumen is obstructed by mucus. Obstruction in the bronchi may give rise to audible snoring or wheezing noises. Obstruction in the larynx or larger bronchi characteristically gives rise to inspiratory noises, while obstruction in the small bronchi and bronchioles produces expiratory wheezing. The latter is heard in bronchitis and asthma (obstructive airways disease). Alternating periods of cessation of respiration and hyperventilation (Cheyne-Stokes respiration) occur in left heart failure and in various cerebral disturbances. The breathing may be characteristic of diseases quite distinct from those of the respiratory system. Examples of this are the stertorous breathing of apoplexy, the hissing expiration of uraemia, and the 'air-hunger' of diabetic keto-acidotic coma, which affects both inspiration and expiration.

Odours. The odours of alcohol and paraldehyde are easily recognizable in the breath. That of alcohol does not mean that the patient's condition is due to alcoholic intoxication, since alcohol may have been administered as a form of resuscitation. The odour of diabetic ketosis has been described as 'sweet and sickly'; that of uraemia as 'ammoniacal or fishy'; and that of hepatic failure as 'mousy', but one should not rely too far on such delicate distinctions.

THE MENTAL STATE

The examination of the mental state (pp. 264–269) is the equivalent in psychiatry of the physical examination in general medicine. The patient's words should be recorded exactly. With mute or otherwise disturbed patients the 'mental state' examination may be merely a description of behaviour. It is assumed that common psychoneurotic symptoms (anxiety, phobias, etc.) will have been asked about in the history taking. The important aspect of the mental state examination are:

General observations. Appearance (appropriate, neat, dishevelled, etc.); manner (friendly, unfriendly, suspicious); unusual movements or mannerisms; speech (normal or abnormal words (neologisms)); rapport and 'contact' with the patient. Confusion (of time, place or persons) is an important sign suggesting organic, rather than psychological, disturbance of the brain.

Attention. Can the patient sustain attention or does his mind wander?

Mood. Elation or depression of mood; appropriateness to the situation.

Thinking. Preoccupations, peculiar 'notions' or ideas, false beliefs (delusions). Ability to understand abstract concepts is often lost in the elderly or demented subject so that errors of judgement occur.

Memory. Impairment of memory for recent or on-going events may not be apparent unless tested for.

Sensations. Unreality feelings (depersonalization); false sensations (hallucinations) commonly of hearing, less commonly vision, taste or smell.

Special attention needs to be paid to the mental state of the *elderly*. The bright and smiling face of an old lady may well mask considerable defects of memory and orientation.

Questions such as 'Where do you live?', 'What place are you now in?', 'What is the day of the week and the date?', 'Who are the other people in the ward or home?' and 'What do they do?' may reveal *disorientation* for place, time and person.

3

The skin, the nails and the hair

Colour and pigmentation
Haemorrhages
Eruptions
Palpation
Distribution of skin lesions
The hair
The nails
Skin manifestations of internal disease
Examination for parasites

For the examination of the skin and its appendages, the patients should be stripped as completely as circumstances permit and should be examined by daylight.

COLOUR AND PIGMENTATION

First notice the colour of the skin. The normal colour is very variable, some persons having a fresh complexion, and others, though quite healthy, a pale one, Pallor is also often seen in a variety of illnesses. It may be seen temporarily in haemorrhage, shock and intense emotion. Anaemic persons are often pale, but not all pale persons are anaemic. The colour of the mucous membrane of the eyelids and mouth is a better indication of anaemia than is the colour of the skin. *Undue redness* is seen in overheating, extreme exertion, sunburn, some fevers, in many of the exanthemata and in skin disease. *Cyanosis* is a bluish or purplish tint, which may be more or less generalized or limited to one or more extremities. It is due to the presence of an excess of reduced haemoglobin resulting from impaired oxygenation or circulation of the blood (p. 183). It is important to note that *methaemoglobinaemia* may produce a blue tint which is less bright and more leaden than cyanosis. Methaemoglobinaemia may be due to poisoning by aniline or nitro-benzene, or to drugs such as phenacetin, sulphanilamide or dapsone.

Jaundice varies from the 'subicteric', 'lemon-yellow', or 'daffodil' tints seen in pernicious anaemia and acholuric jaundice, to various shades of yellow, orange or dark olive green in obstructive jaundice. Jaundice must be distinguished from the yellowness of carotinaemia, due to the presence of an excess of lipid-soluble yellow pigments in the plasma. Carotene does not stain the conjunctivae, which jaundice does. Slight degrees of jaundice cannot be seen in artificial light.

Normal skin contains varying amounts of brown *pigment*. A congenital absence of pigment in the skin which is generalized is known as *albinism*: if it is localized it is known as *piebaldism*. Alternating patches of white and darkly pigmented skin are seen in *leucomelanodermia* or *vitiligo*. A pale skin due to diminished pigment is also characteristic of *hypopituitarism* and *hypogonadism*. Increased pigmentation may be racial, due to sunburn or connected with various diseases. In *Addison's disease* there is a brown or dark brown pigmentation, affecting exposed parts, and parts not normally pigmented such as the axillae and the palmar creases; the lips and mouth should always be examined and may exhibit dark bluish-black areas that have been compared with the stains produced by sucking a pen. Note, however, that mucous membrane pigmentation is a normal finding in a substantial proportion of negroids. More or less generalized pigmentation may also be seen in *haemochromatosis*, where it has a peculiar bronze colour with a metallic sheen; in *chronic arsenic poisoning*, where it is finely dappled and affects covered more than exposed parts; in *argyria*, where the deposition of silver in the skin produces a diffuse slatey-grey hue; and occasionally in the cachexia of advanced malignant disease. In *pregnancy* there may be pigmentation of the nipples and their areolae, of the linea alba and sometimes a mask-like pigmentation of the face (chloasma); it is also seen sometimes in those taking the birth pill. A similar condition, melasma, may be seen in Asian and African males. Localized pigmentation may be seen in *hyperthyroidism, pellagra, rheumatoid arthritis* and a variety of chronic wasting diseases. Localized pigmentation is also seen in scars of various kinds, particularly those due to X-irradiation therapy and those following varicose ulcers of the legs. Vagabond's disease, a pigmentation due to chronic infestation with lice, is now rarely seen. *Erythema ab igne*, a coarsely mottled pigmentation of the legs of women who habitually sit too near the fire, used to be common.

HAEMORRHAGES

Haemorrhages into the skin occur in various forms and in various conditions. If less than 1 mm in diameter they should be referred to as *petechiae*; if from 2 mm to 5 mm in diameter as *purpuric spots*; and if larger as *ecchymoses*. If the haemorrhage is large enough to produce an elevation of the skin, it is referred to as a *haematoma*.

Petechiae and purpuric spots do not disappear when they are pressed on by a glass slide or lens, which serves at once to distinguish them from erythematous spots and from telangiectases, which consist of a small collection of dilated skin vessels. They must also not be confused with senile haemangiomas (de Morgan's spots) or cherry spots, which are common and have no pathological significance. De Morgan spots are unusual among haemangiomas because the blood in them cannot be expressed by pressure.

ERUPTIONS

Next, one should seek the presence of any eruption. If present, inquiry should be made on the lines laid down on p. 53. The exact situation and extent of the eruption should be noted and whether it is symmetrical or confined to one side only. One should then pass to a description of the minute characters of the eruption. In order to do this, it must be remembered that every cutaneous eruption consists of a primary lesion, to which secondary lesions may or may not be superadded.

Primary lesions

Macules (spots).   Macules are an alteration in the colour of the skin which may be seen but not felt. A macule may be small or large. It may be due to dilation of blood vessels as in capillary naevi or telangiectasis or erythemas which blanch on pressure. Purpuric or pigmented macules do not blanch when pressed.

Papules.   Papules are solid projections above the surface, which are not larger than a pea. The term *nodule* is applied to any solid projection from the skin which is larger than a pea, but not larger than a cherry. Anything larger than that is called a *tumour*. Always note whether the top of the papule is rounded as in some forms of eczema, pointed as in acne or flattened as in lichen. As regards the base, observe whether it infiltrates the skin widely or not. The wider the infiltration, the more extensive and severe the inflamation.

If the skin is stretched by applying the tension on either side a papule in the epidermis will retain its prominence, e.g. a wart, while a dermal papule will sink and become less prominent, e.g. a granuloma of tuberculosis, sarcoidosis or a reticulosis.

Vesicles.   Vesicles are elevations of the horny layer of epidermis by transparent or milky fluid, which are not larger than a pea. If larger than this, they should be described as *bullae* or *blebs*. Always note whether or not there is an area of redness around the base of a vesicle, for such redness indicates that the vesicle is planted upon an inflamed base—a fact which may be of diagnostic value. Ruptured vesicles leave transient pits on the skin.

Pustules.   Pustules are small elevations of the skin containing pus. They are often follicular, as in boils and staphylococcal or chemical folliculitis; non-follicular pustules may be a sequel to eczema or may be viral as in the late stage of herpes simplex.

Weals. The lesions of nettle rash or hives or the raised component of the triple response of Lewis are weals. They are slightly elevated portions of the skin, the centre of which is paler than the periphery. Scratch the normal skin of the back with a spatula; an exaggerated weal is characteristic of physical urticaria (dermographism).

Burrows. Burrows are short linear, straight or sinuous lines in the skin, usually dark in colour. They are made by the female scabies mite in the process of laying eggs.

Blackheads. Blackheads are dark horny plugs in the pilosebaceous openings; they are the primary lesions of acne vulgaris.

Plaques. Plaques are circumscribed flat areas of abnormal skin which are raised or sunk below the level of the surrounding skin, e.g. psoriasis or morphoea (the localized type of scleroderma).

Scales. Scaling indicates a disorder of keratinization, e.g. dandruff, psoriasis, ichthyosis, the dry state of eczema, the peeling of scarlet fever.

In moist lesions (vesicles, pustules, bullae) the epidermal cells become glued together by the dried fluid and a scab or crust forms. The scab may be serous, purulent, haemorrhagic or sebaceous according to the nature of the contents of the primary lesions.

Secondary lesions

Next look for *secondary lesions*. These are either produced mechanically or are the result of changes which take place in the primary lesion in the course of its growth or decline. The commonest secondary lesions of mechanical production are *excoriations* due to scratching and *fissures*, which are deep cracks going down to or into the corium, produced by the stretching of the skin after it has become inelastic owing to thickening of any kind. Fissures are often very painful.

The following are the secondary lesions produced by changes in those which are primary:

Infiltration. Infiltration may occur around the primary lesions, leading to a leathery feeling in the skin. This is usually the result of prolonged chronic inflammation.

Lichenification.   Skin which is continually rubbed, as in the chronic stage of atopic eczema, becomes thickened and the normal lines become apparent. This is called lichenification because it resembles the lichen on trees.

Dyschromia.   Inflammation of the skin, especially in those of dark colour often leads to hyperpigmentation or hypopigmentation.

Ulceration.   Ulceration is caused by the breaking-down of the primary lesions and destruction of a part of the true skin.

The points to note in describing an ulcer are: *a.* the nature of the floor of the ulcer and the granulations covering it; *b.* the character of the edge—smooth, raised, undermined, etc.; *c.* the discharge, whether serous, purulent, watery, fetid, etc.; and *d.* the character of the surrounding skin, whether indurated, pigmented, etc. It is also important to examine the lymph nodes that drain the area of the ulcer.

Scar formation.   Scar formation only occurs where the true skin has been involved, i.e. where there has been an ulcer or an equivalent injury. Describe the scar, noting especially whether it is thin or thick, freely movable or adherent to the deeper tissues, pale or livid, pitted or not, surrounded by a zone of pigmentation or not.

Keloids are exaggerated scars with dense hypertrophic fibrous tissue formation. The edges often show 'claw' formation. They may be a sequel to burns but may also arise spontaneously. Persons of black African ancestry are very prone to form keloids.

PALPATION

Proceed now to the palpation of the skin. Pass the hand gently over it, pinching it up between the forefinger and thumb, and note the following points:

Is it smooth or rough, thin or thick, dry or moist? If there is any visible sweating, note whether it is general or local. The *elasticity* of the skin should be investigated. If a fold of healthy skin is pinched up, it immediately flattens itself out again when released. Sometimes, however, it only does so very slowly, remaining for a considerable time in a creased condition. This may be of little or no significance in old persons with loose inelastic skins, but may be an important sign of dehydration in conditions associated with prolonged vomiting and diarrhoea.

The conditions of the subcutaneous tissue should be investigated. The presence of *oedema* is usually recognized by the fact that if the skin is pressed with the finger, especially over a hard body such as a bone, a pit is left which persists for some little time. In some cases, no pitting can be produced, especially when the oedema is of very long standing. The best place to look for slight degrees of oedema in cardiac disease is behind the malleoli of the tibia and fibula in patients who are ambulant, and over the sacrum in those who are confined to bed. The pressure of the finger should be maintained for 20–30 seconds, or small degrees of oedema will be overlooked. Pitting is absent in oedema due to lymphatic obstruction, where the skin is usually thickened and tough.

Subcutaneous emphysema gives rise on palpation to a characteristic crackling sensation. It starts in, and is usually confined to, the neighbourhood of the air passages or air-containing organs. In rare cases it may be due to infection with gas gangrene organisms.

DISTRIBUTION OF SKIN LESIONS

The distribution of an eruption is often of great diagnostic importance. Stand a little way from the patient to assess the pattern and the symmetry of the rash.

In psoriasis the scalp, the knees, the elbows and the small of the back are often involved.

In atopic eczema, after infancy, it is the popliteal and antecubital fossae and sometimes the wrists and face, which are affected.

In pityriasis rosea there is often a large first lesion, the herald patch, and then a crop of lesions which are scaly at the edges on the trunk. The lesions on the back are arranged in an inverted Christmas tree pattern.

The exposed areas are normally most affected in light-induced eruptions, e.g. porphyria, lupus erythematosus, pellagra and photo reactions to drugs such as chlorpromazine and certain tetracyclines. 8-Methoxypsoralen is now being used in the treatment of psoriasis. It sensitizes the skin to long wave ultraviolet light (UVA 320–400 nm). Externally applied substances also photosensitize; these are found in eau de cologne and perfumes, in meadow grass and plants of the parsnip family, in antiseptics used in the recent past, in hair dressings and soaps.

Allergic contact dermatitis to dusts and vapours often affects the exposed parts. The thin-skinned areas, the antecubital and popliteal fossae and the scrotum are often affected as well. Nail varnish seldom produces disease of the nail, it may, however, produce contact dermatitis of the eyelids and sides of the neck.

Swelling of the eyelids is an important sign. Without redness and scaling, bilateral orbital oedema may indicate acute nephritis, nephrosis or trichinosis. If there is irritation, insect bites or angio-oedema may be suspected; these are often unilateral. If there is scaling or weeping and irritation, contact dermatitis is the probable diagnosis. Dermatomyositis often produces swelling, helio-trope erythema and scaling. Cellulitis and erysipelas may also affect the eyelids.

THE HAIR

The hair colour and texture are often genetically determined. The mongol races have black straight hair, the negroids black curly hair and the white caucasoids fair, brown, red or black hair. The hair may be dyed. The colour, the texture and the appearance as well as traces of the natural colour at the hair roots will afford clues to this.

Hypothyroidism produces dry skin and puffiness of the face. The scalp hair thins and the outer part of the eyebrows may be shaded. Hypothyroidism, anaemia and even a low serum iron level may produce diffuse alopecia. Systemic lupus erythematosus may produce hair loss, especially in the temporal regions. Small round or oval bald patches with normal or over-supple scalp skin and sometimes exclamation mark hairs are features of alopecia areata. Similar areas with a slightly scaly scalp skin and short broken off hair stumps are usually the result of ringworm infections. Examination under Wood's light often gives a bright green fluorescence of the hair stumps.

Secondary syphilis may be marked by 'moth-eaten' alopecia.

The secondary sexual hair appears at puberty, if it does not there may be failure of development of the gonads. Facial hirsut-ism in the female is commonly a genetic or familial variant of the normal, but may be a sign of a virilizing tumour. The tendency for 50% of male caucasoids to develop frontal, and in some cases, vertical recession of the scalp hair is the consequence of interaction of circulating male hormones and the inheritance of the balding gene ('Eunuchs, women and children never go bald' Aristotle). A severe insult to the body, such as a fever, haemorrhage or major operation, may cause all or almost all of the scalp hairs to go into the resting phase (telogen). One to three months later new growing phase (anagen) hairs displace the resting hairs and transient diffuse alopecia develops. A somewhat similar process may occur after pregnancy (telogen defluvium). Antimitotic drugs may produce thinning of the skin scalp hair (anagen defluvium).

THE NAILS

The nails should be carefully examined. Clubbing and koilonychia are dealt with elsewhere. Thimble pitting of the nails is characteristic of psoriasis but eczema and alopecia areata may also produce pitting. A severe illness may temporarily arrest the growth of the nails. When growth starts again a transverse ridge develops. These are Beau's lines and can be used to date the time of onset of the fever. Chronic paronychia produces similar changes. The changes described above arise from disturbance of the nail matrix. The nail bed also makes a contribution to the nails. Disturbance of the nail bed may produce thick nails (pachyonychia) or separation of the nail from the bed (onycholysis). This may happen in psoriasis, eczema and other conditions. The nail may be destroyed in severe lichen or epidermolysis bullosa (a genetic abnormality in which the skin blisters in response to minor trauma). Some nails are missing in the nail patella syndrome. Splinter haemorrhages under the nails may result from trauma, psoriasis, rheumatoid arthritis or other 'collagen' diseases, bacterial endocarditis and trichinosis.

SKIN MANIFESTATIONS OF INTERNAL DISEASE

White patches shaped like small ash leaves which are present at birth may be the first sign of tuberous sclerosis. Sometimes they are difficult to see by natural light but show up under the Wood's light. They should be looked for in infants suffering from fits. Patchy depigmented macules which are hypoaesthetic and associated enlargement of the peripheral nerves are features of tuberculoid and borderline leprosy. *Café au lait* patches are often the first sign of neurofibromatosis. The presence of six or more with diameters of at least 1·5 cm and associated axillary 'freckling' make this diagnosis virtually certain. *Paget's disease* of the nipple is a well defined red discoloration which looks like eczema. It is associated in most instances with a duct carcinoma of the underlying breast. *Dermatomyositis* often presents with a heliotrope discoloration and oedema of the eyelids and fixed erythema over the dorsa of the knuckles, fingers and over the bony points. There is usually weakness of the proximal limb muscles. Dermatomyositis in the middle aged is associated in 50% of cases with internal malignancy.

Acanthosis nigricans is brownish thickening of the axillae and groin and the sides of the neck. Sometimes there is thickening of the palms, soles and gums. In the middle aged, acanthosis nigricans is associated with internal malignancy.

Icthyosis (fish skin) is usually present from childhood and is genetic but if icthyosis is acquired in adult life a search should be made for malignancy or other underlying disease. The same is true of acquired epidermolysis bullosa. *Widespread pruritus* without obvious signs may occur naturally in the aged but Hodgkin's disease and internal malignancy should also be considered. *Diabetes mellitus* has a number of skin manifestations: pruritus vulvae, boils, ulcers on the soles or toes from the neuropathy and gangrene of the extremities from arteriosclerosis. *Necrobiosis lipoidica* consists of brown plaques, usually on the shins, with central atrophy of the skin which reveals the vessels in the dermis. There is a significant association with diabetes. *Spider naevi* consist of a central arteriole feeding a leash of vessels around. These, particularly when they arise in childhood, may be genetic. In older age groups pregnancy, the birth pill, the administration of oestrogens and liver disease may be responsible. Liver disease and systemic lupus erythematosus may produce erythema of the thenar and hypothenar emminences.

Xanthomata are yellow or orange deposits of lipid in the skin. They may be the effect of hyperlipoproteinaemia (types I to V, WHO classification) or of diabetes, liver disease, myxoedema or renal disease. Deposits of lipid (arcus senilis) in the cornea may have a similar explanation but may be a normal feature in those of 60 years of more. The flat lipid deposits around the eyes (xanthelasma) may be due to lipid disturbance but are also seen in the middle aged and elderly without any general metabolic upset.

Carotinaemia produces a warm orange yellow colour of the skin, especially of the palms and soles. It occurs in those who eat great quantities of carrots and other vegetables, in hypothyroid persons, in diabetics and also in those taking β-carotene for the treatment of erythropoietic porphyria.

Erythema nodosum is a condition in which tender red nodules occur, usually on the lower legs. The condition may be a response to sarcoidosis or to tuberculosis or streptococcal or other bacterial, as well as fungal or viral infections. It may also occur as a drug eruption.

EXAMINATION FOR PARASITES

Microscopical examination of the skin and its appendages is useful in the diagnosis of some *parasitic diseases*, of which the following are the chief:

Scabies or itch

Scabies or itch is due to the *Acarus (Sarcoptes) scabiei*. The female *Acarus* is larger than the male and forms burrows in the skin, in which the eggs are deposited. These burrows should be looked for between the fingers and on the inner aspects of the wrists. They are recognized with the naked eye as little short dark lines terminating in a shining spot of skin. The eggs lie in the dark line, the insect in the shining spot. It may be picked out by means of a flat surgical needle passed along the black line to the clear spot. The use of a lens aids the operation—which is by no means invariably successful—and makes possible the recognition of the insect. The latter may be placed on a slide under the microscope for more detailed examination.

Pediculosis

Three varieties of pediculosis occur—*Pediculus capitis* on the head, *P. corporis* on the trunk, *P. pubis* on the pubic and axillary hairs. The eggs or 'nits' of *P. capitis* are stuck on the hairs. From their position on the hairs one can judge roughly of the duration of the condition, for they are fixed at first near the root of the hair, and are then carried up with the latter in its growth. The higher up the nits are, therefore, the longer the pediculi have been present. *P. corporis* should be looked for in the seams of the clothes, especially where the latter come into close contact with the skin—e.g. over the shoulders. The bites of the parasite produce haemorrhagic spots, each with a dark centre and a paler areola. Marks of scratching should always be looked for on parts accessible to the patient's nails.

P. corporis is the longest of the three, *P. pubis* is shortest, and *P. capitis* is between the two in size. *P. pubis* is also distinguished from the others by being yellowish-brown in colour. *P. capitis* and *P. corporis* are both greyish in colour, though the latter varies considerably with the colour of the skin of its host. The shape of the thorax and abdomen forms a distinguishing character between these varieties and *P. pubis*.

Fungus infections

Fungus may grow in the skin, nails, or hair and cause disease (ringworm).

Skin.   Between the toes, on the soles of the feet and in the groins are the commonest sites of fungal infection. The lesions may be scaly and vesicular areas tending to spread in a ring form and healing in the centre; scaly erythematous plaques with festooned margins; areas of hyperkeratosis on the parts of the skin which have a thick horny layer (palms and soles); or macerated, dead-white offensive-smelling epithelium in the intertriginous areas such as the toe clefts.

Nails.   Discoloration, deformity, hypertrophy, and abnormal brittleness may result from fungus infection.

Hair.   Ringworm of the scalp is most common in children. It presents as round or oval areas of baldness covered with short, broken-off, lustreless hair stumps. These hair stumps usually give a bright green fluorescence when exposed to long-wave ultraviolet light (UVL filtered through Wood's glass).

Microscopical examination

Scales from the active edge of a lesion are scraped off lightly with a scalpel or the roofs of vesicles are snipped off with scissors. The material is placed in a drop of 10–20% aqueous potassium hydroxide solution on a microscope slide, covered with a cover slip and left for 30 minutes to clear. It is then examined with the 8 mm or 4 mm objective, using low illumination. The mycelium is recognized as branching refractile threads which boldly transgress the outlines of the squamous cells (mycelium which respects the cells' outlines is 'mosaic fungus', an appearance probably produced by intercellular lipoid). Nails are examined in much the same way, but as nail is harder and denser it is necessary to break up the snippings and shavings into small fragments. These are either heated in potassium hydroxide or are left to clear in it overnight before being examined. A scalp lesion is cleaned with 70% alcohol or with 1% cetrimide and infected stumps and scales are removed by scraping with a scalpel. The hairs are cleaned in potassium hydroxide in the same way as skin scales. Examination under the microscope reveals spores on the outside of the hair roots, and mycelium inside the hair substance. The species of fungus responsible may be established by culture on Sabouraud's glucose-agar, or on beerwort-agar medium.

4

The abdomen

THE MOUTH AND THROAT

The examination of the mouth and throat is conducted with the patient sitting up either in bed, with the head resting comfortably back on pillows, or in a chair. A bright torch, a tongue depressor (spatula) and fingercots are essential. The lips, teeth, gums, tongue, palate, fauces and oro-pharynx are then visualized systematically, and finally palpation of the sides of the tongue, floor of mouth and tonsillar regions are carried out.

INSPECTION

The lips

Look closely at the philtrum (the shallow depression running from nose to upper lip) for the tell-tale scar of a repaired cleft lip. When present, particularly if associated with 'nasal speech', inspect the palate carefully for signs of a cleft. Next, look at the corners of the mouth for cracks or fissures (angular stomatitis). The cracks are reddish brown, moist, superficial, linear ulcers radiating from the angles of the mouth. In children their origin is infective (perlèche); they are common in the elderly when ill-fitting or deficient dentures result in over closure of the mouth. Cheilosis is also seen in severe iron-deficiency anaemia; it may provide a clue to the diagnosis of post-cricoid carcinoma in women with dysphagia; and also occurs in vitamin B_2 (riboflavin) deficiency.

Rhagades, white scars at the angles of the mouth indicating previous cheilosis due to congenital or tertiary syphilis, are now very rare. Here, however, the fissures extend into the mouth. A crack in the middle of the lower lip is common in cold weather; although difficult to heal because of constant movement of the lips and moistening by the tongue, such a fissure is of no sinister significance.

Observe any desquamation or inflammation of the lips (cheilitis). This is commonplace and self-limiting in cold weather. Grouped vesicles on the lips on a red base with crusted lesions are seen in herpes simplex labialis commonly associated with coryza. This infection is usually of short duration and the lack of induration and ulceration serve to distinguish it from other more serious conditions. Recurrent actinic cheilitis with small blisters and exfoliation, however, is a pre-malignant condition found in people constantly exposed to the sun and wind, such as farmers and fishermen.

Look for any ulcer on the lips. Carcinoma (epithelioma) usually occurs on the lower lip away from the midline; the ulcer is indolent, flat and shallow, although in time the edge may become heaped up and induration may be felt. Epithelioma has to be differentiated from akerato-acanthoma, pyogenic granuloma and the chancre of primary syphilis. Akerato-acanthoma (molluscum sebaceum) is a lesion due to overgrowth of the stratum granulosum of the skin. It usually presents as a firm, rounded nodule sometimes with ulceration; it is more common on the upper lip and heals spontaneously without treatment. Pyogenic granuloma is a soft red raspberry-like nodule on the upper lip which often follows minor trauma. The upper lip is the commonest site of an extra-genital chancre which appears as a small, round lesion that is firm and indurated. If it ulcerates it forms a serpiginous outline and exudes a stringy non-purulent exudate. In both epithelioma and chancre enlarged painless cervical nodes are commonly felt.

Very occasionally one sees multiple small brown or black spots on the skin around the mouth (circumoral pigmentation) which may also extend onto the lips and buccal mucosa. This pigmentation constitutes one of the triad of cardinal features of the Peutz-Jeghers syndrome and signifies underlying small bowel polyposis, a condition inherited as a Mendelian dominant. On the buccal mucosa the pigmentation may look very like that seen in Addison's disease.

Now gently grasp the lower lip with the index finger and thumb of both hands and evert it fully, to display the mucous surface of the lip. Two lesions are commonly seen in this site: aphthous ulcers and retention cysts. Aphthous ulcers are small superficial painful ulcers with a white or yellow base and a narrow halo of hyperaemia. Such ulcers are also seen on the tongue, buccal mucosa and palate. Retention cysts of the mucous glands of the lips and buccal mucosa appear as round, translucent swellings, elevated from the surface with a characteristic white or bluish appearance. They are also found on the mucous surface of the lower lip.

The teeth

Ask the patient to show his teeth, or if he wears dentures to remove them and then open the mouth widely. Using a tongue depressor to retract first the lips and then the cheeks, note the number of teeth present and look for decay (caries). The tooth most commonly 'missing' is an impacted unerupted third mandibular molar (wisdom). Inspect both the buccal and lingual aspects of the teeth. It is said that lack of teeth may cause indigestion, but many edentulous people suffer no indigestion whether they wear dentures or not. Look for any changes in:

Colour.   Tartar deposition occurs mainly on the lingual aspect of the lower incisor and canine teeth and consists of precipitated calcium salts of saliva which in smokers is stained brown. Children up to the age of eight treated with tetracycline (and children of expectant mothers so treated after the fourteenth week of pregnancy) are at risk of acquiring permanent staining of both the deciduous and permanent teeth. This takes the form of disfiguring horizontal bands, which may be yellow or grey and must not be mistaken for bands of hyperplasia on the enamel due to exanthematous fevers or any serious illness occurring during the development of the crowns. In endemic fluorosis chalk-white patches appear on the teeth or the teeth present a dull, unglazed appearance, sometimes with pitting and brown staining (Maldon teeth).

Shape.   Ill-formed hypoplastic teeth have a broad, concave biting edge, whilst some notching of the incisors is seen in those who persistently bite cotton or hold hairclips between their teeth. They must not be mistaken for Hutchinson's teeth—a manifestation of congenital syphilis, but a very rare finding nowadays. In this condition the two central upper permanent incisors are rounded in section and notched at their biting edge. They may also be broader near the gum than at the crown, so as to be peg shaped. The first permanent molars may be dome shaped. The two central upper incisors are commonly lost in leprosy.

Ridging.   Transverse ridging is sometimes seen in the permanent teeth of those who had vitamin C and D deficiency in infancy.

Enlargement of the lower jaw in acromegaly leads to alteration of the bite, so that the lower teeth may close outside the upper ones.

The gums

Examine the gums at the same time as the teeth. Pink, healthy gums adhere closely to the necks of the teeth and have a sharp border. With increasing age gingival recession occurs so making the teeth appear longer and exposing the cementum below the enamel. This makes it easier for infection to gain a hold.

In *chronic marginal gingivitis*, the gums are retracted, frequently bleed easily and lose their characteristic stippling. Sometimes pus can be squeezed from them *(pyorrhoea alveolaris)*.

Acute herpetic gingivostomatitis due to the simplex virus occurs most commonly in infants and children. Many small vesicles appear on the gums, cheeks, palate, tongue and lips. The vesicles rupture to produce shallow ulcers with a yellowish floor and bright red margins. *Vincent's gingivostomatitis*, an infection due to fusiform sphirochaetes, characteristically destroys the interdental papillae. A thick felted greenish grey slough is formed and halitosis is present. In patients exposed to lead compounds, a stippled blue line can often be observed running along the edge of the gum, especially opposite those teeth showing gingivitis. Similar lines may be produced by bismuth or mercury but these are uncommon signs. The gums in scurvy are swollen, irregular in outline, red, spongy and bleed easily. Hypertrophy of the gums may occur in pregnancy and in patients treated for long periods with phenytoin. Haemorrhages may be observed in the buccal mucous membrane in thrombocytopenic purpura and acute leukaemia.

Pus can form in a carious tooth to form an alveolar or dental abscess with throbbing pain, exacerbated by tapping the affected tooth. Localized swelling of the gum and swelling of the face (if pus has escaped through the lateral alveolar margin) are signs associated with this condition. Ill-fitting dentures can produce a granuloma or an ulcer on the gum at the point of pressure where the denture does not fit properly. Such a lesion has to be differentiated from a carcinomatous ulcer arising in the gum; the latter presents the same macroscopic features as malignant ulcers elsewhere in the mouth.

Epulis is a general term used to describe any swelling arising in the gum of the maxilla or mandible.

The tongue

Ask the patient to protrude the tongue. Inability to do so fully *(ankyloglossia)* is seen, very rarely, in infants due to tongue tie (a congenitally short frenulum linguae) or in advanced malignancy of the tongue involving the floor of the mouth. When carcinoma involves the side of the tongue (the commonest site) and the floor of the mouth, slight deviation towards the affected side may occur. Slight deviation is not uncommon and may be due to asymmetry of the jaws. In hemiplegia, deviation towards the paralysed side may be found. In lesions of the hypoglossal nerve or its nucleus there may be fasciculation of the affected side; later this side may be wasted and deeply grooved (lingual hemiatrophy). The tongue is large in acromegaly, cretinism, myxoedema and lymphangioma.

Tremor of the tongue may be due to nervousness, thyrotoxicosis, delirium tremens or parkinsonism.

Next examine the dorsum of the tongue.

Colour. Is the tongue pale, red or discoloured? Pallor is seen in severe anaemia. Discoloration is most often due to the ingestion of coloured things—e.g. red wine or coloured sweets.

Moistness. The state of the tongue gives some indication of the state of hydration of the body, provided the patient is not a mouth breather. A dry, brown tongue may be found in the later stages of any severe illness, but is found particularly in advanced uraemia and acute intestinal obstruction.

Fur. Furring of the tongue is of little value as an indication of disease. It is found in heavy smokers, mouth breathers, the edentulous and those on soft, milky or otherwise sloppy diets. A brown fur, the 'black hairy tongue', is due to a fungus infection and is of no special significance, though frequently a source of great alarm to its possessor. The tongue of scarlet fever at first shows bright red papillae standing out of a thick white fur. Later the white coat disappears leaving enlarged papillae on a bright red surface—'the strawberry tongue'.

The papillae. Generalized atrophy of the papillae produces a smooth or bald tongue which is characteristic of pernicious anaemia, but may also sometimes be found in iron deficiency anaemia, sprue, other gastro-intestinal disorders and deficiency states, especially pellagra. In severe cases smoothness may be associated with wrinkling of the mucous membrane, which has then to be distinguished from fissuring of the tongue seen in chronic superficial glossitis due to syphilis, now rare in the United Kingdom, and congenital fissuring of the tongue or 'scrotal tongue' which is common and of no pathological significance. In chronic superficial glossitis, areas of leukoplakia (whitish opaque areas of thickened epithelium) are separated by intervening smooth and scarred areas; there are no normal papillae to be seen and the fissures run mainly in a longitudinal direction. In congenital fissuring the papillae are normal but the surface is interrupted by numerous irregular but more or less symmetrical folds which tend to run mainly horizontally. In median rhomboid glossitis a lozenge-shaped area of loss of papillae and fissuring is seen in the mid-line anterior to the foramen caecum. It feels nodular and may be mistaken for a carcinoma. It must also be distinguished from a lingual thyroid but this is situated posterior to the foramen caecum. 'Geographical tongue' is another harmless anomaly characterized by localized irregular red areas of desquamated epithelium and filiform papillae surrounded by a whitish yellow border which change in distribution and give the appearance of a map. The 'false geographical tongue' with a similar appearance occurs chiefly in children with fever.

The sides and undersurface. Ask the patient to open the mouth wide and protrude the tongue fully to one side. Then retract the cheek with a spatula. This displays the side and lateral undersurface well. Some patients find this impossible to do, so wrap a gauze swab around the tip of the tongue and with index finger and thumb gently pull the tongue out and to one side. Benign ulcers in this site are common and may be inflammatory or traumatic in origin, very often due to ill-fitting dentures, or broken carious teeth; such ulcers tend to be painful, superficial and lack induration. However, in an elderly patient any ulcer at this site must be regarded as malignant until proved otherwise by biopsy; it is the most frequent site of carcinoma in the mouth and presents as a hard, indurated ulcer with everted raised edges.

Now ask the patient to retract the tongue fully and slightly elevate the tip with the mouth wide open. This displays the undersurface of the anterior tongue and floor of the mouth. Note the frenulum linguae and the orifice of the submandibular duct opening on either side of the base of the frenulum. The ampulla of each duct lies just proximal to the orifice and is a common site for calculi formed in the sub-mandibular salivary gland to lodge. The calculus is seen as a white or yellow bleb distending an oedematous hyperaemic ampulla.

A small ulcer on the frenulum is sometimes seen in persistent coughing and particularly in whooping cough. Sublingual varicosities are common in the elderly. Two types of cyst may be found in the floor of the mouth: a ranula, which forms a bluish white translucent swelling of variable size and is due to blockage of the duct of a mucous gland, and a sublingual dermoid cyst, a round opaque swelling lying beneath the mucosa either above or below the mylohyoid which is due to sequestration of epidermal tissue beneath the skin along the embryological lines of fusion of the mouth.

The buccal mucosa

Inspect the buccal mucosa. Retract the cheek with a spatula. Note the opening of the parotid duct seen as a tiny swelling opposite the upper second molar tooth. In the catarrhal stage of measles, before the appearance of the rash, small bluish white spots, surrounded by a red areola, may be seen opposite the molar teeth. These are known as Koplik's spots. In the same position irregular areas or dots of slatey grey or blue pigmentation are seen in Addison's disease.

Aphthous ulcers, mucous retention cysts and papillomata present the same appearance on the buccal mucosa as elsewhere in the mouth. White opalescent patches (rather like white paint) of leukoplakia may also be seen on the inner aspect of the cheek; these should be differentiated from lichen planus, an oral manifestation of a skin disease, but in this case look elsewhere, especially on the arms and legs, for similar lesions. Thrush (monilial stomatitis), a fungal infection due to candida albicans, presents as a different sort of white patch. It is seen as small white points raised somewhat above the surrounding surface, which is usually redder than normal. As the infection gains hold so the lesions coalesce and may form extensive sheets throughout the mouth. Patches of thrush are apt to be mistaken for small milk curds, but curds can be easily detached, while thrush patches can only be removed with difficulty and then tend to leave behind a raw surface. Thrush is common in debilitated children, beneath unclean dentures and in patients on cytotoxic or immunosuppressive drugs. It is also seen frequently on surgical wards, especially in ill patients with sepsis in the post-operative period and those treated with broad spectrum antibiotics, which destroy the normal bacterial flora of the mouth and thus allow the fungi to flourish.

The palate, fauces, tonsils and pharynx

Ask the patient to put the head right back and keep the mouth wide open. Inspect the hard and soft palates and note the position of the uvula. Get the patient to say 'ah' which raises the soft palate and increases visibility of the fauces, tonsils and oropharynx. (For abnormalities of movement of the soft palate during phonation see p. 303.)

If a good view of these structures has not been obtained thus far, introduce a spatula to depress the base of the tongue and if necessary another spatula to retract the anterior pillar of the fauces to view the tonsils properly.

Again look for any ulcers, erythema or vesicles. Vesicles confined to one side of the hard palate which progress to painful oval ulcers are characteristic of herpes zoster of the maxillary division of the trigeminal nerve (5th cranial); this disorder usually occurs in older patients and is accompanied by a characteristic skin rash in the corresponding dermatome on the face. Herpes zoster infection of the glossopharyngeal nerve (9th cranial) produces similar lesions in the pharynx.

Malignant ulcers do occur on the hard palate but much less frequently then elsewhere in the mouth, and present the same appearances. Ectopic salivary gland tissue may be present in the mouth, the hard palate being the commonest site. Tumours of this tissue present as a smooth, hard swelling projecting from the surface of the hard palate, sometimes with central ulceration.

If a hole is seen in the hard palate it is usually due to one of the following causes:

1. Imperfect closure or breakdown after repair of a cleft palate.
2. Radionecrosis of bone following radiotherapy for treatment of local carcinoma.
3. Tertiary syphilis with formation of a gumma.

Petechiae on the palate are commonly seen in glandular fever, but they are also features of any form of thrombocytopaenia, rubella and streptococcal tonsillitis. Oral lesions may be the presenting feature of glandular fever: enlarged tonsils are covered with a white exudate which tends to become confluent; there is oedema of the fauces and soft palate and erythema of the oropharynx. This contrasts with the yellow punctate follicullar exudate seen in streptococcal tonsillitis. Whenever a membranous exudate is seen, diphtheria should spring to mind and as in all cases of mouth infection a swab should be taken for bacteriological examination. The membrane in diphtheria varies in colour from white to green and often starts on the tonsil before spreading to the fauces and pharynx.

Finally, look at the pharynx. The presence on its surface of a number of small round or oval swellings, somewhat like sago grains, is so common as to be almost normal in appearance. In pharyngitis these are much increased.

Notice any vesicles or ulcers. In chickenpox (herpes varicella) oral lesions may be apparent before the characteristic rash appears. There is erythema of the pharyngeal and buccal mucosae, followed by vesicles which progress to oval or round ulcers with a white slough. In herpangina (Coxsackie virus infection), which is also common in the young, similar lesions may be seen in the oropharynx, soft palate and uvula.

In the common cold (coryza), muco-pus may be noticed on the posterior wall of the pharynx running down from the nasopharynx. Not very commonly seen nowadays are a peri-tonsillar abscess (quinsy) and retropharyngeal abscess. The latter forms a smooth, tense, tender swelling which bulges forwards from the posterior wall of the oropharynx.

The breath

Carious teeth, infection or ulceration of the gum, stomatitis, retention and decomposition of secretion in the follicles of enlarged tonsils are the commonest sources of offensive breath. Characteristic odours may be recognized: in ketosis, the breath smells of acetone; in uraemia, there is a fishy or ammonical odour; and in hepatic failure, the odour is described as 'mousey'. In suppurative conditions of the lung the breath may have a putrid smell, whilst the odour of bronchiectasis has been compared to that of apple blossom with a hint of stale faeces. Paraldehyde and alcohol also impart their characteristic smell to the breath.

PALPATION

Palpation forms an important, frequently neglected part of the examination of the mouth, particularly in patients who complain of oral symptoms or in whom unexplained cervical lymph-adenopathy is found. Palpation is imperative in anyone with a solitary or suspected ulcer in the oral cavity, and bimanual palpation provides further information about such things as swellings in the floor of the mouth or cheek.

Impress on the patient that you will be as gentle as possible. Put on a disposable glove or fingercot, ask the patient to remove any dentures, and to open the mouth widely. With the tongue elevated and to one side, place the index finger of the right hand beneath the tongue on one side of the frenulum and run the finger back along the floor of the mouth. Even a small calculus can easily be felt in any part of the submandibular duct. Then come forwards, running the finger along the lingual side of the tongue, to the midline and return on the buccal side of the gum towards the lower molar teeth. Now run the finger up the mucosa covering the ascending ramus of the mandible, and examine both palatal and buccal aspects of the gum of the upper jaw.

If an ulcer is present, try and decide whether any induration is present or not. To perform bimanual examination, with the index finger already inside the mouth, place the fingertips of the left hand flat beneath the mandible, or over the cheek, outside the mouth, and exert gentle pressure between your right index finger and the fingers of the left hand.

Now palpate the tongue and feel the dorsum and the lateral and under surfaces with the index finger; it sometimes helps for the patient to protrude the tongue to one or other side to do this, and if necessary the tongue can be held in a gauze swab between finger and thumb of the other hand.

Palpation of the posterior third of tongue, fauces and tonsils is the least pleasant part for the patient as it usually causes gagging, and it is thus left until last. As before, the index finger is used and run over these structures as rapidly as possible. One is concerned with detecting a small or hidden carcinoma in these sites, so feel for irregularity, ulceration and particularly induration.

Any abnormality felt in these sites in a patient with symptoms demands illuminated head lamp and laryngeal examination (p. 398).

THE ABDOMEN

It is helpful for recording in notes or when communicating information to colleagues to think of the abdomen as divided into regions (Fig. 4.1).

The two *lateral vertical* planes pass from the femoral artery below to cross the costal margin close to the tip of the 9th costal cartilage.

The two *horizontal* planes, the sub-costal and inter-tubercular, pass across the abdomen to connect the lowest points on the costal margin, and the tubercles of the iliac crests respectively.

Remember that the area of each region will depend on the width of the subcostal angle and the proximity of costal margin to iliac crest, in addition to other features of bodily habitus which naturally vary greatly from one patient to the next.

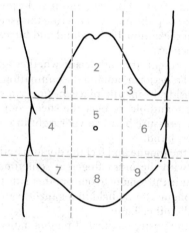

Fig. 4.1 Regions of the abdomen.

1 and 3:	Right and left hypochondrium
2:	Epigastrium
4 and 6:	Right and left lumbar
5:	Umbilical
7 and 9:	Right and left iliac
8:	Hypogastrium or suprapublic

INSPECTION

The patient should be lying flat on his back, arms by his side, on a firm couch or mattress, the head and neck supported by enough pillows, normally one or two, to make him comfortable (Fig. 4.2). A sagging mattress makes examination, particularly palpation, difficult. Make sure there is a good light and a warm room. Stand on the patient's right side and ensure one's hands are warm. A shivering patient cannot relax and vital signs, especially on palpation, may be missed.

The abdomen is exposed by turning down all the bedclothes except the upper sheet. The clothing should then be drawn up to just above the xiphisternum and lastly the sheet folded down to expose the groins and genitalia across the upper thighs. This point is important because many is the patient who presents with intestinal obstruction due to a strangulated femoral or inguinal hernia where the diagnosis is missed initially due to lack of proper exposure of the groins in an effort to save their embarrassment. However, once full inspection has taken place the sheet may be pulled up to the level of the symphysis pubis to allay anxiety.

Inspection is an important and neglected part of abdominal examination. It is well worthwhile spending 30 seconds observing the abdomen from different positions to note the following features.

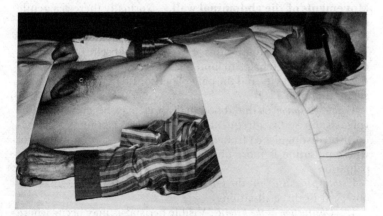

Fig. 4.2 Position of the patient and exposure for abdominal examination. Note that the genitalia must be exposed.

Shape.   Is the abdomen of normal contour and fullness, or distended? Is it scaphoid (sunken)?

Generalized fullness or distension may be due to fat, fluid, flatus, faeces, or fetus. *Localized distension* may be symmetrical as in the case of small bowel obstruction and centred around the umbilicus, or asymmetrical as in gross enlargement of the spleen, liver or ovary. Make a mental note of the site of any such *swelling* or distension; think of the anatomical structures in that region and note if there is any movement of the swelling, either with or independent of respiration.

A *scaphoid* abdomen is seen in advanced stages of starvation and malignant disease, particularly carcinoma of the oesophagus and stomach.

The umbilicus.   Normally the umbilicus is slightly retracted and inverted. Being at the centre of the abdomen one's eyes inevitably come to rest on it at the same time as noting the general shape of the abdomen. If it is everted then an umbilical hernia may be present and can be confirmed by feeling an expansile impulse on palpation of the swelling when the patient coughs. The hernial sac contains omentum, bowel or fluid. A frequent finding in the umbilicus of elderly obese women is a concentration of inspissated desquamated epithelium and other debris (omphalolith).

Movements of the abdominal wall.   Normally there is a gentle rise in the abdominal wall during inspiration and a fall during expiration; the movement should be free and equal on both sides. In generalized peritonitis this movement is absent or markedly diminished, which helps to limit further spread of infection within the peritoneal cavity and the pain of peritoneal irritation (the 'still, silent abdomen').

Visible pulsation of the abdominal aorta may be noticed in the epigastrium and is a frequent finding in nervous, thin patients. It must be distinguished from an aneurysm of the abdominal aorta where pulsation is more obvious and a widened aorta is felt on palpation.

Visible peristalsis of the stomach or small intestine may be observed in three situations.

1.   *Obstruction at the pylorus*. Visible peristalsis may occur where there is obstruction at the pylorus produced either by fibrosis following chronic duodenal ulceration or less commonly by car-

cinoma of the stomach in the pyloric antrum. Peristalsis will be seen as a slow wave passing either across the upper abdomen from left to right hypochondria or, if gross gastric dilation is present, passing down to the suprapubic region and ascending to terminate in the right epigastrium. In pyloric obstruction, a diffuse swelling may be seen in the left upper abdomen but, where obstruction is of long standing with severe gastric distension, this swelling may occupy the left mid and lower quadrants. Such a stomach may contain up to 2 litres of fluid and on shaking the abdomen a splashing noise is usually heard ('succussion splash'). This splash is frequently heard in healthy patients for up to three hours after a meal, so enquire when the patient last ate or drank. In congenital pyloric stenosis of infancy not only may visible peristalsis be apparent but the grossly hypertrophied circular muscle of the antrum and pylorus may be felt as a 'tumour' to the right of the midline in the epigastrium. Both these signs may be elicited more easily after the infant has been given a feed.

2. *Obstruction in the distal small bowel.* Peristalsis may be seen where there is intestinal obstruction in the distal small bowel, or coexisting large and small bowel hold-up produced by distal colonic obstruction, with an incompetent ileocaecal valve allowing reflux of gas and liquid faeces into the ileum. Not only is the abdomen distended and tympanitic (hyper-resonant) but the distended coils of small bowel may be visible in a thin patient and tend to stand out in the centre of the abdomen in a 'ladder pattern'.

3. As a *normal finding* in very thin, elderly patients with lax abdominal muscles or large wide-necked incisional herniae through an abdominal scar.

Skin and surface of the abdomen. In marked distension the skin is smooth and shiny. *Striae atrophicae* or *gravidarum* are white or pink wrinkled linear marks on the abdominal skin. They are produced by gross stretching of the skin with rupture of the elastic fibres and indicate a recent change in size of the abdomen such as is found in pregnancy, ascites, wasting diseases, and severe dieting. Wide purple striae are characteristic of Cushing's syndrome and excessive steroid treatment.

Note any *scars* present, their site, whether they are old (white) or recent (red or pink), linear or stretched (and therefore likely to be weak and contain an incisional hernia). Common examples are given in Fig. 4.3.

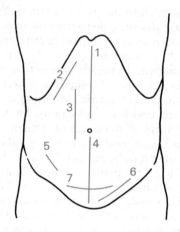

Fig. 4.3 Some commonly employed abdominal incisions.

    1:   Upper midline
    2:   Right subcostal (Kocher's)
    3:   Right paramedian
    4:   Lower midline
    5:   Appendicectomy (Gridiron)
    6:   Left inguinal
    7:   Suprapublic (Pfannensteil)

Look for *prominent superficial veins*, which may be apparent in three situations (Fig. 4.4).

Small, thin veins over the subcostal margins are common and usually of no significance. Distended veins around the umbilicus (caput Medusae) are uncommon but if present signify portal hypertension, whose other signs include splenomegaly and ascites. Distended veins represent the opening up of anastomoses between portal and systemic veins and are seen in other sites as oesophageal varices and piles. In patients who have inferior vena caval obstruction, not only will there be oedema of the limbs, buttocks and groins, but in time distended veins on the abdominal wall and chest wall appear. These represent dilated anastomotic channels between the superficial epigastric and circumflex iliac veins below, and the lateral thoracic veins above, conveying the diverted blood

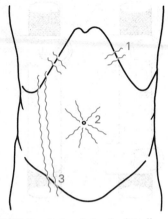

Fig. 4.4 Veins of the abdominal wall.
1: Thin veins over control margin
2: Caput medusae
3: Dilated veins in obstruction of inferior venacava

from long saphenous vein to axillary vein; the direction of flow is therefore upwards. If the veins are prominent enough, try to detect the direction in which the blood is flowing (Fig. 4.5).

Pigmentation of the abdominal wall is seen in the midline below the umbilicus where it forms the linea nigra and is a sign of pregnancy. Erythema ab igne is a brown mottled pigmentation produced by constant application of heat, usually a hot water bottle or heat pad, on the skin of the abdominal wall. It is a sign that the patient is experiencing severe pain.

Finally, inspect both groins, and the penis and scrotum in a male, for any swelling and to ensure that both testes are in their normal position. Then bring the sheet up just to cover the symphysis.

PALPATION

Palpation forms the most important part of the abdominal examination. Tell the patient to relax as best he can, to breathe gently and that you will be as gentle as possible. Enquire for the site of any pain and come to this region last. These points, together with

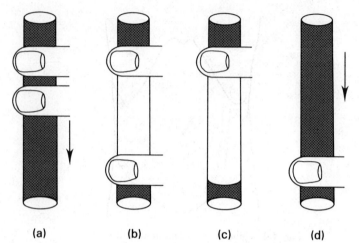

(a)   (b)   (c)   (d)

Fig. 4.5 A way of detecting the direction of blood flow in a vein. (*a*) Place 2 fingers side by side. (*b*) Move the lower finger away thus emptying part of the vein. (*c*) Remove the lower finger; in this example the vein remains empty. (*d*) Replace the lower finger and remove the upper finger; blood will be seen to run down from above.

unhurried palpation with a warm hand will give the patient confidence and enable one to gain the maximum amount of information. It is helpful to have a logical sequence to follow and if this is done as a matter of routine then no important point will be omitted. The scheme below is suggested:

1. Start in the left iliac region palpating lightly and work anti-clockwise to end in the suprapubic region, repeat this using deeper palpation and with both hands if necessary
2. Next feel for left kidney
3. Feel for spleen
4. Feel for right kidney
5. Feel for liver
6. Feel for urinary bladder
7. Feel for aorta and para-aortic glands and common femoral vessels
8. If a swelling is palpable, spend time eliciting its features
9. Palpate both groins
10. Examine the external genitalia

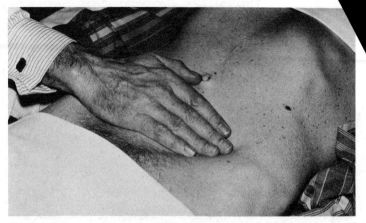

Fig. 4.6 Correct method of palpation. The hand is held flat and relaxed and 'moulded' to the abdominal wall.

Start by placing the right hand flat on the abdomen in the left iliac fossa with the wrist and forearm in the same horizontal plane where possible, even if this means the examiner bending down or kneeling by the patient's side (Fig. 4.6).

The art is to 'mould' the relaxed right hand to the abdominal wall, not to hold it rigid. The best movement is gentle but with firm pressure with the fingers held almost straight with slight flexion at the metacarpophalangeal joints.

At all costs avoid sudden poking with the fingertips (Fig. 4.7). Try and visualize the normal anatomical structures beneath the examining hand, and gently palpate each quadrant of the abdomen noting any area of tenderness or localized rigidity. Palpation is then repeated more slowly and deeply if necessary; in a fat or very muscular patient, putting the left hand on top of the right will enable you to exert increased pressure (Fig. 4.8).

There is no doubt that a small proportion of patients find it impossible to relax their abdominal muscles when being examined. In such cases it may help to ask them to breathe deeply, to bend their knees up or to distract their attention in other ways. No matter how experienced the examiner, he will gain little from palpation of a poorly relaxed abdomen.

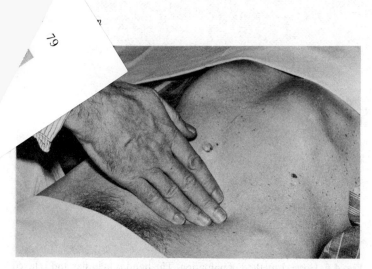

Fig. 4.7 Incorrect method of palpation. The hand is held rigid and mostly not in contact with the abdominal wall.

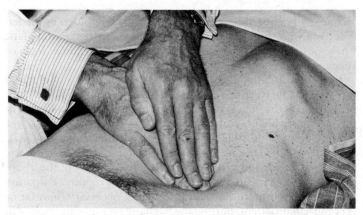

Fig. 4.8 Method of deep palpation in an obese, muscular or poorly relaxed patient.

Left kidney

The right hand is placed anteriorly in the left lumber region whilst the left hand is placed posteriorly in the left loin (Fig. 4.9).

Ask the patient to take a deep breath in, press the left hand

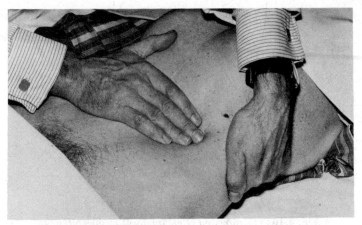

Fig. 4.9 Palpation of the left kidney.

forwards, and the right hand backwards, upwards and inwards. The left kidney is not usually palpable unless either low in position or enlarged. Its lower pole, when palpable, is felt as a rounded firm swelling between both right and left hands (i.e. bimanually palpable) and it can be pushed from one hand to the other.

Spleen

Like the left kidney the spleen is not normally palpable. It has to be enlarged to two or three times its usual size before it becomes so and then is felt beneath the left subcostal margin. It is not sufficiently appreciated that enlargement takes place in a superior and posterior direction before it becomes palpable subcostally. Once the spleen has appeared in this situation, the direction of further enlargement is downwards and towards the right iliac fossa (Fig. 4.10). Place the flat of the left hand over the lowermost rib cage posterolaterally, and the right hand beneath the costal margin way out to the left. Ask the patient to breathe in deeply, press in deeply with the fingers of the right hand beneath the costal margin, at the same time exerting considerable pressure medially and downwards with the left hand (Fig. 4.11). Repeat this manoeuvre with the right hand being moved more medially beneath the costal margin on each occasion (Fig. 4.12). If enlargement of the spleen is

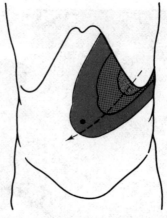

Fig. 4.10 The direction of enlargement of the spleen.

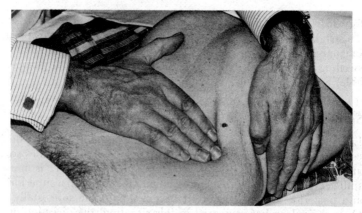

Fig. 4.11 Palpation of the spleen. Start well out to the left.

suspected from the history and it is still not palpable, turn the patient half onto his right side and repeat the examination as above.

In minor degrees of enlargement, the spleen will be felt as a firm swelling with smooth rounded borders. Where considerable splenomegaly is present, its typical characteristics include a firm swelling appearing beneath the left subcostal margin in the left

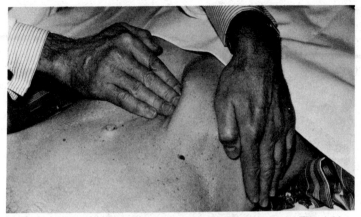

Fig. 4.12 Palpation of the spleen more medially than in Fig. 4.11.

upper quadrant of the abdomen, which is dull to percussion, moves downwards on inspiration, is not bimanually palpable, whose upper border cannot be felt (i.e. one cannot 'get above it') and in which a notch can often, though not invariably, be felt in the lower medial border. The last three features distinguish the enlarged spleen from an enlarged left kidney; in addition there is usually a band of colonic resonance anterior to an enlarged kidney.

Right kidney

Feel for the right kidney in much the same way as for the left. Place the right hand horizontally in the right lumbar region anteriorly with the left hand placed posteriorly in the right loin. Push forwards with the left hand, ask the patient to take a deep breath in and press the right hand inwards and upwards (Fig. 4.13).

The lower pole of the right kidney, unlike the left, is commonly palpable in thin patients and is felt as a smooth rounded swelling which descends on inspiration and is bimanually palpable.

Liver

Sit on the couch beside the patient. Place both hands side by side flat on the abdomen in the right sub-costal region lateral to the rectus with the fingers pointing towards the ribs. If resistance is encountered move the hands further down until this resistance disappears. Ask the patient to breathe in deeply and at the height of inspiration press the fingers firmly inwards and upwards (Fig. 4.14).

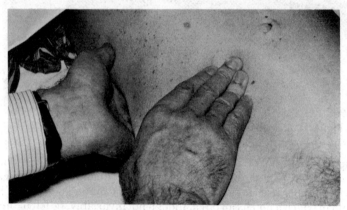

Fig. 4.13 Palpation of the right kidney.

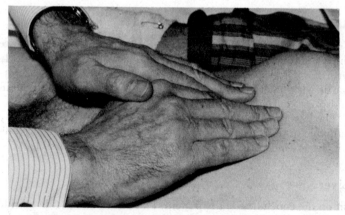

Fig. 4.14 Palpation of the liver: preferred method.

If the liver is palpable it will be felt as a sharp regular border which rides beneath the fingers. Repeat this manoeuvre working from lateral to medial regions to trace the liver edge as it passes upwards to cross from right hypochondrium to epigastrium. Another commonly employed, though less accurate, method of feeling for an enlarged liver is to place the right hand below and parallel to the right subcostal margin. The liver edge will then be felt against the radial border of the index finger (Fig. 4.15). The liver is often palpable in normal patients without being enlarged, whilst in patients with emphysema it is frequently felt. Considerable hepatomegaly is spoken of as being so many 'finger breadths' palpable below the right costal margin. Try and make out the character of its surface, i.e. whether it is soft, smooth and tender as in heart failure, very firm and regular as in obstructive jaundice and cirrhosis or hard, irregular, painless and sometimes nodular as in advanced secondary carcinoma. In tricuspid regurgitation the liver may be felt to pulsate. Occasionally a congenital variant of the right lobe projects down lateral to the gallbladder as a tongue-shaped process, called Reidel's lobe. Though rare, it is important to be aware of this because it may be mistaken either for the gallbladder itself or the right kidney.

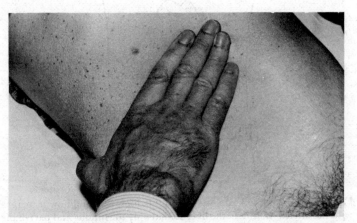

Fig. 4.15 Palpation of the liver: alternative method.

Gallbladder

The gallbladder is palpated in the same way as the liver. The normal gallbladder cannot be felt. When it is distended, however, it forms an important sign, and may be palpated as a firm smooth, round or globular swelling with distinct borders, just lateral to the edge of the rectus abdominis near the tip of the 9th costal cartilage. It moves with respiration. Its upper border merges with the lower border of the right lobe of the liver, or disappears beneath the costal margin and therefore can never be felt (Fig. 4.16). When the liver is enlarged or the gallbladder grossly distended, the latter may be felt not in the hypochondrium, but in the right lumbar or even as low down as the right iliac region.

The ease of definition of the rounded borders of the gallbladder, its comparative mobility on respiration, the fact that it is not normally bimanually palpable and that it seems to lie just beneath the abdominal wall, help to identify such a swelling as gallbladder rather than a palpable right kidney. This distinction may prove difficult however, especially when the gallbladder lies in the mid or lower quadrants.

The gallbladder can usually be palpated in the following clinical situations. In *all* the swelling is painless.

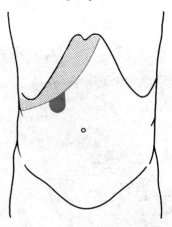

Fig. 4.16 Palpation of an enlarged gallbladder, showing how it merges with the inferior border of the liver so that only the fundus and part of the body can be palpated.

1. In carcinoma of the head of the pancreas and other causes of malignant obstruction of the common bile duct, the ducts above become dilated as does the gallbladder. The patient is also deeply jaundiced.

2. In mucocoele of the gallbladder, a gallstone becomes impacted in the neck of a collapsed empty uninfected gallbladder and mucus continues to be secreted into its lumen. Finally the uninfected wall is so distended that it becomes palpable. In this case the bile ducts are normal and the patient is not jaundiced.

3. In carcinoma of the gallbladder, the gallbladder will be felt as a stony hard irregular swelling, whereas in 1. and 2. it is firm and regular.

Murphy's sign. In acute inflammation of the gallbladder (acute cholecystitis) severe pain is present. Often an exquisitely tender but indefinite mass can be palpated which represents the underlying acutely inflamed gallbladder walled off by greater omentum. Ask the patient to breathe in deeply, and palpate for the gallbladder in the normal way; at the height of inspiration the breath is arrested with a gasp as the mass is felt. This represents Murphy's sign. The sign is *not* found in chronic cholecystitis or uncomplicated cases of gallstones.

The urinary bladder

Normally the urinary bladder is not palpable. When it is full and the patient cannot empty his bladder (retention of urine) a smooth firm regular oval shaped swelling will be palpated in the suprapubic region and its dome (upper border) may reach as far as the umbilicus. The lateral and upper borders can be readily made out, but it is not possible to feel its lower border, i.e. the swelling is 'arising out of the pelvis'. The fact that this swelling is symmetrically placed in the suprapubic region beneath the umbilicus, that it is dull to percussion, that pressure on it gives the patient a desire to micturate together with the signs above, confirm such a swelling as the bladder (Fig. 4.17).

In women, however, the swollen bladder has to be differentiated from a gravid uterus (firmer, mobile side to side and vaginal signs different), a fibroid uterus (may be bosselated, firmer and vaginal signs different) and an ovarian cyst (usually eccentrically placed to left or right side).

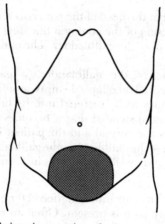

Fig. 4.17 Physical signs in retention of urine: smooth firm regular swelling arising out of the pelvis which cannot be palpated from below and is dull to percussion.

The aorta and common femoral vessels

The aorta is not readily felt but with practice it can usually be palpated a little above and to the left of the umbilicus; however, palpation has to be deep, so warn the patient of this. Palpation of the aorta is one of the few times that the fingertips are allowed as a means of palpation. Press the extended fingers of both hands, held side by side, deeply into the abdominal wall in the position shown in Fig. 4.18; make out the left wall of the aorta and note its pulsation. Remove both hands and repeat the manoeuvre an inch or so over to the right. In this way the pulsation and width of the aorta can be estimated. It is difficult to detect small aortic aneurysms; where a large one is present, its width may be assessed by placing a finger on either side of it and its expansile character noted by the fact that when pulsation occurs the width between each finger increases.

The common femoral vessels are found just below the inguinal ligament at the midpoint between anterior superior iliac spine and symphysis pubis. Place the pulps of the right index, middle and ring fingers over this site in the right groin and palpate the wall of the vessel. Note the strength and character of its pulsation and

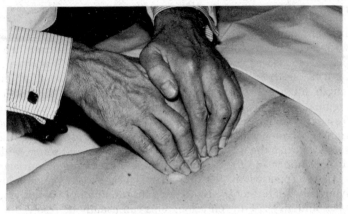

Fig. 4.18 Palpation of the abdominal aorta.

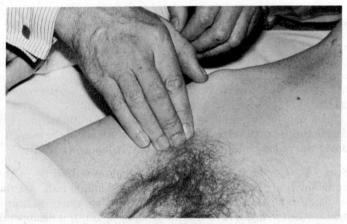

Fig. 4.19 Palpation of the right common femoral artery.

then compare it with the opposite femoral pulse (Fig. 4.19).
Nodes lying along the aorta (para-aortic) are palpable only
when considerably enlarged. They are felt as rounded, firm, often
confluent, fixed masses in the umbilical region and epigastrium
along the left border of the aorta.

Causes of confusion on palpation

In many patients, especially those with a thin or lax abdominal wall, faeces in the colon may simulate an abdominal mass. The pelvic colon is frequently palpable, particularly when loaded with hard faeces. It is felt as a firm tubular structure some 12 cm in length situated low down in the left iliac fossa, parallel to the inguinal ligament. The caecum is often palpable in the right iliac fossa as a soft, rounded swelling with indistinct borders. The transverse colon is sometimes palpable in the epigastrium. It feels somewhat like the pelvic colon but rather larger and softer, with distinct upper and lower borders and a convex anterior surface.

In the epigastrium, the muscular bellies of rectus abdominis lying between its tendinous intersections can mimic an underlying mass and give rise to confusion. This can usually be resolved by asking the patient to tense the abdominal wall, when the 'mass' may be felt to contract.

What to do when an abdominal mass is palpable

When a swelling in the abdomen is palpable make sure first that it is not a *normal* structure, as described above. Next consider whether it could be due to enlargement of the liver, spleen, right or left kidney, gallbladder, urinary bladder, aorta or para-aortic nodes.

Now palpate the swelling again. The aim of examination is to decide the organ of origin and pathological nature of the mass. In doing this it is helpful to bear in mind the following points:

Site. First make sure that the swelling does indeed lie in the abdominal cavity and not in the anterior abdominal wall. Ask the patient to lift his head and shoulders off the pillow and press firmly against the forehead. Now feel the swelling again. If it disappears or becomes much less obvious then it lies within the peritoneal cavity, whereas if it remains the same size it must be within the layers of the abdominal wall.

Note the region which the swelling occupies. Think of the organs that normally lie in or near this region and consider whether the swelling could arise from one of these organs. For instance, a swelling in the right upper quadrant most probably arises from the liver, right kidney, hepatic flexure of colon, or gallbladder.

Now, if the swelling is in the upper abdomen, try and determine if it is possible to 'get above it' and, similarly, if it is in the lower abdomen whether one can 'get below it'. By this is meant that one cannot feel the upper, or lower border of the swelling as it disappears above the costal margin or into the pelvis respectively. If one cannot 'get above' an upper abdominal swelling, a hepatic, splenic, renal or gastric origin should be suspected. If one cannot 'get below' a lower abdominal mass the swelling probably arises in the bladder, uterus, ovary or occasionally upper rectum.

Size and shape. As a general rule, gross enlargement of the liver, spleen, uterus, bladder or ovary present no undue difficulty in diagnosis. On the other hand swellings arising from the stomach, small or large bowel, retroperitoneal structures such as pancreas, or the peritoneum (see under mobility), may be difficult to diagnose. The larger a swelling arising from one of these structures, the more it tends to distort the outline of the organ of origin. For example, the characteristic reniform outline of the kidney is retained early on, but when there is a large renal mass this outline is lost and recognition becomes difficult.

Surface, edge and consistency. The pathological nature of a mass is suggested by a number of features. A swelling that is hard, irregular in outline and nodular is likely to be malignant, whilst a regular, round, smooth, tense swelling is likely to be cystic and benign, but remember degeneration and softening with cyst formation occurs in malignant tumours not infrequently. A solid, ill defined and tender mass suggests an inflammatory lesion as in Crohn's disease of the ileocaecal region.

Mobility and attachments. Considerable information can be gained from eliciting the mobility or fixity of an abdominal mass. Swellings arising in the liver, spleen, kidneys, gallbladder and distal stomach all show downward movement during inspiration, due to contraction of the diaphragm. One cannot, however, move such structures with the examining hand. In contrast, swellings originating in structures that have a mesenteric or other broad base of attachment are uninfluenced by respiratory movements but *can* be made to move freely by palpation, e.g. tumours of the small bowel and transverse colon, cysts in the mesentery, and large secondary deposits in the greater omentum.

When, on the other hand, the swelling is completely fixed it signifies usually one of three things: a mass of retroperitoneal origin, e.g. pancreas; part of an advanced tumour with extensive spread to the anterior or posterior abdominal walls or abdominal organs; or, a swelling resulting from severe chronic inflammation involving other organs, e.g. diverticulitis of the sigmoid colon or a colo-vesical attachment or fistula.

In the lower abdomen, the side to side mobility of a fibroid or pregnant uterus rapidly establishes such a swelling as uterine in origin and as not arising from bladder or ovary.

Is it bimanually palpable or pulsatile?   Bimanually palpable swellings in the lumbar region are usually renal in origin. Just occasionally, however, a posteriorly situated gallbladder or a mass in the posteroinferior part of the right lobe of the liver may give the impression of being bimanually palpable.

Finally, try to decide whether a swelling exhibits *pulsation*. It is often difficult to be certain whether a swelling in the upper abdomen that is pulsatile is merely transmitting pulsation from the underlying aorta or whether it is truly expansile in nature. The best way to determine this is to place two fingers on the swelling and observe what happens to them in systole. If the fingers remain parallel, then the pulsation is transmitted. If, however, the fingers tend to separate, then true expansile pulsation is present and the swelling is an aneurysm.

PERCUSSION

Details of how to percuss correctly are given on page 175. In the abdomen only light percussion is necessary—a resonant (tympanitic) note is heard throughout except over the liver where the note is dull. Whilst the technique is of limited value it can nevertheless provide important information.

Defining the boundaries of abdominal organs and masses

Liver.   The upper and lower borders of the right lobe of the liver can be mapped out accurately by percussion. Start anteriorly, at the 4th intercostal space, where the note will be resonant over the lungs, and work vertically downwards. In the normal liver the upper border is found at about the 5th intercostal space where

the note will become dull; this dullness extends down t
border found at or just below the right subcostal m
normal dullness over the upper part of the liver is redu
emphysema, in the presence of a large right pneumothor ax
when there is gas or air in the peritoneal cavity. The latter,
occurring in a patient with severe abdominal pain, indicates perforation of a viscus (unless the patient has recently undergone
laparotomy). This sign, however, is not one that should be relied
on as there has to be a large volume of air or gas present to reduce
the normal liver dullness, and this is not usually the case.

Spleen. Percussion over an enlarged spleen provides rapid
confirmation of the findings detected on palpation (p. 81 and Fig.
4.10). Dullness extends from the left lower ribs into the left
hypochondrium and left lumbar region. The lower border of an
enlarged spleen is readily mapped out; splenic dullness gives way
to the resonance of surrounding bowel.

Bladder. The findings in a patient with retention of urine are
usually unmistakable on palpation alone (p. 87 and Fig. 4.17). The
dullness on percussion provides reassurance that the swelling is
cystic or solid and not gaseous; its superior and lateral borders can
be readily defined from adjacent bowel, which is resonant.

Other masses. The boundaries of any localized swelling in the
abdominal cavity, or in the wall of the abdomen, can sometimes be
defined more accurately by percussion than palpation. The dullness of a solid or cystic mass contrasts with the tympanitic note of
surrounding loops of bowel.

Detection of ascites and its differentiation from ovarian cyst and intestinal obstruction

Three common causes of diffuse enlargement of the abdomen are:

1. The presence of free fluid in the peritoneum (ascites)
2. A massive ovarian cyst
3. Obstruction of the large bowel, distal small bowel, or both

Percussion rapidly distinguishes between these three as can be
seen in Fig. 4.20. Other helpful symptoms or signs that are usually
present are also listed below.

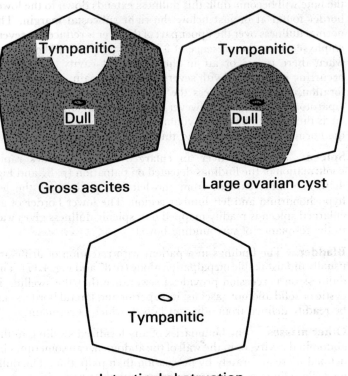

Fig. 4.20 Diffuse enlargement of the abdomen.

Gross ascites: dull in flanks; umbilicus is transverse and/or hernia present; shifting dullness positive; fluid thrill positive.

Large ovarian cysts: resonant in flanks; umbilicus is vertical and drawn up; large swelling felt arising out of pelvis which cannot be palpated from below.

Intestinal obstruction: resonant throughout; colicky pain; vomiting; constipation; complete bowel sounds.

It is unwise and difficult to diagnose *ascites* unless there is sufficient free fluid present to give generalized enlargement of the abdomen. Two signs, shifting dullness and a fluid thrill, present either singly or together, make the diagnosis of ascites certain. Useful as these two signs are, they can only be elicited in about half the cases of ascites. Absence of shifting dullness or of fluid thrill or both does *not* exclude a diagnosis of ascites.

To demonstrate *shifting dullness*, lie the patient supine and, on percussion, note dullness in the flanks and lower abdomen with a central area of resonance at and above the umbilicus. Now turn the patient on his right side. Allow time for the intestines to float upwards and the free fluid to gravitate down and percuss again. Note that whereas before the left flank was dull it is now resonant and that the height of the dullness on the lower side has risen. Now repeat this, turning the patient onto his left side.

To elicit a *fluid thrill* the patient is again laid on his back. Place one hand flat over the lumbar region of one side, get an assistant to put the side of his hand firmly in the midline of the abdomen, and then flick or tap the opposite lumbar region (Fig. 4.21). A fluid thrill or wave is felt as a definite and unmistakable impulse by the watching hand held flat in the lumbar region. The purpose of the assistant's hand is to dampen any impulse that may be transmitted through the fat of the abdominal wall. As a rule a fluid thrill is only present when there is a large amount of ascites present which is under tension.

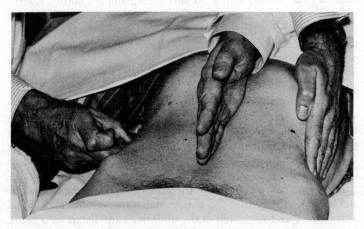

Fig. 4.21 Eliciting a fluid thrill.

AUSCULTATION

Auscultation is a useful way of listening for bowel sounds and deciding whether they are normal, increased or absent, and of detecting bruits in the aorta and main abdominal vessels.

The stethoscope should be placed on one site on the abdominal wall (just to the right of the umbilicus is best) and kept there until bowel sounds are heard. It should not be moved around from site to site. Normal bowel sounds are heard as intermittent low or medium pitched gurgles interspersed with an occasional high pitched noise or tinkle.

In simple acute mechanical obstruction of the small bowel the bowel sounds are excessive and exaggerated. Frequent loud low pitched gurgles (borborygmi) are heard, often rising to a crescendo of high pitched tinkles and occurring in a rhythmic pattern with peristaltic activity. The presence of such sounds occurring at the same time as the patient experiences bouts of colicky abdominal pain is pathognomonic of small bowel obstruction. In between the bouts of peristaltic activity and colicky pain, the bowel is quiet and no sounds are heard on auscultation.

In an obstructed loop of bowel, when strangulation and later gangrene supervene, however, peristalsis ceases, and the bowel sounds rapidly become less frequent and stop altogether. In *generalized peritonitis* bowel activity rapidly disappears and a state of *paralytic ileus* ensues, with gradually increasing abdominal distension. The abdomen is 'silent' but one must listen for several minutes before being certain that such a state exists. Frequently towards the end of this period, a short run of faint, very high pitched tinkling sounds are heard. This represents fluid spilling over from one distended gas- and fluid-filled loop to another and is characteristic of ileus.

A *succussion splash* may be elicited by palpation (p. 77) but also on auscultation. It may be heard in pyloric stenosis, advanced intestinal obstruction with grossly distended loops of bowel and in paralytic ileus. Place the stethoscope on the abdomen and with the free hand quickly depress the abdominal wall. A splashing noise is heard.

Bruits may also be heard in the abdomen. Press the bell of the stethoscope deeply into the abdominal wall over the abdominal aorta above and to the left of the umbilicus and listen for a bruit. Do likewise over each iliac artery in the corresponding iliac fossa, and over the common femoral arteries in each groin. If a bruit is heard it is a significant finding which indicates stenosis in the underlying vessel. Very occasionally bruits may be heard in the epigastrium when there is stenosis of the coeliac axis or superior mesenteric artery, or on either side of the midline in the mid-abdomen with patients with hypertension due to stenosis of the renal artery (see Chapter 13).

THE GROINS

Once the groins have been inspected (p. 73), ask the patient to turn his head to one side and cough. Look at both inguinal canals for any expansile impulse. If none is apparent, place the left hand in the left groin so that the fingers lie over and in line with the inguinal canal; place the right hand similarly in the right groin (Fig. 4.22). Now ask the patient to give a loud cough and feel for any expansile impulse with each hand. When a patient coughs, the muscles of the abdominal wall contract violently and this imparts a definite, though not expansile, impulse to the palpating hands which is a source of confusion to the inexperienced. Trying to differentiate this normal contraction from a small, fully reducible inguinal

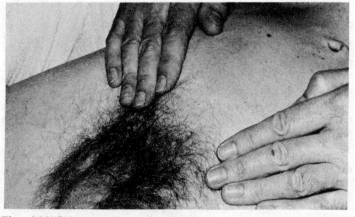

Fig. 4.22 Palpating the groins to detect an expansile impulse on coughing.

hernia is difficult, and the matter can usually only be resolved when the patient is examined standing up.

The femoral vessels have already been felt (p. 88 and Fig. 4.19) and auscultated (p. 96). Now palpate along the femoral artery for enlarged inguinal nodes, feeling with the fingers of the right hand, and carry this palpation medially beneath the inguinal ligament towards the perineum. Then repeat this on the left side. If the patient complains of a lump in the groin he should be examined lying down *and standing up*.

THE MALE GENITALIA

It is not always possible to avoid causing some discomfort, particularly in very sensitive patients, so always warn the patient what is about to happen. Tell him that the examination will be as gentle as possible and aim to make it so. Make sure the patient is warm; palpation is much more difficult, and therefore more likely to hurt a cold patient.

Ask the patient to separate his legs slightly, which allows one to deliver the scrotum to an accessible position.

If there is any suspicion of venereal infection put on disposable gloves.

INSPECTION

Note the distribution of pubic hair, the appearance and size of the penis, the presence or absence of a prepuce, and the site of the external urethral orifice. Look at the scrotal skin for any redness, swelling, oedema or ulceration. If any swelling is present, observe whether it appears to extend into the groin, and note whether both testes are in the scrotum. Lift up the scrotum to inspect its posterior surface.

PALPATION

The penis

Lift up the penis and palpate the corpora cavernosa, feeling for any induration, and the urethra, lying on the ventral aspect of the penis, from the glans to the perineum. If the patient is uncircumcised establish that the prepuce can be readily retracted by gently withdrawing it over the glans penis. This allows inspection of the inner lining of the prepuce, the glans penis, the coronal sulcus and the external urethral orifice (meatus). Always remember to draw the prepuce forwards, otherwise *paraphimosis*, painful oedema of the glans due to constriction by a retracted prepuce, may ensue. The internal male genitalia (prostate and seminal vesicles) are examined per rectum (p. 106).

Abrasions or small superficial sores on the outer surface of the prepuce or penile shaft are commonly due to trauma following intercourse. A *primary syphilitic chancre* is usually found on the inner aspect of the prepuce adjacent to or in the coronal sulcus. It commences as a small red papule which gradually hardens and erodes in the centre; a painless ulcer forms and typically the margins and base feel densely indurated. Retraction of the foreskin may reveal a *carcinoma* which presents the characteristic features of a malignant ulcer with raised everted edges and an indurated base. It is almost unknown in those circumcised before puberty.

Phimosis is narrowing of the preputial orifice so preventing retraction of the foreskin. This commonly results in recurrent episodes of infection of the glans penis (balanitis) and of the prepuce (posthitis), which are termed *balanoposthitis*. *Hypospadias* is a congenital anomaly where the external urethral orifice opens not at the tip of the glans penis but on its ventral surface in the midline, anywhere from the glans to the shaft or even in the perineum. It is much more common than a similar opening situated on the dorsal surface of the penis, called *epispadias*.

In the skin of the scrotum, *sebaceous cysts* are common and often multiple, presenting as round, firm, whitish nodules. *Malignant ulcers* (epitheliomata) are still occasionally seen in those workers who constantly wear heavily oil-stained clothes. Ulceration can also occur as a result of fungation from an underlying tumour of the testis or from a gumma. Sinuses on the scrotal skin are uncommon now in this country, but may occur as a result of tuberculous epididymo-orchitis in its advanced stages.

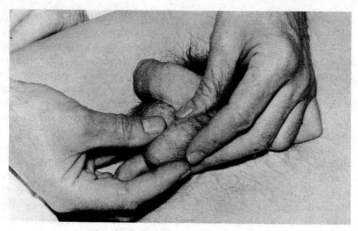

Fig. 4.23 Palpation of the left testis.

The testis

Now place the right hand below the scrotum and palpate first the
testis. Arrange the hands and fingers as shown in Fig. 4.23; this
'fixes' the testis so that it cannot slip away from the examining
fingers. The posterior aspect of the testis is supported by the
middle, ring and little fingers of each hand, the right hand being
inferior. This leaves the index fingers and thumb of each hand free
to palpate. Gently move the index finger and thumb over the
anterior surface of the body of the testis, feel the lateral border with
the index finger and the medial border with the pulp of each
thumb. Note the size and consistency of the testis and any nodules
or other irregularities. Now very gently approximate the fingers
and thumb of the left hand (the effect of this is to move the testis
inferiorly which is easily and painlessly done because of its great
mobility inside the tunica vaginalis). In this way the upper pole of
the testis can be readily felt between the approximated index finger
and thumb of the left hand. Next move the testis upwards by
reversing the movements of the hands and gently approximating
the index finger and thumb of the right hand, so enabling the lower
pole to be palpated.

The epididymis

Now palpate the epididymis. The head is found at the upper pole of the testis on its posterior aspect and is felt between the left thumb anteriorly and the index and middle fingers posteriorly. The epididymus is a soft nodular structure about 1 cm in length. The tail lies on the posterolateral aspect of the inferior pole of the testis and is felt between the thumb and fingers of the right hand. The tail too is soft, but unlike the head its coiled tubular structure can usually be made out.

The spermatic cord

Finally palpate the spermatic cord (Fig. 4.24) with the left hand. Exert very gentle downward traction on the testis, place the fingers of the right hand behind the neck of the scrotum, and with the thumb placed anteriorly press forward with the fingers of the right hand. The spermatic cord will be felt between the fingers and thumb; it is about 1 cm in width. The only structure that can be positively identified within it is the vas deferens, which feels like a thick piece of string. Having examined the testis, epididymis and cord on one side repeat the examination on the other side.

A lump in the groin or scrotum is a common clinical problem in all age groups. Most lumps in the groin are due either to herniae or

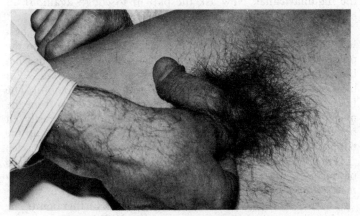

Fig. 4.24 Palpation of the left spermatic cord.

enlarged inguinal nodes; inguinal herniae are considerably more common than femoral with an incidence ratio of 4:1. In the scrotum hydrocoele of the tunica vaginalis or a cyst of the epididymus are common causes of painless swellings; acute epididymo-orchitis is the most frequent cause of a painful swelling.

Examination of the groins and scrotum is only part of a general examination and must not be conducted in isolation. Generalized diseases such as lymphoma may present as a lump in the groin.

Usually the diagnosis of a lump in the groin or scrotum can be made simply and accurately. Remember that the patient should be examined not only lying down, but also standing up.

What to do if a patient complains of a lump in the groin

Ask the patient to stand in front of you, get him to point to the side and site of the swelling and note whether it extends into the scrotum. Get him to turn his head to one side and give a loud cough; look for an expansile impulse and try to decide whether it is above or below the crease of the inguinal ligament. If an expansile impulse is present on inspection, it is likely to be a hernia, so move to whichever side of the patient the lump in the groin is on. Stand beside and slightly behind the patient. If the right groin is being examined place the left hand over the right buttock to support the patient, the fingers of the right hand being placed obliquely over the inguinal canal. Now ask the patient to cough again. If an expansile impulse is felt then the lump must be a hernia.

Next decide whether the hernia is inguinal or femoral. The best way to do this is to determine the relationship of the sac to the pubic tubercle. To locate this structure push gently upwards from beneath the neck of the scrotum with the index finger (Fig. 4.25) but not invaginating the neck of the scrotum as this is painful. The tubercle will be felt as a small bony prominence 2 cm from the midline on the pubic crest. In thin patients the tubercle is easily felt but this is not so in the obese. If difficulty is found, follow up the tendon of adductor longus which arises just below the tubercle.

If the hernial sac passes *medial to and above* the index finger placed on the pubic tubercle, then the hernia must be inguinal in site; if it is *lateral to and below*, then the hernia must be femoral in site.

If it has been decided that the hernia is inguinal then further points one needs to know are:

1. *What are the contents of the sac?* Bowel tends to gurgle, is soft and compressible, whilst *omentum* feels firmer and is of a doughy consistency.

2. *Is the hernia fully reducible or not?* It is best to lie the patient down to decide this. Ask the patient whether the hernia is reducible and if so then get him to reduce it himself to confirm this. It is more painful if the examiner reduces it.

3. *Is the hernia direct or indirect?* Again, it is best to lie the patient down to decide this. Inspection of the direction of the impulse is often diagnostic, especially in thin patients. A direct hernia tends to bulge straight out through the posterior wall of the inguinal

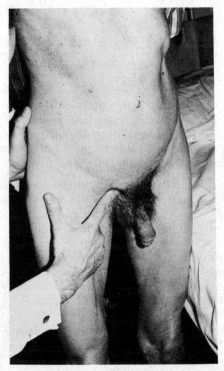

Fig. 4.25 Locating the pubic tubercle. *Note* the position of the examiner, at the side of the patient, with one hand supporting the buttock.

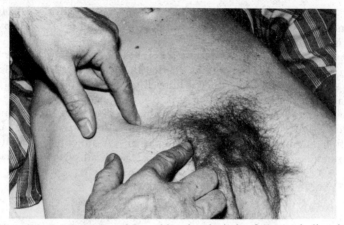

Fig. 4.26 *Left* Palpation of the pubic tubercle: index finger occluding the deep inguinal ring, *right* index finger on the pubic tubercle.

canal, whilst in an indirect hernia the impulse can often be seen to travel obliquely down the inguinal canal. Another helpful point is to place one finger just above the mid-inguinal point over the deep inguinal ring (see Fig. 4.26). If a hernia is fully controlled by this finger then it must be an indirect inguinal hernia.

Apart from a femoral hernia, *the differential diagnosis of an inguinal hernia* includes a large hydrocoele of the tunica vaginalis, a large cyst of the epididymis (one should be able to 'get above' and feel the upper border of both of these in the scrotum), an undescended or ectopic testis (there will be an empty scrotum on the affected side), a lipoma of the cord, and a hydrocoele of the cord in a male, or a hydrocoele of the canal of Nuck in a female.

In considering *the differential diagnosis of a femoral hernia*, one must think not only of an inguinal hernia but of a lipoma in the femoral triangle, an aneurysm of the femoral artery (expansile pulsation will be present), a sapheno-varix (the swelling disappears on lying down, has a bluish tinge to it, there are often varicose veins present and there may be a venous hum), a psoas abscess (the mass is fluctuant, and may be compressible beneath the inguinal ligament to appear above it in the iliac fossa) and an enlarged inguinal lymph node. Whenever the latter is found, the feet, legs, thighs, scrotum, perineum, and the pudendal and peri-anal areas must be carefully scrutinized for a source of infection or primary tumour.

The examination is completed by following the same scheme in the opposite groin.

What to do when the patient complains of a swelling in the scrotum

It is easier and better to examine the patient first lying down and afterwards standing up. Inspection, palpation and trans-illumination are the three keys to rapid, accurate diagnosis. After inspection of the scrotum and groins, try and answer the following questions.

1. *Can I 'get above' the swelling?* Palpate the neck of the scrotum between the fingers and thumb (see Fig. 4.24). If fingers and thumb cannot be approximated so that only the spermatic cord is palpable, then the swelling in question is not confined to the scrotum, but is descending from the groin and is therefore an inguino-scrotal hernia, i.e. one 'cannot get above' it. (Very rarely an infantile hydrocoele occurs which leads to the same signs though the testis is impalpable.) If fingers and thumb can be approximated so that one 'can get above' the swelling, that swelling can only be arising from the cord, the epididymis or the testis.

2. *Is the swelling cystic or solid? Is the testis palpable separate from the swelling?* Palpate the swelling in the same way as the testis and scrotal contents (p. 100) which will give a good indication whether the swelling is cystic or solid. *Now transilluminate the swelling*; tense the scrotal skin gently over the swelling and place a bright torch *behind* the swelling. If it conducts light then it must be a cystic swelling and is either a *cyst of the epididymis* (a spermatocoele) or a *hydrocoele of the tunica vaginalis*. The former lies above and a little behind the testis and the testis is palpable separate from the swelling. In the latter the testis is not palpable separate from the swelling, i.e. it is enclosed within the tunica vaginalis and therefore surrounded by fluid.

If the swelling is not translucent then its consistency is solid. Palpate the epididymis and testis again. Enlargement of the epididymis is found in inflammation (epididymitis): if it is tender it is acute; if it is painless, it is chronic (and usually tuberculous). Enlargement of the testis is found in orchitis (usually acute) when it is therefore tender, or rarely as a result of malignancy.

Finally stand the patient up. A swelling that is not apparent on lying down but appears on standing and which feels soft and rather like palpating a bag of worms is a *varicocoele*, i.e. varicosity of the veins of the pampiniform and/or cremasteric plexi.

RECTAL EXAMINATION

Few other regions of the body reveal such a wealth of physical signs and diagnoses on inspection and digital examination as the perianal area, anus, anal canal and rectum.

The left lateral position is best for routine examination of the rectum (Fig. 4.27). Make sure that the buttocks project over the side of the couch with the knees drawn well up, and that a good light is available. Put a disposable glove on the right hand and stand slightly behind the patient's buttocks, facing the patient's feet. Tell the patient what you are about to do and that you will be as gentle as possible.

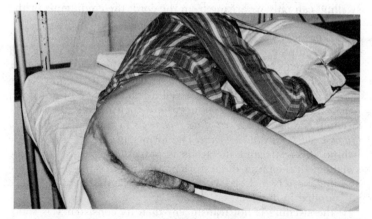

Fig. 4.27 Left lateral position for rectal examination.

INSPECTION

Separate the buttocks and carefully inspect the perianal area and anus. Note the presence of any *pruritus ani*, which may vary in appearance from mild erythema to a raw, red, moist, weeping dermatitis, or in chronic cases thickened white skin with exaggeration of the anal skin folds. The latter form *anal skin tags*, which may not only follow severe pruritus but also occur when prolapsing piles have been present over a period of time. Tags should not be confused with *anal warts* (condylomata acuminata) which are sessile or pedunculated papillomata with a red base and a white surface. Anal warts may be so numerous as to surround the anal verge, and even extend into the anal canal. Note any 'hole' or dimple near the anus with a telltale bead of pus or granulation tissue surmounting it which represents the external opening of a *fistula-in-ano*. It is usually easy to distinguish fistula-in-ano from a *pilonidal sinus*, where the opening lies in the midline of the natal cleft but well posterior to the anus.

The following acutely painful anorectal conditions can usually be diagnosed readily on inspection. An *anal fissure* usually lies directly posterior in the midline. The outward pathognomonic sign of a chronic fissure is a tag of skin at the base (sentinel pile). The fissure can easily be demonstrated by gently drawing apart the anus to reveal the tear in the lining of the anal canal.

A *perianal haematoma* (thrombosed external pile) occurs as a result of rupture of a vein of the external haemorrhoidal plexus. It is seen as a small (1 cm), tense, bluish swelling on one aspect of the anal margin and is exquisitely tender to the touch. In *prolapsed strangulated piles*, there is gross swelling of the anal and perianal skin, which look like oedematous lips, with a deep red or purple strangulated pile appearing in between, and sometimes partly concealed by, the oedema of the swollen anus. In a *perianal abscess*, an acutely tender, red fluctuant swelling is visible which deforms the outline of the anus. It is usually easy to distinguish this from an *ischiorectal abscess* where the anal verge is not deformed, the signs of acute inflamation are often lacking and the point of maximum tenderness is located midway between the anus and ischial tuberosity.

Note the presence of any ulceration. Finally, if *prolapse* is suspected, ask the patient to bear down and note whether any pink rectal mucosa or bowel appears through the anus, or whether the perineum itself bulges downwards.

PALPATION

Put a generous amount of lubricant on the gloved index finger of the right hand, place the *pulp* of the finger (not the tip) flat on the anus (Figs 4.28 and 4.29) and press firmly and slowly in a slightly

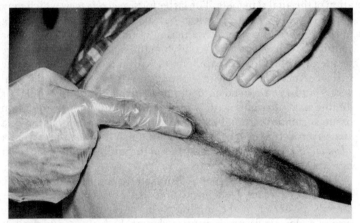

Fig. 4.28 Correct method for insertion of index finger in rectal examination. The pulp of the finger is placed flat against the anus.

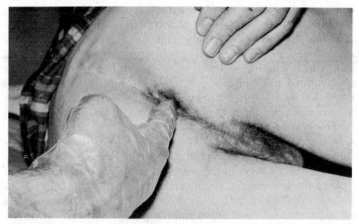

Fig. 4.29 Incorrect method of introduction of finger into anal canal.

backwards direction. After initial resistance the anal sphincter relaxes and the finger can be passed into the anal canal. If severe pain is elicited attempting this manoeuvre then further examination should be abandoned as it is likely the patient has a fissure and unnecessary pain will be caused.

Rotate the finger through 360° in the anal canal and feel for any thickening or irregularity of the wall of the canal. Assess the tone of the anal musculature; it should normally grip the finger firmly. If there is any doubt ask the patient to contract the anus on the examining finger. In the normal patient the contraction will be readily appreciated, whilst in the old and infirm with anal incontinence or prolapse almost no appreciable contraction will be felt. With experience it is usually possible to feel a shallow groove just inside the anal canal which marks the dividing line between the external and internal sphincter. The anorectal ring may be felt as a stout band of muscle surrounding the junction between the anal canal and rectum.

Now pass the finger into the rectum. The examiner's left hand should be placed on the patient's right hip and later it can be placed in the suprapubic position to exert downward pressure on the sigmoid colon. Try to visualize the anatomy of the rectum, particularly in relation to its anterior wall. The rectal wall should be assessed with sweeping movements of the finger through 360°, 2, 5 and 8 cm inwards or until the finger cannot be pushed any higher into the rectum. Repeat these movements as the finger is being withdrawn. In this way it is possible to detect malignant ulcers, proliferative and stenosing carcinomas, polyps and villous adenomas. The hollow of the sacrum and coccyx can be felt posteriorly. Laterally, on either side, it is usually possible to reach the side walls of the pelvis. In men one should feel anteriorly for the *rectovesical* pouch, *seminal vesicles* and the *prostate*. Normally the rectovesical pouch and seminal vesicles are not palpable. In a patient with a pelvic abscess, however, pus gravitates to this pouch which is then palpable as a boggy, tender swelling, lying above the prostate. If the pouch contains malignant deposits, hard irregular nodules may be felt. In infection of the seminal vesicles, these structures become palpable as firm, almost tubular swellings deviating slightly from the midline just above the level of the prostate.

Assessment of the *prostate gland* is important. It forms a rubbery, firm swelling about the size of a large chestnut. Run the finger over each lateral lobe, which should be smooth and regular. Between the two lobes lies the median sulcus which is palpable as a faint depression running vertically between each lateral lobe. Though one can say on rectal examination that a prostate is enlarged, accurate assessment of its true size is not possible. In carcinoma of the prostate, the gland loses its rubbery consistency and becomes hard, whilst the lateral lobes tend to be irregular and nodular and there is distortion or loss of the median sulcus.

In women, the cervix is felt as a firm rounded mass projecting back into the anterior wall of the rectum. This is often a disconcerting finding for the inexperienced. The body of a retroverted uterus, fibroid mass, ovarian cyst, malignant nodules or a pelvic abscess may all be palpated in the pouch of Douglas (rectouterine pouch) which lies above the cervix. This aspect of rectal examination forms an essential part of pelvic assessment in female patients.

On withdrawing the finger after rectal examination look at it for evidence of mucus, pus and blood. If in doubt wipe the finger on a white swab. Finally make sure to wipe the patient clean before telling him or her that the examination is completed.

THE FEMALE GENITALIA

It goes without saying that any examination of the female genitalia must be performed with gentleness and consideration, otherwise the patient will not be relaxed and vital signs may be missed. A good light is essential and a chaperone should be present. Ask the patient to empty the bladder immediately prior to examination as this makes bimanual examination easier; little information can be gained with a full bladder.

Ask the patient to lie in the left lateral position (see p. 106). Put on a pair of disposable gloves.

INSPECTION

Look carefully at the external genitalia, perineum, anus and inner thigh regions. Using both hands, separate the inner thighs to display the labia majora adequately (in an obese patient this will be made easier by asking the patient to raise the right leg slightly).

A swelling commonly seen in the posterior part of a labium majus is a Bartholin's cyst produced by blockage of the duct of Bartholin's gland; if infection supervenes an abscess develops. In *kraurosis vulvae* the labia are atrophic, the skin is white and rather thin and the introitus narrowed. In *leukoplakia of the vulva* white plaques, like white paint, are seen over the labia and perineum. Small wart-like papillary growths (condylomata acuminata) may be seen scattered over the vulva; these are due to a virus and not to syphilitic infection.

Hold the right buttock and thigh up slightly with the left hand, separate the labia minora with the index finger and thumb of the right hand and display the clitoris, urethral orifice and introitus of the vagina. The urethral orifice is seen as a small slit. In elderly women who complain of frequent painful micturition it is not uncommon to find an *urethral caruncle*, easily visible as a small, red polypoid lesion, rather like a tiny cherry, distorting the urethral orifice.

Note whether the hymen is intact. If it is, then digital examination per vaginum is not carried out; further information is gained by rectal examination and when necessary by vaginal examination under anaesthesia. Note any discharge at the introitus, its colour and amount. Inspection is completed by asking the patient to cough or bear down, at the same time observing the urethral orifice together with the anterior and posterior walls of the lower vagina. A small dribble or spout of urine issuing from the urethral orifice is apparent in *stress incontinence*. Bulging of the anterior vaginal wall backwards so that it appears to occlude the vaginal lumen is termed a *cystocoele* and is due to prolapse of the urinary bladder. A large forward bulge in the posterior vaginal wall is a *rectocoele*. Finally, the cervix may appear at the introitus in uterine prolapse (procidentia uteri). The common aetiology of these conditions is stretching and laxity of the pelvic muscles and ligaments following childbirth.

PALPATION

Put lubricant jelly on the right index and middle fingers. Gently insert the index finger into the vagina, pressing towards the perineum. When the pelvic floor muscles are felt to relax, introduce the middle finger with the thumb raised forwards over the symphysis but held away from the urethral orifice and clitoris. Push up gently with both fingers extended and feel for the cervix. Note the direction in which the cervix points, its contour, size, mobility and any irregularity of its surface. Now place the tips of the fingers in each fornix-anterior, right, lateral, left lateral and posterior (pouch of Douglas) in turn, and feel for any induration, swelling or mass that may be present. By gentle pressure in each lateral fornix it is usually possible to reach the side walls of the pelvis.

Whilst bimanual palpation may be carried out in the left lateral position, more information will be gained if it is conducted with the patient lying supine, the knees drawn up and allowed to fall apart, and the heels together.

Uterus

The lubricated index and middle fingers are introduced into the vagina, and the cervix and fornices reassessed. Now place the fingers of the left hand in the midline in the suprapubic region of the abdomen and press firmly downwards; the uterus will be pushed down towards the fingers of the right hand. Try to approximate the fingers of both hands; the fundus of the uterus will be felt and the position, size, contour and mobility of the uterus can be made out. Normally the uterus is palpable as a firm, non-tender, mobile swelling in the midline. In obese or poorly relaxed patients, however, this is not an easy thing to do.

Try to decide whether the uterus is *anteverted* or *retroverted* (Fig. 4.30). In the normal anteverted uterus, the cervix points backwards to make an angle of about 45° with the vagina; and the fundus and upper part of the body of the uterus are easily palpable. If the uterus is retroverted, the cervix will be felt either pointing in the long axis of the vagina or anteriorly, and the fundus will not be palpable suprapubically.

When the uterus is enlarged, symmetrical and soft, either pregnancy or carcinoma should be suspected. When it is enlarged, firm, mobile and nodular, such a finding is typical of fibroids. Fibroids may grow to a large size and may be palpable on abdominal examination as a swelling 'arising out of the pelvis'. When uterine mobility is reduced or the uterus is fixed and tender, there is usually an inflammatory cause. This is especially likely when there is associated induration in one of the vaginal fornices.

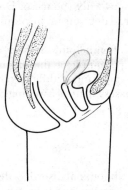 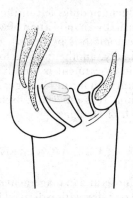

Normal anteverted uterus   Retroverted uterus

Fig. 4.30 The uterus.

Adnexa

It is often not possible to feel the ovaries, Fallopian tubes and parametrium unless they are enlarged or diseased. To palpate the adnexa, move the left hand to one side of the midline suprapubically and press down firmly whilst pushing gently upwards with the index and middle fingers of the right hand in the appropriate lateral fornix. Each fornix is palpated in this way and in the normal patient they should be soft and supple.

A normal ovary, if palpable, will be felt as a firm swelling about the size of a walnut, that is slightly mobile and tender.

An ovarian cyst is a common abnormality and often attains great size. It distorts the vaginal vault and is palpable as a swelling in the fornices, which has to be differentiated from fibroids or other uterine swelling. If sufficiently large, the cyst will be palpable through the abdomen as a swelling 'arising out of the pelvis' when it should be differentiated from a distended bladder, a fibroid uterus or ascites (p. 87).

As the normal Fallopian tube is not palpable, any thickening or induration that is palpable in the lateral fornix is abnormal. Such thickening is usually indicative of local inflammation or malignant spread from carcinoma of the cervix. Firm, painless, discrete or confluent nodules felt in the posterior fornix (pouch of Douglas) are usually an indication of widespread deposits in the peritoneum (carcinomatosis peritonei).

Finally, another satisfactory and often helpful method of deep pelvic assessment is simultaneous palpation of the vagina and rectum with the index finger in the vagina and middle finger in the rectum. It is especially useful for assessment of swellings in the pouch of Douglas.

THE ACUTE ABDOMEN

Diagnosis and management of acute abdominal disorders depends both on information derived from the history, and from the examination.

HISTORY

The patient usually presents with acute abdominal pain. In considering this symptom, its site, severity, radiation, character, time and circumstances of onset, and any relieving features are all important.

Site.   Ask the patient to point to the site of maximal pain with one finger. If pain is experienced mostly in the *upper abdomen* think of perforation of a gastric or duodenal ulcer, cholecystitis or pancreatitis. If pain is located in the *mid-abdomen*, disease of the small bowel is likely. Pain in the *right iliac fossa* is commonly due to apendicitis and pain in the *left iliac fossa* to diverticulitis. In women *low abdominal pain* of acute onset is often due to salpingitis, but rupture of an ectopic pregnancy should also be considered; the menstrual history is thus important. The coexistence of *severe back and abdominal pain* indicates a ruptured abdominal aneurysm or a dissecting aneurysm. When the parietal peritoneum is irritated, pain is felt at the site of the affected organ but when the visceral peritoneum is predominantly involved pain is often referred in a somatic distribution. For example, in acute appendicitis pain is felt near the umbilicus at first but later, with parietal peritoneal involvement, the pain moves towards the site of the appendix, usually in the right iliac fossa.

Severity.   Try to assess how severe the pain is. Ask the patient whether it keeps him awake. In women, compare the severity with labour pains. Sometimes comparison to the pain of a fractured bone is useful.

Radiation. If pain radiates from the right subcostal region to the shoulder or to the interscapular region, inflammation of the gall-bladder (cholecystitis) is a likely diagnosis. If pain begins in the loin but then is felt in the lumbar region a renal stone or renal infection should be considered. Pain beginning in the loin and radiating to the groin is likely to be due to a ureteric calculus and umbilical pain radiating to the right iliac fossa is usually due to appendicitis. Central upper abdominal pain, later radiating through to the back, is common in pancreatitis.

Character and constancy. Constant severe pain, felt over many hours, is likely to be due to infection. For example, diverticulitis or pyelonephritis can present in this manner. *Colicky pain* on the other hand, i.e. *pain lasting a few seconds or minutes and then passing off, leaving the patient free of pain for a further few minutes*, is pathognomonic of small bowel obstruction. If such pain is suddenly relieved after a period of several hours of severe pain, perforation of a viscus should be considered. Large bowel obstruction produces a more constant pain than small bowel obstruction, but colic is usually prominent.

Mode of onset. In obstruction from mechanical disorders such as that due to biliary or ureteric stone, or obstruction of the bowel from adhesions or volvulus, the onset of colicky pain is usually sudden. It is often related to activity or movement in the previous few hours. In infective and inflammatory disorders the pain usually has a slower onset, sometimes over several days, and there is no relation to activity. Recent ingestion of a rich heavy meal often precedes pancreatitis. Alcohol excess, or the ingestion of aspirin or steroid therapy are often observed as precipitating features in patients presenting with perforated peptic ulcer or with haematemesis.

Relieving features. Abdominal pain relieved by rest suggests an infective or inflammatory disorder. If the patient cannot keep still and rolls around in agony then ureteric or biliary colic are likely diagnoses.

Vomiting. A history of vomiting is not in itself very helpful because vomiting occurs as a response to pain of any type. However, effortless projectile vomiting often denotes pyloric stenosis or high small bowel obstruction. In peritonitis the vomitus is usually small in amount but vomiting is persistent. There may be a faeculent smell to the vomitus when there is low small bowel obstruction. Persistent vomiting with associated diarrhoea strongly suggests gastroenteritis. (See Examination of Vomit.)

Bowels. Constipation is the rule in the great majority of abdominal emergencies, whether inflammatory or obstructive. Absolute constipation occurs when there is complete intestinal obstruction. Absence of faecal matter occurs first and then the patient observes that the passage of flatus ceases and that abdominal distension has occurred. Diarrhoea occurring in the natural history of an acute abdominal disorder is evidence against a surgical cause. Alternating diarrhoea and constipation is seen in patients with diverticulitis or subacute intestinal obstruction. Sometimes a patient will be aware that the bowel sounds have become very noisy and frequent, which is evidence of chronic incomplete intestinal obstruction, probably in the colon.

The examination of the faeces is discussed in Chapter 5.

Micturition. Increased frequency of micturition occurs both in urinary tract infections and in other pelvic inflammatory disorders as well as in patients with renal infections or ureteric stones. In the latter haematuria commonly occurs.

Appetite and weight. In patients with a chronic underlying disorder, such as abdominal cancer, there may be a history of anorexia and weight loss, although weight loss also occurs in a variety of other disorders. Sudden loss of appetite clearly indicates a disorder of sudden onset.

Other features. It is important to note whether there have been previous episodes of abdominal pain and whether or not they have been severe. A tendency to improvement or worsening of the patient's symptoms after the onset is also important in deciding on management. The patient may have noticed swellings at the site of a hernial orifice indicating the likelihood of an obstructed hernia or there may be a history of blunt or penetrating abdominal trauma. Sometimes the patient may be aware of increasing abdominal distension, a phenomenon indicating intestinal obstruction or paralytic ileus probably associated with an inflammatory or infective underlying bowel disorder. Food poisoning may be suggested by history of ingestion of unusual foods such as shell fish or a meal in an unfamiliar surrounding. The menstrual history should never be forgotten particularly in relation to the possibility of an ectopic pregnancy. Enquiry should always be made as to a purulent vaginal discharge indicating salpingitis or of discharge of mucus, pus or blood from the rectum, suggesting ulcerative colitis.

EXAMINATION

A detailed explanation of the findings in the very large number of causes of an acute abdomen are out of place in this book. The student should consult an appropriate textbook of surgery. What is intended here is a very brief explanation of the terms used and of the findings on palpation in acute inflammatory conditions of the peritoneum. The physical signs found on inspection (p. 73) and on auscultation (p. 96) have already been discussed.

Guarding. Guarding is an involuntary reflex contraction of the muscles of the abdominal wall overlying an inflamed viscus and peritoneum, producing localized rigidity. It indicates localized peritonitis. What is felt on examination is spasm of the muscle, which prevents palpation of the underlying viscus. Guarding is seen classically in uncomplicated acute appendicitis. It is very important to distinguish this sign from voluntary contraction of muscle.

Rigidity. Generalized or 'board-like' rigidity is an indication of diffuse peritonitis. It can be looked upon as an extension of guarding, with involuntary reflex rigidity of the muscles of the anterior abdominal wall. It is quite unmistakable on palpation, as the whole abdominal wall feels hard and 'board-like', precluding palpation of any underlying viscus. The least downward pressure with a palpating hand in a patient with generalized rigidity produces severe pain. It may be differentiated from voluntary spasm by getting the patient to breathe: in voluntary spasm the abdominal wall will be felt to relax during expiration.

Rebound tenderness. Rebound tenderness is elicited by palpating slowly and deeply over a viscus and then suddenly releasing the palpating hand. If rebound tenderness is positive, then the patient experiences pain. This sign is explained by the fact that gradual stretching of the abdominal wall by deep palpation followed by sudden release of this pressure stimulates the parietal peritoneum which, if inflamed, produces pain. Rebound tenderness is not always a reliable sign and should be interpreted with caution, particularly in those patients with a low pain threshold.

EXAMINATION OF VOMIT

The character of the vomit varies with the nature of the food ingested and the absence or presence of bile, blood or intestinal obstruction. In pyloric stenosis the vomit is apt to be copious and sour smelling, contains recognizable food eaten many hours before and exhibits froth on the surface after standing. The presence of much mucus gives vomit a viscid consistency. The appearance of the vomit in haematemesis varies in relation to the site and severity of the bleeding. If bleeding is copious the vomit may present the appearance of pure blood, or it may be dark red and contain clots. Such bleeding may come from a gastric ulcer or from the oesophageal varices of portal hypertension. More commonly the blood is altered to a blackish or dark brown colour by being in contact with gastric juice. The dark brown colour is due to the conversion of haemoglobin into haematin. The altered blood gives to the vomit an appearance often compared to that of 'coffee grounds'. The taking of preparations of iron or red wine may produce a similar appearance in the vomit. Vomit which contains dark green bile may resemble vomit which contains blood; however, on diluting with water the green colour of the bile becomes more apparent while blood remains dark. Remember that blood in vomit may have come from the nose or lungs and been swallowed; bright red blood that is 'vomited' nearly always originates from the naso- or oropharynx and not from the stomach. Faeculent vomit, characteristic of advanced intestinal obstruction, is brown in colour, rather like vomited tea. Its main hallmark, however, is its typically faecal odour. Vomit containing formed faeces is rare but indicates a communication between the stomach and transverse colon, i.e. gastrocolic fistula.

ASPIRATION OF PERITONEAL FLUID

Aspiration of peritoneal fluid (paracentesis abdominis) is undertaken for diagnostic and therapeutic purposes. It is essential first to make sure that the bladder is empty; if there is any doubt a catheter should be passed before paracentesis is attempted.

The patient should be lying flat or propped up at a slight angle. An abdominal binder or many-tailed bandage should be placed in position around the patient's back before paracentesis is begun. The aspiration is usually performed in the right iliac fossa, a little outside the midpoint of a line drawn from the umbilicus to the anterior superior iliac spine.

With suitable sterile precautions, the skin at the point chosen should be infiltrated with local anaesthetic and the anaesthetic then injected down to the parietal peritoneum. If the puncture is made simply for diagnostic purposes, a 10 ml syringe and a suitable needle can be used. If it is intended to drain the peritoneum, a trocar and flanged cannula (which can be fixed to the skin with adhesive tape) should be employed. A tiny incision should be made in the anaesthetized area of the skin and then the trocar and cannula inserted. A resistance is felt as the trocar perforates the parietal peritoneum. The trocar is then withdrawn from the cannula and the fluid drained into a bottle via a tube connecting the cannula to the bottle. The binder is then secured over the abdomen which helps to promote drainage. The rate of flow, which should not be too fast, can be controlled by means of a clip on the tubing. When aspiration is complete, the cannula should be withdrawn. The puncture wound is sealed with a plastic dressing and a dry dressing applied. Therapeutic drainage should, however, be avoided if possible as diuretics are preferable.

The fluid withdrawn is sent for bacteriological and cytological examination and chemical analysis. Transudates, such as occur in heart failure, cirrhosis and nephrosis, normally have a specific gravity less than 1·018 and a protein content under 25 g/litre. Exudates occurring in tuberculous peritonitis or in the presence of secondary deposits usually have a specific gravity above 1·018 and more than 23 g/litre of protein. The distinction, however, is somewhat unreliable. Tubercle bacilli may be demonstrated in the fluid in tuberculous peritonitis; blood-stained fluid strongly suggests metastases. Malignant cells may also be demonstrated in the latter condition and in malignant ascites the fluid recurs rapidly after paracentesis.

THE GASTRO-INTESTINAL TRACT

Under this heading common and important methods of examining the *stomach* and *duodenum*, *small* and *large intestine*, the *liver*, *gall bladder* and *pancreas* will be described.

STOMACH AND DUODENUM

Intubation.   Intubation is used more for therapeutic than diagnostic purposes. In the former case it aids: *a*. gastric decompression in intestinal obstruction and following abdominal surgery; *b*. tube feeding in patients unable to swallow, or unconscious; and *c*. gastric washouts prior to surgery in patients with pyloric holdup. Intubation is, however, a necessary preliminary to studies of gastric acid production.

The nasogastric tubes are now made of soft plastic (Portex). The blind gastric end is round and weighted with metal to render it radiopaque. The lubricated tube is passed via a nostril and then swallowed. For gastric acid studies it should lie in the most dependent part of the stomach and this should be confirmed by screening. If required the tip can usually be passed into the duodenum by lying the patient on his right side and tilted forwards.

Gastric acid studies.   The patient should neither eat, drink nor smoke for eight hours before the study. After the tip's position has been confirmed by screening, all resting fluid should be removed by gentle manual suction with a syringe. The patient should then either sit up or lie on his left side, whichever is more comfortable. Constant manual suction is performed gently with a 20 ml syringe. It is usual to measure the basal acid output (BAO) and the maximum acid output (MAO), though the second is the more informative.

The basal acid output is measured after all resting fluid in the stomach has been removed. The basal secretion is then collected over the next one hour by continuous aspiration. In normal persons it is no more than a few millilitres per hour, containing up to 10 mEq of hydrogen ions.

The maximum acid output is measured after the administration of the synthetic peptide (Pentagastrin) of the hormone gastrin.

After the basal secretion has been measured for one hour, a dose of 6·0 μg/kg body weight of pentagastrin is given by subcutaneous injection. This causes a maximal acid secretion. After the injection, the juice is collected for one hour. The total acid secreted in this hour is the MAO. In normal subjects this may reach a maximum of 27 mEq/hour in males and 25 mEq/hour in females. Patients with duodenal ulcer have normal or raised values (up to 50 mEq/hour), whilst those with gastric ulcer and carcinoma have normal or low values.

The insulin test. The insulin test consists of an injection of insulin which produces hypoglycaemia and thus stimulates the nucleus of the vagus in the brain stem. Impulses then run down an intact vagal nerve and stimulate the production of a small amount of acid in the stomach. This does not happen after a complete vagotomy. Measurement of gastric acid production after an injection of insulin thus tests the completeness of a vagotomy. This investigation is particularly helpful when a patient develops a recurrent ulcer following vagotomy for duodenal ulceration. The blood sugar has to fall below 45 mg/100 ml for the test to be valid and it is measured before and after insulin is injected by slow i.v. infusion 0·04 units/kg/hour. Aspiration is then carried out for 120 minutes. The patient should be watched carefully and given intravenous glucose if severe hypoglycaemia occurs. A rise of acid secretion to 20 mEq/hour or more above basal unstimulated values probably indicates incomplete vagotomy.

Plain radiographs. Plain radiographs of the abdomen (Plate XIV) with the patient supine and in the erect position are of great value in cases of suspected peritonitis due to perforation of a gastric or duodenal ulcer, when gas may be seen under the diaphragm, usually on the right side.

Barium meal. The barium meal is a radiographic investigation in which the patient swallows a suspension of radiopaque barium sulphate, while the radiologist observes its passages on a fluorescent screen or on the TV monitor of an image intensifier. Films are taken to provide a permanent record of any abnormality discovered, but, as in all barium examinations of the alimentary tract, screening is important. The barium meal is principally used in the diagnosis of gastric and duodenal ulcer and of gastric carcinoma.

The barium-filled crater of a chronic gastric ulcer may be seen in the stomach as a projection from the wall ('profile view') or as a rounded deposit ('en face' view) with in either case mucosal folds radiating towards the crater. A duodenal ulcer is usually seen en face with a stellate appearance of the mucosal folds. Often no definite crater is seen, but the cap is deformed as a result of scarring, characteristically producing a trefoil deformity, sometimes with pseudo-diverticula. In cases of pyloric stenosis there is an increased amount of resting juice present and a grossly enlarged stomach which empties extremely slowly. Polypoid gastric carcinomas cause filling defects in the barium-filled organ. Malignant ulcers may be difficult to differentiate from simple ulcers, and the radiologist therefore pays particular attention to the mucosal folds and mobility of the wall in the region of the ulcer. Infiltrating tumours produce a rigid conical shape to the stomach with absence of peristalsis and no ulceration. Carcinomas involving the cardia and pylorus cause obstruction and, if small, may be difficult to differentiate from simple lesions.

Endoscopy and biopsy.   Flexible fibreoptic gastroscopes allow rapid and safe examination under out-patient conditions with the aid of local anaesthesia and light sedation (diazepam). By the use of suitable forward-viewing and side-viewing instruments it is possible to see the whole of the oesophagus, stomach and duodenum. The instruments carry a channel through which biopsy forceps or a brush can be introduced to obtain specimens for histological and cytological examination. Such instruments are of great value in differentiating benign from malignant lesions, assessing the response to treatment of benign gastric and duodenal ulcers, and in the rapid diagnosis of upper gastrointestinal bleeding.

SMALL INTESTINE

Estimation of faecal fats.   Faecal fat analysis is useful in the demonstration of steatorrhoea (see Chapter 5).

Barium meal follow-through X-rays.   The small intestine may be studied by taking films of the abdomen at intervals after a barium meal. Abnormalities in the transit time to the colon and in small bowel pattern, e.g. dilatation, narrowing, increase in transverse barring or flocculation, may be demonstrated in malabsorption states. Areas of narrowing with proximal dilatation, fistulae and mucosal abnormalities may be produced by Crohn's disease. Small bowel diverticula or neoplasms may also be demonstrated. The 'small bowel enema' is an alternative to the barium meal and follow-through examination. This involves intubating the duodenum and passing small quantities of a non-flocculating barium suspension down the tube. This method is particularly valuable for detecting isolated focal lesions.

Biopsy. Biopsy of the small intestinal mucosa can be performed using a spring loaded capsule (the Crosby capsule). This capsule, about 1·5 cm long and 7 mm in diameter, contains a cutting blade which excises a small piece of intestinal mucosa when negative suction is applied to the thin polythene tube to which it is attached. The capsule is swallowed, and a small amount of radiopaque dye is injected, to check that it has passed through the pylorus. Its position in the small intestine can then be checked radiologically. After the biopsy has been taken the capsule is pulled up and the specimen placed on a small piece of card in a preservative solution. It should be examined immediately by the pathologist under a low power microscope, to assess the general appearance of the intestinal villi.

Biopsy must always be preceded by a barium meal and follow-through examination, as the technique might be dangerous if the capsule were to lodge in a duodenal or jejunal diverticulum.

The small intestinal biopsy is of particular importance in diagnosis of the malabsorption syndrome, where a flat mucosa is seen in place of the usual multiple villi. For further tests of intestinal function, such as the xylose and lactose absorption tests, special textbooks should be consulted.

COLON, RECTUM AND ANUS

Proctoscopy. The anal canal and lower rectum can be readily visualized with a proctoscope. Place the patient in the position described for rectal examination and gently pass the lubricated instrument to its full depth. Remove the obturator and inspect the mucosa as the instrument is slowly withdrawn. Piles are seen as reddish/blue swellings which bulge into the lumen of the instrument. The internal opening of an anal fistula, an anal or low rectal polyp and a chronic anal fissure are other abnormalities that may be seen.

Sigmoidoscopy.   It is often necessary to examine the rectum and colon more fully than is possible by proctoscopy, and in such cases the sigmoidoscope is employed. Sigmoidoscopy requires skill and experience. In accomplished hands the instrument can be passed for 30 cm. The procedure causes little discomfort and anaesthesia is unnecessary.

Proctitis, polyps and carcinomas may be seen and biopsies taken. Sigmoidoscopy is particularly useful in the differential diagnosis of diarrhoea of colonic origin.

In suspected amoebic dysentery, the mucous membrane may be inspected and portions of mucus and scrapings from the ulcer may be removed and examined microscopically for amoebic cysts.

Barium enema.   Barium suspension is introduced via a tube into the rectum as an enema and manipulated around the rest of the colon to fill it. Screening is performed by a radiologist and films taken. The barium is then evacuated and further films taken. By this means, obstruction to the colon, tumours, diverticular disease, fistulae and other abnormalities can be recognized (Plate XIV).

If, following evacuation, air is introduced into the colon, detailed study of the mucosa is facilitated. This method is especially valuable for detecting small lesions such as polyps and early tumours.

Colonoscopy.   The use of flexible fibreoptic colonoscopes requires considerable skill and should be restricted to experts. It is frequently possible to inspect the whole of the colonic mucosa round to the caecum. Biopsies can be taken and pedunculated polyps removed by the use of diathermy snare loops, which thus do away with the need for laparotomy to excise such polyps.

THE LIVER

Biochemical tests of liver function are used in the differential diagnosis of jaundice, to detect liver cell damage in other disorders and to monitor the results of surgery of the biliary system and pancreas.

Isotope scan. A radio-isotope of technetium or colloidal gold is injected i.v. and is taken up by the reticuloendothelial system. A gamma camera is used to show the size and shape of the liver. Areas which do not take up the isotope appear as filling defects, and examples are primary or secondary hepatic tumours, abscesses and cysts.

Ultrasound scan. A probe, emitting ultrasonic pulses, is passed across the liver and surrounding areas. Echoes detected from within the patient are received with a transducer, amplified and suitably displayed. The technique is of particular value in the diagnosis of fluid-filled lesions such as cysts and abscesses and in detecting dilated intrahepatic bile ducts.

CAT scanning. Computerized axial tomography can be used to produce cross-sectional images of the liver. However, the place of this investigation in clinical practice is, as yet, undefined.

Exploration of liver for liver abscess. Liver abscesses due to *Entamoeba histolytica* are nearly always found in the right lobe. When suspected clinically, their presence and position may be demonstrated and localized radiologically or by isotope or ultrasound scanning. Metronidazole (Flagyl) 800 mg three times a day for ten days is now the first line of treatment and cures the great majority of cases. Where there is a lack of response to treatment after five days, exploration by needle aspiration for diagnostic and therapeutic purposes may be performed.

The procedure is conducted under local anaesthesia and strict asepsis. A needle of wide enough bore to admit thick pus (a stout, old fashioned lumbar puncture needle is suitable) is selected and a piece of adhesive tape is wound around it 9 cm from its point. The needle is entered either at the site of maximum tenderness or in the right 8th, 9th or 10th intercostal space in the midaxillary line, and passed medially in a horizontal plane to a maximum depth of 9 cm. By this means the whole of the right lobe of the liver may be explored. When pus is encountered, strong suction has to be employed to remove as much of the pus as possible and this is done with the aid of a two-way syringe. As the pus is removed, it may be replaced by a suitable volume of air (about half the volume of pus removed). The patient is then X-rayed in several positions to determine the exact site and size of the abscess, and to allow the effect of treatment to be followed.

Needle biopsy of liver.   For many years needle biopsy was the standard method used in the diagnosis of liver abscess. In the last few decades it has been used to obtain material for histological study. Whilst needle biopsy can be conducted under mild sedation and local anaesthesia, it should only be carried out in hospital under supervision and blood should be available for transfusion if necessary. Generally the method is safe and reliable, but there is a tiny but definite mortality from the procedure due to leakage of bile and/or blood into the peritoneal cavity from the puncture site. The procedure should therefore always be regarded as a potentially dangerous investigation and should only be performed by those well trained in the technique. Contra-indications include patients with a bleeding diathesis, deep obstructive jaundice or ascites.

Selective angiography of coelic axis and hepatic artery. Angiography is not commonly employed in the investigation of hepatic disease, since it is an invasive technique that demands considerable skill on the part of the radiologist. A catheter is passed retrogradely up the aorta from a femoral puncture; its tip is manipulated into the coelic axis and thus into the hepatic artery. Radio-opaque contrast material may then be injected to demonstrate the hepatic vasculature. The technique is occasionally valuable in demonstrating abnormal vascular patterns in isolated lesions, particularly in malignant disease, when other methods have failed.

Gallbladder and bile ducts

The main functions of the gallbladder are to concentrate and store hepatic bile, and to empty this bile into the duodenum after appropriate stimuli. The organ is investigated by performing *oral cholecystography*. This procedure depends on the fact that certain iodine-containing compounds, when absorbed from the gastrointestinal tract, are excreted by the liver and concentrated in the gallbladder, thus rendering it opaque.

Apart from a non-functioning gallbladder, radiolucent stones, abnormalities of the wall of the gallbladder, anatomical variations and failure to contract in response to a fatty meal, may also be demonstrated.

Intravenous cholangiography. Intravenous cholangiography is used to demonstrate the bile ducts. The technique depends on the fact that an intravenously administered iodine-containing compound, is excreted by the liver in the bile in such a concentration that it is radio-opaque, and therefore does not depend on the concentrating power of the gallbladder as in cholecystography. As with cholecystography it cannot be performed in the jaundiced patient.

Of particular interest are the width of the common bile duct (usually less then 10 mm), the presence of stones seen as radiolucent filling defects, and the entry of dye into the duodenum. A dilated duct nearly always signifies an abnormality.

Percutaneous transhepatic cholangiography. Percutaneous transhepatic cholangiography is a very useful investigation in patients with jaundice due to obstruction of the main bile ducts. The site of the obstruction due to tumours of the head of the pancreas, or iatrogenic and malignant bile duct strictures can be accurately localized and differentiated. The information gained prior to laparotomy is of great value to the surgeon.

ERCP (endoscopic retrograde cholangiopancreatography). The development of a side-viewing fibreoptic duodenoscope meant that the duodenal papilla could be readily identified. Biopsy and brushings of the papilla can be taken for histological and cytological examination. The papilla may be cannulated and then injected with dye to display the common bile ducts and pancreatic duct and thus demonstrate abnormalities in their outline or lumen. The technique is particularly useful in the rapid diagnosis and localization of the different causes of jaundice due to obstruction of the main bile ducts, in demonstrating the bile ducts where intravenous cholangiography has failed, and in the speed with which obstruction may be eliminated as a cause of jaundice in those patients with cholestasis.

THE PANCREAS

Lundh test. The Lundh test relies on an assessment of tryptic activity in pancreatic juice collected following duodenal intubation and indirect stimulation of the pancreas by prior ingestion of a meal. Where the mean tryptic activity is less than 6 iu/litre, exocrine insufficiency is present. The test is reliable in experienced hands and is cheap and simple to perform.

Triple test. The triple test is so called because it consists of three parts. A special double lumen tube is swallowed and then screened into position in the duodenal loop. It has a weighted bulbous end and contains two sets of holes, one for duodenal and the other for gastric aspiration. The latter set of holes prevents contamination of the duodenal aspirate.

1. *Exocrine function.* After a short period allowed for stabilization, secretin is injected and duodenal aspirate collected continuously over the next 30 minutes. Pancreozymin (cholecystokinin) is then injected and the process repeated. The volume of aspirate and concentration and output of bicarbonate, amylase, lipase and trypsin are then measured and calculated. Patients with carcinoma of the pancreas, particularly of the head, produce low volumes of low enzyme levels. Patients with chronic pacreatitis secrete low volumes, the juice containing low levels of bicarbonate and normal or low enzyme levels.

2. *Cytology.* Fresh aspirate is examined for malignant cells stained by the Papanicoloau method. Interpretation, however, is difficult and requires an experienced cytologist.

3. *Hypotonic duodenography.* When the first two parts of the test are completed, an anti-spasmodic drug (Buscopan) is injected which paralyses the duodenum. A small amount of barium is injected down the duodenal lumen of the tube followed by 100 ml of air. This delineates the wall of the distended duodenum; ampullary carcinomas, and irregularity and distortion of the medial wall due to infiltration by a carcinoma of the head of the pancreas, may be visualized.

The triple test is more complex, and more unpleasant for the patient than the Lundh test. In experienced hands the procedures should be regarded as valuable screening methods for pancreatic disease, especially where the following more sophisticated investigations are not available.

ERCP. The ERCP procedure (p. 427) can display the entire pancreatic duct system. It is therefore valuable not only in the diagnosis of chronic pancreatitis but also in defining those cases which surgery could benefit.

After stimulation with secretin, pure pancreatic juice uncontaminated with duodenal content may be collected from the duct and cytological examination performed. This provides a better success rate (about 50%) in the diagnosis of pancreatic carcinoma than the similar examination in the Triple test. The procedure should not be performed in patients with acute pancreatitis or those with suspected pseudopancreatic cysts.

5

The excreta

The urine
The faeces
Intestinal parasites

THE URINE

Sir Robert Hutchison used to say that the ghosts of dead patients that haunt us do not ask why we did not employ the latest fad of clinical investigation; they ask 'Why did you not test my urine?' or 'Why did you not put a finger in my rectum?'

To the risk that the urine may not be tested at all, new dangers have been added, in that urine testing is increasingly delegated to non-medical persons, who may be inadequately trained in the performance and interpretation of the tests they use and unaware of their importance. All doctors and students should be thoroughly conversant with urine testing, which is an essential part of any medical examination.

Urine passed into a clean vessel is suitable for routine urine testing. Special methods of collection, designed to reduce urethral and other contamination, are desirable for microscopical examination (p. 146) and essential for bacteriological examination (p. 150).

The urine should be examined physically, chemically, microscopically and bacteriologically.

PHYSICAL EXAMINATION

Attention should be paid to the following points: quantity; colour and transparency; specific gravity; and naked-eye characteristics of the deposit.

Quantity

The normal quantity of urine passed daily varies widely, from 700 to 2500 ml, depending on the fluid intake. Normally, very much more urine is excreted during the day than during the night. An *increased excretion* of urine occurs *physiologically* after food or drink, and after exposure to cold. Conversely, *diminished excretion* occurs when little food or drink has been taken, and after heat-induced sweating.

A *pathological increase (polyuria)* occurs in diabetes mellitus and insipidus, during the elimination of oedema fluid and may be evident in renal failure. *Nocturnal polyuria*, usually shortened to the term *nocturia*, is often the first manifestation of failure of the concentrating power of the kidney, and is commonly the first symptom of chronic renal failure.

Abnormal reduction of urine output may be due to salt and water depletion from diarrhoea, vomiting, fever or excessive sweating; the sudden lowering of blood pressure; severe heart failure; or acute diffuse disease of the kidney tissue such as occurs in post-streptococcal glomerulonephritis.

Complete cessation of urine output (*anuria*) is uncommon and most often results from an obstruction in the urinary tract itself.

Colour and transparency

Urochrome and uroerythrin are pigments which give normal urine its characteristic colour. The exact tint varies widely, and it darkens on standing due to the oxidation of colourless urobilino-gen to coloured urobilin. The concentration of urine cannot be reliably estimated from its appearance.

Small quantities of blood give urine a smoky appearance; larger quantities make it brownish or red. Haemoglobin in large amounts, as in blackwater fever, gives it a colour varying from dark red (when it may be confused with the colour resulting from excessive consumption of beetroot) to brownish black or even almost black.

Bile pigment causes the urine to appear brown, with a green tint at the surface when viewed in the specimen glass against the light; it produces a yellow froth when the urine is shaken in a test tube.

The urine is abnormally pale when it is very dilute, i.e. with specific gravity of about 1·002, and in renal failure, when the normal colouring matter is greatly diminished or absent.

The taking of drugs may also lead to discoloration of the urine. Some examples are tetracyclines (yellow); anthracene purgatives (orange); desferrioxamine (reddish brown); phenindione (pink); nitrofurantoin, furazolidone and niridazole (brown); rifampicin and pyridium (red); methylene blue, present in some proprietary pills (green); and methyldopa and iron sorbitol (grey or black).

Normal urine is quite transparent when freshly passed but it may be *opalescent* from the presence of various substances in suspension, of which the most important are pus, bacteria and phosphates. Phosphates dissolve on adding acid. If the opalescence persists after filtration, it is due to the presence of bacteria. Clear urine may become cloudy when cooled to room temperature; this is probably due to the precipitation of urates, which dissolve when the urine is re-warmed to body temperature.

Specific gravity

The concentration of urine is best expressed as its *osmolality*, which depends on the number of osmotically active solute particles per unit of solvent, and this may be determined by measuring its freezing point.

Although less accurate, it is often helpful, and usually more practicable, to measure the *specific gravity* with a *urinometer*. The specific gravity depends on the type as well as on the number of solute particles. To obtain satisfactory results certain precautions must be taken. The glass-ware used should be clean and free from detergents, and the urinometer should float freely in the measuring cylinder. The reading at the bottom of the meniscus is the relevant one. As the instrument is calibrated at 16°C, a falsely low reading will be obtained if urine is tested whilst warm, so it should be allowed to cool to room temperature. Otherwise 0·001 should be added to the specific gravity recorded for every 3°C by which the urine temperature exceeds 16°C. If there is insufficient urine for the urinometer to float freely, the urine should be diluted with an equal volume of distilled water and the last two figures of the urinometer reading doubled. Randomly measured, the normal specific gravity varies from 1·002 to 1·025, depending on the state of hydration and the time of day. It may occasionally rise to 1·035 even in health.

In normal urine the specific gravity is proportional to the urinary concentration of urea and sodium.

Approximate correlations between specific gravity and osmolality are as follows:

Specific gravity	Osmolality (mOsm/kg)
1·002	100
1·010	285
1·020	750
1·030	1200
1·035	1400

However, unusually high specific gravities compared with osmolalities may be found in urine containing many different heavy particles, e.g. radiographic contrast medium, glucose (as in diabetes mellitus) or protein. 2·7 g per litre of glucose, or 4 g per litre of protein cause the specific gravity to rise by 0·001. In diabetes insipidus, on the other hand, the specific gravity may fall almost to that of distilled water, and this may also happen in compulsive water drinking.

Normally, the concentration of the urine, as reflected by its specific gravity, varies considerably from time to time. As renal failure develops the kidneys progressively lose their ability to concentrate and dilute urine, whose specific gravity approximates more and more to 1·010 (the specific gravity of the glomerular filtrate) until eventually the urine is isotonic with plasma water. This is a simple and useful test of renal function. The specimen passed on rising should be tested for this purpose, as it is normally the most concentrated that is passed in the day. If the specific gravity of this, or any other sample of urine, exceeds 1·018 it can be assumed that renal concentrating power is normal. A period of fluid deprivation longer than overnight is required to achieve maximum concentration, but care must be taken that the patient does not become too dehydrated.

Naked-eye characteristics of the deposit

Normal urine is perfectly clear and transparent when voided. After it has stood for some time a deposit of 'mucus' appears in it. This forms a woolly cloud, which usually settles to the bottom of the glass, but if the urine is of high specific gravity it may be in the middle or at the top. If traces of blood are present in the urine, the cloud of 'mucus' may have a brownish tint.

Phosphates, urates and uric acid may precipitate in normal urine. Phosphates produce a white deposit when the urine is alkaline; warming increases their deposition because the urine becomes more alkaline due to loss of carbon dioxide. They dissolve after acidification with acetic acid. Urates and uric acid form faintly pink deposits, particularly if the urine is concentrated or highly acidic; they disappear on warming or adding sodium hydroxide. Although usually of no significance, they may appear when purine breakdown is increased, as in myeloproliferative disorders, especially after treament, when they may cause renal colic or even urinary obstruction.

Abundant leucocytes and bacteria may give the urine a turbid appearance; a gross deposit of yellow-white pus may rarely be formed. Gross haematuria may produce a red deposit.

CHEMICAL EXAMINATION

Many of the traditional chemical tests for urinary constituents have been replaced for routine purposes by commercial tablet or reagent 'stick' or 'strip' tests. Some of these will be described briefly, but for full details the manufacturer's literature should be consulted. This is especially necessary when a 'combination' indicator strip, which tests for several different constituents of urine, is used because it is easy to confuse the colour bands, or to read the individual indicator areas at the wrong time. *Failure to follow the manufacturer's instructions exactly, or failure to keep the reagents in a satisfactory condition, will result in incorrect deductions.* The indicator ends of reagent strips should not be handled, and urine for testing should be collected in clean containers, free from antiseptics or detergents.

pH

It is customary to test the reaction of the urine with pH indicator papers, but the result is rarely important except when a drug has been given with the intention of altering the pH for therapeutic purposes. Normal urine is nearly always acid. Rarely is it repeatedly neutral or alkaline, when the patient is not taking alkalis, and this may indicate impairment of the ability of the tubules to eliminate acid. This can be confirmed by accurate measurement of the pH of the urine after giving ammonium chloride to the patient (p. 154).

Proteins

Before doing the 'traditional' tests for protein, it is essential that the urine should be absolutely clear and it may therefore be necessary to filter it. If the urine remains turbid after it has been filtered more than once, bacteria are probably present and the protein concentration is best tested with commercial reagent strips. If the turbidity is due to urates, it will disappear when the urine is heated; if due to phosphates it will disappear after acidification.

Commercial reagent strips. Commercial reagent strips (e.g. Albustix) are impregnated with buffered tetrabromophenol blue, and change from yellow to various shades of green depending on the concentration of protein in the urine. The colour of the indicator area on the strip is compared with the colours on the manufacturer's chart immediately after the strip has been transiently dipped in the urine. The test is most sensitive for albumin, and the amount of albumin present in normal urine (up to 20 mg/100 ml) may be indicated on the strip as a trace. Fluorescent light may make appreciation of the colour change difficult. The test is best used for screening, a positive result being followed by the salicylsulphonic acid or boiling tests. False positive results may occur if the urine is very alkaline, contaminated with certain detergents, and during treatment with phenothiazines. The test may give a negative result with urine containing Bence Jones protein.

The salicylsulphonic acid test. The salicylsulphonic acid test for protein is very reliable, semi-quantitative and does not require heat. Filter the urine if cloudy. To 5 ml in a test tube add 20% salicylsulphonic acid, drop by drop. The presence of protein is indicated by a cloudy precipitate, best seen against a black background, but up to 25 drops may be required before it forms. Continue to add salicylsulphonic acid until no more precipitate occurs. For ordinary purposes it is sufficient to express the amount present as a haze, cloud or granular precipitate, a haze of protein representing about 20 mg per 100 ml; a heavier deposit may be allowed to settle and the quantity expressed as the proportion of the total urine volume occupied by the deposit. If this proportion is one half, the urine contains about 1 g protein/100 ml. False positive results may be due to the presence of radiographic contrast medium; they may also occur with the urine of patients treated with sulphonamides, tolbutamide, para-aminosalicylic acid or large doses of penicillin, or if the urine contains a lot of uric acid.

The boiling test. The boiling test is a satisfactory test for protein but is less convenient than the salicylsulphonic acid test.

Fill a small test tube two-thirds full of urine. If the urine is alkaline, add a small piece of indicator paper to the urine, then add 10% acetic acid, drop by drop, mixing thoroughly after each drop, until pH 5 is reached. Incline the tube at an angle, boil the top 2 cm over a flame while holding the bottom of the tube and examine against a dark background. A cloudiness indicates the presence either of protein or of phosphates which have precipitated because loss of carbon dioxide on boiling has made the urine more alkaline. If the precipitate disappears on adding acid it was due to phosphates; if it persists protein is present. If more than a light cloud persists boil all the urine, acidifying until no more protein is precipitated. Allow to settle and express semiquantitatively as described for the salicylsulphonic acid test. The boiling test is comparable in sensitivity to the latter test.

Treatment with tolbutamide, large doses of penicillin or the presence of radiographic contrast medium may result in false positive results.

If proteinuria is detected by either the salicylsulphonic acid or boiling test, but not by Albustix, the presence of Bence Jones proteinuria should be suspected. This is confirmed if a precipitate forms as the urine is heated to about 45°C, only to disappear on boiling and re-precipitate during cooling; however, more sophisticated laboratory tests may be needed to detect it.

Esbach's albuminometer.   Urine protein concentration can be measured more accurately, but simply, using Esbach's albuminometer. The method is not often used. In it, picric and citric acids are added to the urine and the amount of coagulum depends on the type as well as on the amount of protein, the result is only approximate, and the method is perhaps best used for the serial assessment of protein concentration in an individual patient.

The instrument consists of a thick graduated glass tube. Make up Esbach's reagent by dissolving 10 g picric acid and 20 g citric acid in about 900 ml boiling water; allow to cool and make up to 1 litre with water. Filter the urine if not clear, and if alkaline, render slightly acid with acetic acid. If the specific gravity is 1·010 or more it should be reduced to about 1·008 with water, the dilution factor being noted so that subsequent correction of the measured protein concentration can be made. Fill the tube with urine up to the mark 'U'. Pour in the reagent up to the mark 'R'. Close the tube with the rubber stopper and gently invert it several times to mix. Leave for 24 hours, then read off the upper level of the coagulum against the scale, whose figures represent grams of protein per litre of urine.

If the protein concentration exceeds 4 g per litre greater accuracy can be obtained by repeating the test after dilution of the urine. However, protein concentrations of less than 1 g per litre cannot be properly measured.

Significance of proteinuria. Normally less than 150 mg protein is excreted in the urine over a 24-hour period, and random samples contain less than 20 mg per 100 ml. This rarely produces more than a trace reaction with commercial reagent sticks. It should be remembered that all these tests estimate protein concentration, not excretion rate, and consideration should be given to the amount of urine passed on the day of the test. One third of protein in normal urine is albumin, identical with plasma albumin and apparently filtered through the glomerulus. Two-thirds consists of globulins, some of which are derived from plasma globulins, some originating in the renal tubules, and others from the lower urinary tract, e.g. prostatic and urethral secretions and semen; Tamm-Horsfall protein is the major proteinaceous noncellular constituent of casts.

Fever and exercise may transiently increase protein concentration in otherwise healthy people. Orthostatic proteinuria denotes the finding of protein in urine collected during the day, but not in the first urine passed after rising; it is usually of no importance save that it causes confusion. Persistent proteinuria usually indicates the presence of renal disease, but the amount does not indicate the severity of the disease. Proteinuria may also be due to extrarenal disease, such as congestive heart failure. Diseases affecting the lower urinary tract usually cause only slight proteinuria.

Blood and its derivatives

Whole blood may appear in the urine (*haematuria*) or blood pigment may appear without corpuscles (*haemoglobinuria*). Both conditions give positive chemical tests for haemoglobin, but can be differentiated by microscopy of the urine deposit for red cells.

Very small numbers of red cells, such as may be found for several days after an attack of renal colic, and in bacterial endocarditis, cause no discoloration of the urine. Larger numbers give it a peculiar opaque appearance to which the term 'smoky' is applied, and more still produce a brown or red colour, the cells often settling to form a similarly coloured deposit.

Reagent strips.   A commercial reagent strip, e.g. Haemastix, is momentarily dipped in a fresh uncentrifuged well-mixed sample of urine and the test area of the strip examined thirty seconds later. A colour change from cream to blue indicates the presence of blood, haemoglobin or myoglobin. The test depends on the oxidation of orthotolidine to a blue pigment, the reaction being catalysed by the globin. Therefore the use of stale or infected urine (containing peroxides produced by proliferating bacteria) or the presence of other oxidants (e.g. sodium hypochlorite antiseptic solution) may give a false positive reaction; and reducing agents (as in patients taking ascorbic acid) a false negative one.

Occultest.   One drop of urine is placed in the centre of the test paper provided and one Occultest tablet is placed on the resulting moist area. Two drops of water are run on to the tablet. The presence of blood in the urine is indicated by the appearance of a diffuse blue colour on the paper round the tablet within two minutes of the addition of the water. The colour of the tablet itself is irrelevant. The occultest is not available in the UK.

Significance of blood and blood pigments in urine.   Menstrual contamination is the most common cause of blood in the urine. Otherwise this is usually due to disease of kidney, ureter, bladder or urethra, although exercise may occasionally cause haematuria in healthy persons. The site of bleeding cannot be determined by examination of the urine unless the red cells form casts, which implies that there is bleeding within the renal parenchyma.

Haemoglobinuria may occasionally follow strenuous exertion in normal people but in disease may be due to haemolysis within blood vessels (as after mismatched blood transfusion) or in urine (as when blood cells lyse in dilute urine). Myoglobinuria is uncommon; it too can be produced by hard exercise, and by muscle damage, such as found in crash injuries.

Urine which contains blood or haemoglobin must contain some protein, and it is often difficult to say whether the blood is sufficient to account for all the protein present or whether proteinuria exists in addition. If human blood is added to normal urine in an amount sufficient to produce distinct smokiness, the quantity of protein amounts to merely a trace. Even when the quantity added is sufficient to render the urine distinctly red, the amount of protein is only about 0·5%.

Sugars

Several reducing sugars may appear in the urine. Glucose is by far the most important of these. In normal people it occurs in amounts too small to be detected by the usual methods employed, but if it is so detected its presence may be regarded as pathological. Glycosuria may be due to excessive blood glucose levels as in diabetes mellitus or to defective renal tubular reabsorption— 'renal' glycosuria. If the glycosuria is accompanied by undoubted symptoms of diabetes mellitus the diagnosis is not in doubt. If no symptoms are present, it is often simplest to resort immediately to a glucose tolerance test.

The other reducing sugars which may be found in urine include lactose, fructose, pentose and galactose. Lactosuria occurs in late pregnancy and during lactation. Pentosuria, like galactosuria and fructosuria, is usually due to a rare inborn error of metabolism, but may follow the eating of large quantities of certain fruits, such as plums, cherries and grapes. It should be noted that sucrose is a sugar, but not a reducing one.

Reducing substances which are not sugars may occasionally be found in the urine. Thus homogentisic acid (present in alcaptonuria, a rare inborn error of metabolism) and treatment with ascorbic acid, cephalosporins, nalidixic acid or aspirin may give a positive result with tests for reducing sugars.

The presence of a *reducing substance* in the urine may be detected using Benedict's test or Clinitest tablets. Clinistix and Diastix strips are specific tests for glucose, so non-glucose reducing substances do not affect them.

Benedict's test.   To 5 ml of Benedict's reagent add 8 drops of the urine, boil for 2 minutes and allow to cool. If a reducing substance is present, a precipitate will appear, varying from a light green turbidity to a red precipitate. If the reduction is due to glucose, the test gives approximately quantitive results:

Light green turbidity	0·1–0·5% sugar
Green precipitate	0·5–1·0% sugar
Yellow precipitate	1·0–2·0%
Red precipitate	2·0% sugar or over

Clinitest.   This is a convenient modification of Benedict's test, in which the ingredients are present in a tablet and the necessary heat is provided by the interaction of sodium hydroxide and citric acid. Five drops of urine are placed in a test tube with the dropper provided. The dropper is rinsed and 10 drops of water are added. One Clinitest tablet is dropped into the tube and the resulting reaction observed. Effervescence occurs, followed by boiling. Fifteen seconds after the boiling has ceased, the tube should be shaken gently and the colour of the contents compared with the colour scale provided. If the solution turns blue, the result is negative. When a reducing substance is present, the copper sulphate in the solution is converted to cuprous oxide, causing the colour to change through green (0·5%) to orange (2%). If a transient orange 'flash' is seen during effervescence it indicates that the urine contains at least 2 g reducing substance per 100 ml irrespective of the final colour.

Clinistix. This test is specific for glucose, but is less easy to quantify than Clinitest. The reagent strip is dipped transiently in the urine and the colour of the test area is compared with the makers' colour chart 10 seconds later. A change from red towards purple indicates that the urine contains an abnormal amount of glucose.

Clinistix strips have a test area impregnated with a mixture of glucose oxidase, peroxidase and a chromogen system. In the presence of glucose oxidase, glucose is oxidized by atmospheric oxygen to gluconic acid and hydrogen peroxide. The latter, in the presence of peroxidase, oxidizes the chromogen system to a shade of purple. This test is highly sensitive unless inhibited by a high concentration of ascorbic acid in the urine, such as may occur with the oral administration of some tetracycline preparations. False positive reactions may be given by strong oxidizing agents in certain antiseptics, bleaches and detergents.

Diastix. Diastix is a modification of the Clinistix strips above. The results are semi-quantitative. The colour should be read after 30 seconds.

Glucose tolerance test. The usual method for performance of the glucose tolerance test is as follows. The patient, who has been allowed no food since the previous evening, has blood taken for determination of fasting blood glucose concentration and empties his bladder. He then drinks 50 g of glucose dissolved in 100 ml of water. Further specimens of blood are withdrawn and further samples of urine collected at the end of three-quarters of an hour and two hours (or after ½, 1, 1½ and 2 hours).

Under normal conditions the fasting blood glucose is between 80 and 120 mg/100 ml. The blood glucose should not rise to more than 160 mg/100 ml, and by two hours should have fallen to less than 120 mg/100 ml. The corresponding specimens of urine contain no glucose, since glucose does not pass into the urine in detectable quantities in normal persons until the blood glucose reaches 180 mg/100 ml—the so-called 'renal threshold'. A diagnosis of diabetes mellitus can be confidently made if the fasting blood level exceeds 120 mg/100 ml or the two hour level exceeds 150 mg/100 ml.

In renal glycosuria the blood glucose curve is normal, but glucose is found in one or more of the specimens of urine.

The glucose tolerance test is employed in the diagnosis of diabetes mellitus. For this purpose it is essential that the patient should have been eating a normal amount of carbohydrate during the previous week. Normal persons on a low carbohydrate diet may show abnormal blood glucose levels after a test dose of glucose, and hence be misdiagnosed as cases of mild diabetes, if this precaution is not observed.

Ketone bodies

Aceto-acetic acid and acetone (as well as hydroxybutyric acid, which is not a ketone) may appear in the urine of patients with severe diabetes mellitus, and after starvation or prolonged vomiting. The ketones may be detected using Rothera's nitroprusside test or one of its modifications such as Ketostix or Acetest, all of which are very sensitive. Severe degrees of ketonuria may be tested for using the ferric chloride (Gerhardt) test.

Rothera's test. The urine must be fresh and unboiled because aceto-acetic acid is easily decomposed. 10 ml of urine is saturated with ammonium sulphate by adding an excess of the crystals; 3 drops of a strong freshly prepared solution of sodium nitroprusside and 2 ml of strong ammonia solution are then added. A deep permanganate colour is produced. This test is given both by acetone and aceto-acetic acid but by no other substances that may occur in fresh urine. If Rothera's test is negative, ketone bodies are absent.

Acetest.   This is a modification of Rothera's test in tablet form. One droop of fresh urine is allowed to fall on an Acetest tablet on a clean white surface. A purple discoloration of the tablet 30 seconds later indicates the presence of aceto-acetic acid or acetone, and the amount can be estimated roughly by comparison with the makers' colour chart.

Ketostix.   A ketostix reagent strip is dipped momentarily in the fresh urine. A mauve colour of the test end of the strip after 15 seconds constitutes a positive result. Keto-Diastix reagent strips combine a semi-quantitative test for glucose with the test for ketones.

Gerhardt's test.   10% ferric chloride solution is added drop by drop to 5 ml of urine in a test tube. A precipitate of ferric phosphate usually forms, but disappears again when more ferric chloride is added. The solution becomes brownish-red if aceto-acetic acid is present.

Aspirin and other salicylates, phenothiazines, phenol and some other drugs give a similar colour with ferric chloride. Boiling for about 5 minutes (before adding the ferric chloride) destroys aceto-acetic acid, but the other substances which react similarly with ferric chloride are unaffected. If, therefore, urine which has been boiled still gives the ferric chloride reaction, it may be inferred that the reaction was not due to aceto-acetic acid. Boiling after adding ferric chloride destroys the colour, whether this is due to aceto-acetic acid or to other substances.

A positive ferric chloride reaction is obtained only if aceto-acetic acid is present in considerable amount. If the urine reacts to Rothera's test but not to ferric chloride, it may be inferred that only small quantities of ketone bodies are present. If both are positive, the patient has a ketosis of considerable severity, demanding urgent treatment.

Bile

Bilirubin.   Bilirubin is the end product of metabolism of haem, contained in proteins such as haemoglobin and myoglobin, which are formed mainly in reticuloendothelial cells. Normally haem is transported in plasma in an unconjugated form, which is lipid soluble and strongly bound to protein, and therefore not excreted in the urine. Bilirubin is conjugated to form diglucuronide during its secretion into bile. This compound is water-soluble and less tightly bound to albumin, and can potentially pass across the glomerulus. In health bilirubin is not found in urine because it does not normally circulate in this form.

The finding of bilirubinuria in a jaundiced patient suggests that the jaundice is due to the appearance of conjugated bilirubin in the plasma, resulting from hepatocellular damage or hepatic obstruction. Jaundice due solely to unconjugated bilirubin, as in intravascular haemolysis, is not associated with bilirubinuria.

Urobilinogen and urobilin. Bilirubin secreted by the liver into bile is reduced by intestinal bacteria to urobilinogen, some of which is reabsorbed into the portal circulation to be excreted into bile by the liver again (enterohepatic circulation). A small amount reaches the systematic circulation and is excreted into urine. The colourless urobilinogen oxidizes to the pigmented urobilin on standing, and, if present in quantity, colours the urine orange. Estimation of the urinary urobilinogen may be useful in several circumstances. Absence of urinary urobilinogen in a patient with obstructive jaundice indicates that the obstruction is so complete that no bile pigment is reaching the intestine. In a patient without jaundice, urobilinogenuria may imply that a normal liver is unable to cope with an unduly large load of urobilinogen or that a damaged liver is unable to excrete the normal amount of urobilinogen coming to it via the enterohepatic circulation. The first circumstance is found during haemolysis of red cells which may be insufficient to cause clinical jaundice and which does not produce bilirubinuria. The second occurs in the pre-icteric stage of infective hepatitis and in diffuse diseases of the liver such as severe cirrhosis when it may be accompanied by bilirubinuria.

Bile pigment makes the urine yellow or brownish in colour but this is not specific for bile. A crude test for its presence is to shake the urine in a test tube: a positive result is given by the formation of a stable yellow froth, the stability of which is due to the presence of bile salts and the colour to bilirubin. Ictotest is a more sensitive and reliable test for bilirubin.

Ictotest. Five drops of urine are placed on the test mat provided. One Ictotest tablet is placed in the centre of the moistened area. Two drops of water are placed on the tablet and allowed to flow onto the mat. If bilirubin is present the mat around the tablet turns bluish purple. A pink or red colour should be ignored as should any discoloration of the tablet. Chorpromazine in large quantities may produce a false positive result.

Ehrlich's aldehyde test and Urobilistix. An excess of urobilinogen in the urine can be detected by Ehrlich's aldehyde test or by the 'Urobilistix' modification of this reaction. Colourless urobilinogen condenses with Ehrlich's aldehyde reagent in acid solution to form red dyes which can be extracted by a mixture of amyl and benzyl alcohols. The test must be performed on fresh urine because on standing urobilinogen undergoes spontaneous oxidation to urobilin, which does not give the reaction. Porphobilinogen (which is excreted in the urine in certain types of porphyria and condenses to porphyrins on standing, giving stale porphyric urine a port wine colour) also produces a red colour in the test; but the colour is not extracted into the alcohol phase.

1 ml of fresh urine at room temperature is mixed with 1 ml of Ehrlich's aldehyde reagent (2 g paradimethylamino-benzaldehyde, dissolved in 100 ml of 5% hydrochloric acid). After 1·5 minutes 2 ml saturated aqueous sodium acetate are added and mixed, followed by 2 ml of a 3 : 1 (v/v) mixture of amyl alcohol and benzyl alcohol. The test tube is stoppered and its contents are shaken gently for one minute. After the phases have separated a red colour of the upper (organic) phase indicates that urobilinogen is present, whilst a similar colour in the lower (aqueous) phase denotes porphobilinogen. Fresh urine normally contains a little urobilinogen which may be sufficient to produce a slight pink discoloration in the test. Urine diluted 10 times with water will not do so.

In the *Urobilistix* test, the reagent strip is dipped momentarily into fresh urine and the colour change in the test area compared with the makers' chart 60 seconds later. Positive reactions are also produced by porphobilinogen and para-amino salicylic acid.

MICROSCOPICAL EXAMINATION

It is customary to examine with a microscope the deposit from urine which has been centrifuged at 1000–1500 rpm for about three minutes; a cover slip should be used. This is useful for qualitative examination, and mid-stream urine (see 'Bacteriological Examination') is generally suitable for the purpose. However, it should be remembered that fragile items, such as casts, may be disrupted by prolonged or rapid centrifugation. Cells and casts disintegrate rapidly if urine is allowed to stand, and it is essential to examine fresh urine if red, white and epithelial cells are to be distinguished. Unstained cellular elements, especially casts, are not very refractile. They are best seen if the microscope diaphragm is partially closed and the condenser racked down.

Quantitative examination of the cellular deposit is best done on uncentrifuged urine in a haemocytometer chamber.

Red blood corpuscles (Plate II)

Typically erythrocytes appear as roughly circular elements of about 7 μm diameter with clear yellowish centres. If the urine is concentrated they are shrunken and crenated, but in dilute urine they become larger and their biconcave shape changes to a more spherical one. Normal urine contains no more than 3 red cells/mm^3 of uncentrifuged urine or less than 1 per high power field (hpf) of centrifuged urine. Red cells may be confused with droplets of oil from fingers or catheter lubricant. However, oil droplets are easily differentiated by their variable size, their higher refractive index and the fact that they are more circular.

The detection of microscopic haematuria may be very important in diagnosis, particularly in patients with systemic diseases which may affect the kidney, e.g. subacute bacterial endocarditis. Small numbers of red cells do not discolour the urine, and may not give a positive chemical test for haemoglobin (Haemastix) especially if the urine is fresh.

Leucocytes (Plate III)

Leucocytes are slightly larger than red cells and can usually be recognized by their round shape, lobed nuclei and refractile granular cytoplasm. Their structure is more easily seen if the urine is acidified with a few drops of glacial acetic acid (which will cause the red cells to disintegrate) but, without the use of phase contrast microscopy or of special stains, they cannot be differentiated reliably from renal tubular epithelial cells. When numerous, they tend to form clumps. They degenerate in a matter of hours and must be sought in fresh urine. More than 10 leucocytes/ml of uncentrifuged mid-stream urine is abnormal in adult women, between 3 and 10 being of doubtful significance; more than 3 leucocytes/ml is abnormal in men. This difference between men and women is a result of contamination of the urine by vaginal secretions. Centrifuged urine should not contain more than 5 leucocytes per high power field.

An increase in the number of leucocytes suggests that the urine is infected with bacteria, although it may occur without detectable infection, e.g. in patients with renal calculi. If pus cells are repeatedly found in apparently sterile urine, tuberculosis of the urinary tract must be considered. The diagnosis of bacterial urinary infection ultimately rests on culture, not microscopy, for infection can be present without any increase in urinary leucocytes.

Epithelial cells

Transitional epithelial cells from bladder or ureters appear as large oval cells with single nuclei. Sheets of polygonal squamous cells come from urethral or vaginal secretion; if present in quantity in urine collected from women such sheets suggest that the specimen is contaminated and probably unsuitable for culture.

Spermatozoa

Spermatozoa occur at times in urine from males and females where their characteristic appearance makes it easy to recognize them. They have no pathological significance.

Prostatic threads

Prostatic threads are found when there is chronic inflammation of the prostate, especially after gonorrhoea. They are much larger than casts, being visible readily enough to the naked eye as they float in the urine or on its surface.

Casts (Plate III)

The precipitation of mucoprotein in renal tubules is thought to result in the formation of hyaline casts. On this basic material erythrocytes (forming red cell casts), leucocytes (forming white cell casts), or tubular epithelial cells (forming epithelial casts, or if they contain fats, fatty casts) may be deposited. Disintegration of the cellular elements of a cast changes its appearance to that of a granular or waxy cast. Very broad casts (called 'renal failure' casts) are so shaped because they are formed in tubules which are large and dilated through severe parenchymal disorganization.

Hyaline casts themselves are normal. The finding of the more complex casts indicates that the cells concerned come from the kidney, and therefore that the kidneys are diseased.

Casts are easily missed if the microscopic illumination is too bright and disintegrate if the urine has been centrifuged too rapidly or for too long. They should be looked for towards the edges of the cover slip. They are distinguished from other objects which may be mistaken for them—such as hairs, wool, cotton, masses of urates, prostatic threads, and rolled-up epithelial cells—by their shape and sharply defined outline. They are always cylindrical, and may have rounded ends, or one end may be ragged as if fractured. Hyaline casts are pale, transparent and homogeneous, and may be difficult to distinguish from the background unless phase contrast microscopy is used; they may be long and narrow with a tapering end and then are sometimes called cylindroids. Cellular casts are recognized by their constituent cells. Granular casts contain fine or coarse granules.

Crystals

Alkaline urine often contains crystals of ammonium magnesium phosphate (triple phosphate). Calcium oxalate crystals are normal in acid urine.

Amorphous or urate debris frequently obscures interesting cellular material, and dissolves on acidification or gentle warming respectively. Crystals are usually of no pathological significance, but occasionally are of diagnostic importance, e.g. cystine crystals, indicative of cystinuria.

Micro-organisms

Bacteria, especially if motile, may be seen during high power microscopy of unstained, uncentrifuged urine, but they are more easily seen by Gram-staining the centrifuged deposit. Their finding on microscopy indicates that they are present in very large numbers and, if the urine is fresh and uncontaminated, strongly suggests a urinary infection. Urine from women may contain *Trichomonas vaginalis* or yeasts, which usually result from contamination with vaginal secretion. The former are pear-shaped or round parasites about twice the size of leucocytes and with unipolar flagellae that may be seen with difficulty. Yeasts are slightly smaller than red cells, and may be confused with them, with air bubbles, or with oil droplets.

Bilharzia

Schistosoma haematobium is best looked for in the last few millilitres of a stream of urine passed in mid-morning. The ova (Plate IV) measure about 0·12 mm by 0·44 mm. A spine projects at one pole. The ova of *Schistosoma mansoni* are less often found in urine and have a lateral spine.

BACTERIOLOGICAL EXAMINATION

Collection of samples

It is rarely necessary to catheterize a patient for the purpose of obtaining urine for culture. A mid-stream urine specimen, collected after the vulva or glans penis has been cleaned with tap water, is suitable for most bacteriological purposes. Antiseptic solutions should not be used for cleaning, because enough antiseptic to interfere with the growth of bacteria during culture may get into the urine.

In women the labia are separated by patient or nurse and the vulva is cleaned twice in an anteroposterior direction with swabs soaked in tap water and then finally with a dry swab. Whilst the labia are still held apart some urine, perhaps 20–50 ml, is passed into a toilet or bowl, but the next portion ('mid-stream urine') is collected into a clean wide-mouthed jar. Urine collected in this way is unsuitable for culture if the patient is menstruating heavily, but reasonably satisfactory specimens can be collected after insertion of a vaginal tampon if menstruation is light.

Sometimes it is important to obtain a specimen free from urethral contaminants. This can be done by suprapubic aspiration of urine. The patient is asked not to micturate for several hours before attending the clinic, so that her bladder is full; if necessary she can be given water to drink on arrival. After bladder distension has been confirmed by percussion, the suprapubic area is shaved and cleaned with antiseptic. An 'intramuscular' needle is inserted at right angles to the skin surface immediately above the symphysis pubis and urine aspirated; it may be necessary to use a longer needle if the patient is fat. The technique is safe and, with slight modification, may be used in pregnant women and infants.

The most satisfactory specimen for culture is the one collected first after arising from sleep, for any bacteria in the bladder have been able to multiply undisturbed for several hours. This should be cultured as soon as possible (and certainly within two hours of collection) or refrigerated at 4°C immediately, in order to prevent contaminant bacteria from multiplying so much that they may be misinterpreted as pathogens. Mid-stream urines, and those obtained by catheretization, should be cultured quantitatively. The most accurate quantitative culture techniques, in which known volumes of serial dilutions of urine are mixed with molten agar or spread over solid agar, and the colonies of bacteria which grow are counted, are time-consuming and expensive. There are several simpler techniques which are less accurate but satisfactory for routine use. In the dipslide method a plastic graticule coated with agar on both sides is dipped momentarily into the urine, which because of surface tension leaves a thin film of approximately constant volume on the agar surface. The slide is incubated and the individual bacterial colonies counted in the normal way: the concentration of bacteria in the original urine can be estimated from the slide count. The technique is especially useful in that the patient can inoculate the slide herself at home, as instructed by a doctor, and post it to a laboratory for incubation.

Significance of bacteriuria

In general the finding of over 100 000 bacteria/ml of mid-stream urine indicates the presence of urinary infection. However, contamination without infection may sometimes produce counts above this figure and urinary infection may sometimes be present with lower counts. It is therefore advisable to culture several mid-stream specimens and to discuss the results in doubtful cases with a bacteriologist. In such cases culture of a suprapubic aspirate may be helpful; any growth in such a specimen, other than a few skin contaminants, indicates that there is infection within the urinary tract.

ESTIMATION OF RENAL FUNCTION

One of the main functions of the kidneys is to rid the body of the waste products of metabolism which are presented to them in the blood stream. This they do by the excretion of waste products into the urine and by the retention of those substances which are not waste. The former is carried out primarily by the glomeruli, which filter off the contents of the plasma except those of high molecular weight or which are tightly bound to plasma protein. The tubules then reabsorb certain solutes, excrete others and reabsorb most of the filtered water. Progressive damage to the kidney by chronic renal disease is usually associated with destruction of, or cessation of function in, a large number of glomeruli. This leads to a reduction in the overall glomerular filtration rate which, if marked, causes a rise in the plasma urea concentration. At the same time there is a much greater flow of urine through the remaining tubules, which overloads the diluting and concentrating mechanisms at the distal ends of the tubules. The result is a progressive diminution in the ability of the kidneys to concentrate and dilute urine, as renal destruction progresses, until finally the specific gravity becomes fixed at 1·010.

Plasma concentration of urea and creatinine

The plasma concentration of urea depends on a balance between its production from exogenous and endogenous protein and its excretion by the kidneys. Its level thus varies with protein intake and may also be raised in conditions such as fever and haemorrhage into the gastrointestinal tract, which increase endogeneous production but where there is no renal involvement. In spite of these objections the plasma concentration of urine is widely used by clinicians as a crude indicator of renal function, and high levels correlate fairly well with the clinical picture of 'uraemia'. The normal range is usually given as 15–40 mg/100 ml (2·5–6·6 mmol/litre). Raised levels may indicate renal failure due to disease of the kidneys themselves, their obstruction or their disturbance in conditions such as hypotension, saline depletion or heart failure which affect blood flow to or within the kidneys. The height of the urea is no guide to the cause of the renal failure and levels of 300 or 400 mg/100 ml, occasionally more, may be found.

Creatinine (normal 0·7–1·4 mg/100 ml or 62–124 μmol/litre) is derived almost entirely from endogenous sources, but is more difficult to measure accurately than urea. Its plasma concentration correlates with the glomerular filtration rate better than does that of urea. Levels as high as 20 mg/100 ml may be reached in advanced renal failure.

The relationship between plasma urea and creatinine concentrations on the one hand, and glomerular filtration rate on the other, is hyperbolic not linear, and glomerular filtration must fall considerably before urea and creatinine concentrations become abnormal. For both clinical and research purposes it may be necessary to measure impairment of renal function short of that which produces a rise in plasma urea and to measure individual renal functions. Numerous methods are available and the subject is a complicated one. We shall describe here the estimation of the glomerular filtration rate (GFR) and tests of the renal concentrating and acidifying abilities.

Estimation of glomerular filtration rate

The reference method of estimating the glomerular filtration rate (GFR) is that of inulin clearance. The renal clearance of a substance is the smallest volume of plasma from which the amount of that substance excreted in the urine each minute could have been obtained at the time of the test. It is calculated from the expression UV/P, where U is the concentration of the substance in the urine (in micromol/litre), V is the volume of urine produced (in ml/minutes) and P is the plasma concentration of the substance (in micromol/litre).

If a substance is excreted by glomerular filtration, and is neither secreted nor reabsorbed by the tubules, its clearance is equal to the glomerular filtration rate. Although inulin clearance is considered to be an accurate measure of GFR there are practical difficulties in performing the test and other methods are preferred for routine use.

The clearance of endogenous creatinine is popular as a reasonably good index of GFR, but it over-estimates GFR at low filtration rates and in patients with the nephrotic syndrome. In order to minimize inaccuracies due to errors in the timing and measurement of urine collections, such collections should be made over 24 hours. It is not necessary to catheterize patients for the test. Urea clearance does not correlate well with GFR and should no longer be used for this.

GFR can also be estimated by methods which do not require urine collections. It can be derived mathematically from the plasma creatinine concentration. The rate of disappearance of ^{51}Cr–EDTA or certain other isotopes from the circulation may be used to measure GFR accurately. The normal figure of about 120 ml/minute may be reduced by up to two-thirds before the plasma urea concentration becomes elevated.

Renal concentrating ability

The concentration of the urine, best measured as its osmolality, may be as low as 50 mosmol/kg after water loading, or as high as 1300 mosmol/kg after fluid deprivation. Specific gravity, as discussed earlier, is affected by the nature as well as by the number of osmotically active particles in solution. However, if a random specimen of urine has a specific gravity greater than 1·018 it can be assumed that concentrating ability is normal. Fluid deprivation for prolonged periods, or injection of vasopressin, may be used to provide more accurate tests of concentrating ability; a urine osmolality of at least 750 mosmol/kg, or a specific gravity of 1·020 should be attained if concentrating power is normal. In order to produce maximum concentration, fluid depletion for 24–36 hours may be necessary. This is unpleasant and may result in excessive dehydration if concentrating power is poor; it is a slightly more effective stimulus to concentration than vasopressin.

Renal acidifying ability

If the pH of a random specimen of urine is below 5·5, it can be assumed that renal acidifying ability is normal. In chronic glomerular disease the kidneys usually retain the ability to reduce urine pH below 5·5 until renal failure is advanced. In certain diseases affecting predominantly the renal tubules the urine cannot be adequately acidified, even when glomerular filtration rate is normal. In order to test for this, ammonium chloride capsules (0·1 g/kg body weight) are given orally; normally the urine pH is reduced to less than 5·4. The test should not be carried out if the patient is already acidotic. Renal tubular acidosis is a cause of renal calculi and nephrocalcinosis, the investigation of which is the most frequent reason for the test being performed.

OTHER INVESTIGATIONS

Excretion urography

This depends on the excretion by the kidney of certain radio-opaque organic compounds of iodine. After a plain film of the whole abdomen has been taken the contrast medium is injected intravenously, and X-ray films of the kidneys, ureters and bladder are taken after various time intervals, the last after the patient has emptied the bladder. This investigation provides evidence concerning the anatomy and function of the kidneys and their outflow tracts. It is important in the investigation of renal failure and of suspected urinary obstruction or other surgical abnormalities, and is often done in the investigation of hypertension. When renal function is poor the kidneys are more easily seen if tomographs and large doses of contrast medium are used.

Micturating cystography

In this investigation a similar radio-opaque medium is instilled into the bladder through a catheter passed with strict aseptic precautions. Cineradiograms are taken of the bladder, its outflow tract and the ureters, as the patient voids the dye. This test may be important in the investigation of the bladder outflow tract.

Cystography and urethroscopy

The interior of the bladder and urethra may be inspected through a cystoscope and urethroscope respectively. The main value of these procedures is in diagnosis of tumours of the lining epithelium of the bladder and in assessment of the effects of disease of the prostate. It is possible to insert fine catheters through the cysto-scope into the ureters, enabling urine from each kidney to be collected separately; by instilling contrast medium, radiographs of ureters, pelves and calyces can be taken.

Renal biopsy

By means of a special needle inserted into the back, biopsy speci-mens of the kidney may be obtained. Considerable skill is required and there is a small but definite risk to the patient. The method is of most clinical value in predicting the likely outcome and response to steroid therapy of certain patients with the nephrotic syndrome. It may also be valuable in the investigation of acute renal failure and in the diagnosis and assessment of systemic disorders such as amyloidosis and systemic lupus erythematosus.

THE FAECES

Examination of the faeces is an investigation of great importance all too easily omitted. No patient with bowel disturbance has been properly examined until the stools have been inspected. The white surface of a bedpan makes an ideal background for the detection of blood, pus and mucus.

NAKED-EYE INSPECTION

The following points should be noted:

The amount.   It is sufficient to state whether the stools are copious or scanty.

Colour.   *Black* stools may be produced by the ingestion of iron or bismuth. In haemorrhage occurring high up in the intestine the altered blood makes the stools dark, tarry-looking and very offen-sive, and all chemical tests for blood are strongly positive. *Pallor* of the stools may be due to lack of entrance of bile into the intestine, as in obstructive jaundice; to dilution and rapid passage of the stool through the intestine as in diarrhoea; or to an abnormally high fat content as in malabsorption.

Odour.   The stools in jaundice are often very offensive. Cholera stools, on the other hand, contain very little organic matter, and are almost free from odour. The stools of acute bacillary dysentery are almost odourless, while those of amoebic dysentery have a characteristic odour, something like that of semen.

Form and consistency. In constipation the stools may be drier and harder than normal, and sometimes resemble sheep's stools. In all forms of diarrhoea they are more fluid than normal, and may be watery. Slimy stools are due to presence of an excess of mucus.

Abnormal ingredients. Abnormal ingredients can be detected by placing the stool on a fine sieve and adding a large quantity of water. The whole is shaken and stirred up till the soluble parts are all washed away. The residue is then examined. The head of a tapeworm can best be seen if this residue is strained through black muslin. The head is about as large as that of a large pin, and the neck about as thick as a stout thread.

Watery stools are found in all cases of profuse diarrhoea, and after the administration of purgatives. To the stools of cholera the special name of *rice-water* stools is applied. Such a stool is colourless, almost devoid of odour, alkaline in reaction and contains a number of small flocculi consisting of shreds of epithelium and particles of mucus. Purulent or pus-containing stools are found in severe dysentery or ulcerative colitis, or in cases where an abscess has found its way into the intestines. Slimy stools are due to the presence of an excess of mucus, and point to an affection of the large bowel. The mucus may envelop the faecal masses, or may be intimately mixed with them. Bloody stools vary in appearance according to the site of the haemorrhage. If the bleeding takes place high up, the stools look like tar. In an intussusception they may look like red-currant jelly. If the haemorrhage is from the large intestine, the blood is less intimately mixed with the faecal matter, and may even be of a bright colour. In haemorrhage from the rectum or anus it may merely streak the faecal masses. The stools of bacillary dysentery consist at first of faecal material mixed with blood and pus, later of blood and pus without faecal material. Those of amoebic dysentery characteristically consist of fluid faecal material, mucus and small amounts of blood. The stools of steatorrhoea are very large, pale and putty-like or porridge-like and sometimes frothy. They are apt to stick to the sides of the lavatory pan and are difficult to flush away. If formed, they usually float.

CHEMICAL EXAMINATION

Tests for occult haemorrhage

Since benzidine ceased to be available, on account of a high incidence of carcinoma of the bladder in those who made it, orthotolidine has taken its place.

Orthotolidine test.   A portion of faeces the size of a pea is suspended in 5 ml of distilled water and boiled for 5 minutes. A 4% stock solution of orthotolidine in 95% ethyl alcohol is prepared. A 1 in 5 solution is made in glacial acetic acid. 1 ml of this reagent, 0·25 ml of the faecal suspension and 0·25 ml of the hydrogen peroxide (20 vol. strength) are mixed in a test tube, and the result read in three minutes. A strong positive is indicated by a dark green colour and a weak positive by a pale green. This is a moderately sensitive test, and to avoid false positives the patient should have been on a meat-free diet for three days before the test and should not have been taking aspirin.

Haematest tablet test.   These tablets contain orthotolidine and strontium peroxide. A blue colour is produced when a wetted tablet is in contact with faeces containing blood.

A thin smear of faeces is made on the test paper provided. A tablet is placed in the centre of the smear, and two drops of water are run on to the tablet. The water overflows on to the smear of faeces. A slight blue colour on the tablet is of no significance, but a blue colour developing in the smear at the edge of the tablet within two minutes is a positive result.

This test is relatively insensitive. It can therefore be used on patients on a normal diet, but will not detect small amounts of gastrointestinal bleeding.

Both tests are of value in indicating the presence of gastrointestinal bleeding, but both may be negative in the presence of lesions which bleed intermittently or slightly, particularly those situated in the upper gastrointestinal tract. Spectroscopic methods and isotopic methods using radioactive chromium labelled red cells are also available.

Haemastix.   As described under urine (p. 140), this can be used as a rough screening test for blood in faeces.

Fats in faeces

Fat is present in food as neutral fat or triglyceride. It is split to greater or lesser degree by lipases, mainly of the pancreas, into glycerol and fatty acids. Some of the fatty acids, if unabsorbed, combine with bases to form soaps. Fat may, therefore, be found in the faeces as neutral fat, fatty acids and soaps.

The estimation of the proportion of split and unsplit fats present has been found unreliable as a method of distinguishing pancreatic from non-pancreatic steatorrhoea because of the effects of bacterial activity on neutral fats.

For the estimation of the fat in the stools, the patient may be placed on a diet containing 50 g of fat per day. The fat present in the stools collected over three or better five days is then estimated and should not exceed 6 g/day (or 12 g in three days). It has been found that equally reliable results are obtained if the patient eats a normal diet provided a three to five day collection is made.

MICROSCOPICAL EXAMINATION

See Protozoa (p. 163).

INTESTINAL PARASITES

The parasites which occur in the intestinal tract include worms and protozoa. Some of the nematode and cestode worms will be described.

NEMATODA

The commonest of all internal parasites is the threadworm, *Enterobius vermicularis*, whose presence is associated with considerable itching about the anus. It inhabits the large intestines, caecum and appendix, and female specimens can often be seen wriggling about in the recently passed motion of their host. To the naked eye they look like small white threads, 0·5 to 1 cm in length. Under the microscope the female may be distinguished by her much larger size, by the large uterus filled with ova, and the pointed posterior end. For appearance of ovum, see Plate IV.

Ascaris lumbricoides, the roundworm, has a general resemblance to an earthworm. It usually measures up to 25 cm but may be up to

33 cm long. The ova, which can occasionally be found in the faeces, have brownish-yellow granular contents, and in many cases the shell is surrounded by an irregular sheath (Plate IV).

Ankylostoma duodenale, the hookworm, is an important cause of anaemia and debility in the tropics, where heavy infestations may occur. It is no longer indigenous in Great Britain, but may be found in immigrants. It lives for the most part in the upper part of the jejunum, and its presence there is probable when, in an infested district, severe anaemia, otherwise inexplicable, sets in. The diagnosis is confirmed by the discovery of ova in the motions (Plate IV). They exhibit a segmented yolk enclosed in a thin shell, and are sufficiently numerous to be readily detected. The adult worm, which is rarely seen before therapeutic agents have been employed, is about 1 cm long, and the mouth is provided with four claw-like teeth.

Trichinella spiralis gains access to the body as the result of the eating of infested pork. Trichiniasis is rare when pork is eaten cooked, but small outbreaks and sporadic cases have been reported in Great Britain and in the USA. When man ingests the muscle trichinellae of the pig, larvae are set free in the small intestine, giving rise to the symptoms of the first stage of the illness—abdominal pain, vomiting and diarrhoea. The adult female, 3 mm long, penetrates the intestinal wall and discharges embryos into lymph spaces, whence they migrate into muscles. In this second stage of the illness the patient has fever and high eosinophilia and the muscles swell and become hard and tender. Rarely death may occur at the height of the myositis. Otherwise the embryo undergoes no further development, and its capsule becomes calcified. Unlike cysticerci, described below, calcified trichinellae are not visible in X-rays.

CESTODA

Many different kinds of tapeworm have been found as parasites in man, but the most important are *Taenia saginata*, *T. solium* and *Echinococcus granulosus*. Besides its occurrence in the fully developed state, *T. solium* may be present in the tissues in the form of a cysticercus; *T. saginata* is never found in this condition in man; whilst *E. granulosus* always occurs in the cystic stage, and has never been found in the mature condition in the human intestinal tract.

The presence of an adult tapeworm in the bowel is generally revealed by the passage of ripe proglottides in the stools, and after the administration of antihelmintics, the head may be detected by the method previously described (p. 157).

Taenia saginata (mediocanellata) is the beef tapeworm. Infestation occurs as a result of consuming insufficiently cooked beef infested with the embryo of the worm. The adult parasite reaches a length of 4–8 m and consists of about 2000 segments. The ripe proglottides measure 13 by 6 mm. The head is quadrate, measures 2 mm in diameter, has 4 suckers, but is devoid of hooklets. The terminal gravid segments of the worm become separated from time to time and the ova may be then ingested by the bullock or cow, in the muscles of which the larva develops. It becomes a bladder worm, *Cysticercus bovis*, measuring 10 by 16 mm and containing an invaginated head which possesses in miniature the characteristics of the adult scolex. *Cysticercus bovis* is never found in human muscle tissue or brain. For appearance of ovum, see Plate IV.

Taenia solium, the pork tapeworm, is not encountered in Britain but is endemic wherever infested pork is eaten raw or insufficiently cooked. It measures 2 to 4 m in length; a ripe proglottis is 10 by 5 mm. The head measures 1 mm in diameter and in addition to 4 suckers has a rostellum with 32 hooklets. The ova in the terminal proglottides may be ingested by the pig, in the muscles of which the bladder worm *Cysticercus cellulosae* develops. Occasionally persons in infected areas become infested with *Cysticercus cellulosae* from eating food contaminated with the ova of the parasite. The muscles of the human host are then infested by cysticerci, which are palpable through the skin as tense ovoid swellings 10 by 5 mm and of almost cartilaginous hardness. About four years after infestation they become calcified and may then be demonstrated radiologically. The thigh muscles are those in which cysticerci are most easily demonstrated. Cysticerci may also occur in the brain and are a cause of epilepsy.

Echinococcus granulosus. The adult worm, which consists of a head and three segments, and whose length is only 3 to 8 mm, need not be fully described, since it is not found in man. The *cystic stage* is very important, as it gives rise to serious disease in man in many of the viscera and especially in the liver. The cysts of this are not simple, but produce from their inner surface one or two generations of secondary vesicles, on which the brood capsules, containing the cestode heads, are formed. During the period in which this process is going on, the primary vesicle dilates to accommodate its increasing contents, and may eventually reach the size of a coconut. The vesicles may rupture spontaneously, and their contents may escape by the lungs, by the bowel or by the urinary passages. Specimens may be obtained by aspiration or after surgical interference.

The diagnosis of suspected hydatid disease may rest upon the recognition of the nature of fluid withdrawn, of hooklets or scolices, or the appearance of parts of the ectocyst, which are sometimes coughed up from the lungs. The Casoni intradermal test may be of some assistance, though cross reactions may occur in infestation with other cestodes.

The *fluid* is clear, alkaline, devoid of protein, and contains abundance of sodium chloride and traces of glucose. Its density is low, being generally under 1010. The *scolex*, if it is obtained in a perfect condition, is about 0·3 mm in diameter, and a number of them often spring in a group from one brood capsule. They have 4 suckers and a crown of hooklets. Portions of the *ectocyst* appear as whitish-yellow shreds, which can be recognized under the microscope by their lamination and by their pectinate markings on the laminae.

Diphyllobothrium latum (Dibothriocephalus latus), the fish tapeworm, is encountered in Sweden, Finland and Michigan. The adult worm measures from 3 to 10 m or more and has a total of 3000 segments. The scolex is small, spatula-shaped and possesses two deep suctorial grooves. The first larval host is a water flea and the second the pike, perch or salmon trout. Human infestation takes place from eating raw or undercooked fish. In a tiny proportion of cases, a vitamin B_{12} deficiency anaemia may be produced.

TREMATODES

Schistosomes or blood flukes are the most important trematode parasites of man. They are found in three varieties, and produce the disease known as schistosomiasis or bilharziasis. *Schistosoma japonicum* and *Schistosoma mansoni* inhabit the portal blood stream, and the ova (Plate IV) are passed in the faeces. *Schistosoma haematobium* characteristically inhabits the vesical plexus, so that the ova (Plate IV) are passed in the urine (p. 150). They may occasionally also be found in the faeces. *Schistosoma mansoni* is found in Africa and South America; *Schistosoma haematobium* in Africa and the Near East, particularly in Egypt; and *Schistosoma japonicum* in the Orient.

PROTOZOA

A number of protozoa, many of them non-pathogenic, have been found in the faeces. Of these the most important clinically is *Entamoeba histolytica* (Plate IV), which causes amoebic dysentery (as opposed to bacillary dysentery) and sometimes tropical abscess of the liver. *Entamoeba coli* (Plate IV) is non-pathonogenic.

Entamoeba histolytica is found in the stools in two forms. In acute attacks vegetative amoebae can generally be found, whilst in the more quiescent stage cysts are passed. So-called 'small' and 'large' races of *Entamoeba histolytica* have been described. It is likely that both are pathogenic.

If amoebic dysentery is suspected, a stool should be passed into a clean bedpan; this must be free from antiseptics, and the stool must not be mixed with urine. It should be taken immediately to the laboratory so that it is examined whilst warm.

With a platinum loop, select a piece of blood-stained mucus, or failing this, a small particle of faeces; emulsify it with a drop of warmed (37°C) normal saline and apply a cover-slip.

The diagnosis of vegetative *Entamoeba histolytica* depends for practical purposes on the demonstration of actively motile amoebae, which contain red cells. The slide must be examined on a heated stage, or, if this is not available, it may be kept warm by applying coins pre-heated in a Bunsen flame, on each side of the cover-slip. Care must be taken not to overheat it. Motile amoebae are readily seen under the low power, and can be studied further under the 16 mm objective. Iodine will kill the amoebae, and must not be used.

Cysts can be seen under the low power as small round refractile bodies. They are seen even better if the stool is emulsified in 1% aqueous eosin, when, provided the stool is fresh, they show as white bodies against a pink background. The characteristic chromatoid bodies of *E. histolytica* are well shown by this method. Globules of oil or fat, which may be present in the faeces of patients who have been given oil as an aperient, may resemble them, and, if numerous, may make any attempt at further examination useless. Oil droplets vary in size, are structureless, and their edges cannot be sharply focused. If cysts are present, iodine should be used for their further identification. Make a further preparation using 1% Lugol's iodine. Find a suspected cyst under the low power. Apply the 16 mm objective and centre the cyst in the middle of the field. Rack up the microscope tube, apply a small drop of oil to the cover slip without moving it, and carefully lower the oil-immersion objective into the drop. The main differences between *E. histolytica* and *E. coli* and their cysts are shown in Tables 5.1 and 5.2.

Table 5.1.   *ENTAMOEBA HISTOLYTICA* AND *ENTAMOEBA COLI*: VEGETATIVE FORMS

	Entamoeba histolytica	*Entamoeba coli*
Occurrence	Fairly abundant, when present in amoebic dysenteric stools	Never abundant. Occasionally seen in dysenteric stools
Size	Variable, average 20 to 30 μm	Less variable. Generally larger than *E. histolytica*
Motility	Active. Large pseudopodia. These become larger as activity diminishes before death	Sluggish. Small cone-shaped pseudopodia
Cytoplasm	Homogeneous and 'ground-glass like'. Differentiation of ectoplasm and endoplasm clearly seen. Red blood corpuscles often seen	Appearance porcellanous. Ectoplasm less plentiful, line of demarcation between it and endoplasm inconspicuous. Endoplasm granular. Abundant food vacuoles with usually bacterial inclusions. Red blood corpuscles never present
Nucleus	Karyosome, not seen in unstained preparations, small and *central*. Periphery marked by ring-like layer of regular sized chromatin granules	Distinct. Karyosome usually large, irregular and *nearly always eccentric*. Ring-like layers of peripheral granules more pronounced and irregular in size and shape

Table 5.2. *ENTAMOEBA HISTOLYTICA* AND *ENTAMOEBA COLI:* CYSTS

Entamoeba histolytica	*Entamoeba coli*
When mature, 4 nuclei, with nuclear karyosomes central. Peripheral chromatin often semilunar	When mature, 8 nuclei, with nuclear karyosomes usually eccentric
Size slightly smaller on average, varying from 10 to 20 μm	Size slightly larger, varying from 10 to 20 μm
Glycogen less abundant	Glycogen more abundant
Refractility moderate	Refractility considerable
Rod-shaped 'chromidial bodies' usually seen in fresh specimen	'Chromatoid bodies' not often present: thread-like or in bundles when seen
Cyst wall rather thinner	Cyst wall rather thicker

Besides *E. coli*, there are three other non-pathogenic amoebae, which must not be mistaken for *E. histolytica*. They are *Endolimax nana*, *Iodamoeba bütschlii* and *Dientamoeba fragilis*. In the diagnosis of the vegetative forms this mistake will be avoided if it is remembered that *E. histolytica* alone is actively motile and contains red cells. The cysts of *Iodamoeba bütschlii* (Plate VIII) contain a single small nucleus, an eccentric karysome and a very large compact mass of glycogen.

Giardia lamblia is a flagellate protozoon, which inhabits the duodenum and may be found in the stools of patients with diarrhoea in both cystic and vegetative form (Plate IV). There is some doubt whether or not it is pathogenic. The fact that a course of mepacrine will eradicate it, sometimes with relief of the diarrhoea, suggests that it is.

Trichomonas hominis (Plate IV) is another flagellate protozoon, which may be seen in the stools in diarrhoea. It is probably non-pathogenic. Similar if not identical trichomonas may be found in the vagina in leucorrhoea and in the mouth in oral sepsis.

Isospora belli (I. hominis) (Plate IV), one of a group of parasites which may produce coccidiosis in man, animals and birds, has occasionally been described as the cause of acute diarrhoea in man, particularly in the eastern Mediterranean.

Balantidium coli (Plate IV) is a large ciliate protozoon which is found in the intestine of pigs. It occasionally infects man, and may rarely cause severe diarrhoea or frank dysentery.

6

The respiratory system

ANATOMICAL LANDMARKS

Lobes of the lungs.   It is important to know the limits of the individual lobes. A line from the second thoracic spine to the sixth rib in the mammary line corresponds to the upper border of the lower lobe (the major interlobar fissure). A horizontal line on the right side from the sternum at the level of the fourth costal cartilage, drawn to meet the first, marks the boundary between the upper and middle lobes (the minor interlobar fissure). The greater part of each lung, as seen from behind, is composed of the lower lobe, only the apex belonging to the upper lobe; while the middle and upper lobes on the right side, and the upper lobe on the left, occupy most of the area in front. In the axillary regions, parts of all the lobes are accessible.

The bifurcation of the trachea corresponds in front with the lower border of the manubrium sterni, that is with the angle of Louis, and behind, with the disc between the fourth and fifth thoracic vertebrae.

The twelfth rib cannot always be felt and so it is not wise to count the ribs from below upwards. These are best counted downwards from the second costal cartilage. This cartilage articulates with the sternum at the extremities of the angle of Louis, a transverse bony ridge at the junction of the body and the manubrium which is easily felt beneath the skin.

Anatomy of the bronchi.   The two main bronchi each give off four main branches: on the right, one to the upper lobe, one to the middle lobe, one·to the dorsal lobe (the upper and posterior part of the lower lobe), and one to the remainder of the lower lobe; and on the left, one to the upper lobe proper, one to the lingular process of the upper lobe (which represents the middle lobe on the left side), and a dorsal and lower lobe bronchus as on the right side. These main bronchi then divide into segmental bronchi, which supply individual segments of lung. It is useful to know about these segments, because it is often possible from the signs and X-ray appearance to determine which segment and which segmental bronchus is affected by disease. The accompanying diagrams (Figs 6.1–6.3) give a simplified scheme of the anatomy of the segmental bronchi and indicate the 'respiratory districts' or bronchopulmonary segments supplied by them.

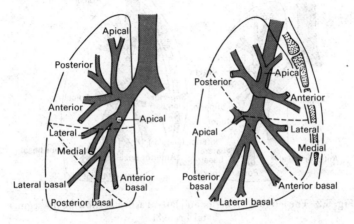

Fig. 6.1 The right lung (anterior and lateral aspects) showing the segmental bronchi.

Upper lobe $\left\{\begin{array}{l}\text{Apical bronchus and segment}\\\text{Posterior bronchus and segment}\\\text{Anterior bronchus and segment}\end{array}\right.$

Middle lobe $\left\{\begin{array}{l}\text{Lateral bronchus and segment}\\\text{Medial bronchus and segment}\end{array}\right.$

$\left\{\begin{array}{l}\text{Apical bronchus and segment}\\\text{Medial basal bronchus and segment}\\\text{(bronchus not shown)}\end{array}\right.$

Lower lobe $\left\{\begin{array}{l}\text{Anterior basal bronchus and segment}\\\text{Lateral basal bronchus and segment}\\\text{Posterior basal bronchus and segment}\end{array}\right.$

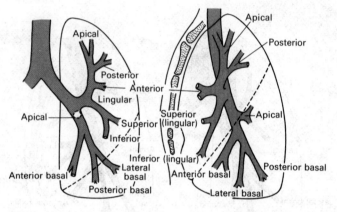

Fig. 6.2 The left lung (anterior and lateral aspects) showing the segmental bronchi.

Upper lobe	Upper division bronchus	Apical bronchus and segment
		Posterior bronchus and segment
		Anterior bronchus and segment
	Lingular (lower division) bronchus	Superior bronchus and segment
		Inferior bronchus and segment
Lower lobe	Apical bronchus and segment	
	Anterior basal bronchus and segment	
	Lateral basal bronchus and segment	
	Posterior basal bronchus and segment	

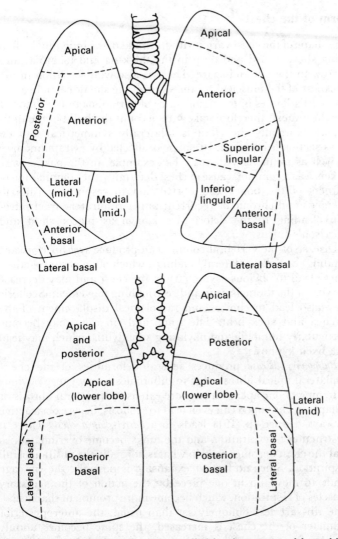

Fig. 6.3 The respiratory districts supplied by the segmental bronchi. *Above*, anterior aspect. *Below*, posterior aspect.

INSPECTION

Form of the chest

The shape of the chest varies with the build of the individual, often being short, broad and deep in the thick-set and long, flat and narrow in the tall and spare. There is also wide variation in the thickness of the muscles and the slope of the shoulders in healthy people. Estimates of the significance of variations in the shape of the chest must, therefore, take into account the build of the individual. Normally the chest is bilaterally symmetrical and on cross-section is elliptical. Its shape is affected by extrapulmonary as well as pulmonary disease. For example, in the past, severe rickets was a common cause of chest deformity, the combination of softness of the bones and obstruction to respiration (due to adenoids and chronic or recurrent upper respiratory tract infection) leading to the deformities known as pigeon-chest and Harrison's sulcus.

Disease of the vertebral column can produce *kyphosis* (forward bending) or *scoliosis* (lateral bending), which often occur together. These lead to obvious asymmetry of the chest and may decrease the size of the thoracic cage and restrict lung movement. Scoliosis may also lead to clinical and radiological displacement of the trachea and apex beat. The spine and rib cage may become particularly immobile in ankylosing spondylitis, which may lead to a fixed kyphosis.

Pulmonary disease produces several deformities of the chest. Unilateral apical fibrosis due to tuberculosis may cause obvious flattening of one apex, whilst more extensive unilateral fibrosis or collapse in childhood can even lead to scoliosis. Severe obstructive airways disease (p. 191) leads to a *barrel-shaped chest*. There is obstruction to expiration, and the lungs become overinflated, so that the chest becomes fixed in what is normally the position of full inspiration. Since no further expansion is possible, the rib cage tends to move up in one piece by the action of the accessory muscles of respiration, which become more prominent than usual. The ribs are less obliquely set than usual, the anteroposterior diameter of the chest is increased, the spine becomes unduly concave forwards and the sternum is more arched than usual, with a prominent angle of Louis.

Movements of the chest

The *rate of respiration* for a normal adult is about 14–18 beats/ minute, but can increase up to 22 if the patient is nervous under examination. An increased rate of respiration or *tachypnoea* is a sign of pulmonary disease which is frequently missed owing to lack of observation or inaccurate counting. Increased rate may result from exertion, nervous excitement, fever or hypoxia. Such hypoxia may be due to cardiac, pulmonary, bronchial or laryngeal causes, to alteration in the oxygen-carrying power of the blood or to interference with the normal reflex control of respiration. Tachypnoea may also rise from the association of pain with breathing, as in pleurisy and peritonitis, when the breathing becomes shallow and must therefore be more frequent to make up for the slighter expansion.

The *rhythm* varies very considerably even in health and if the breathing is performed consciously it may become irregular. Study it, therefore, when the patient is off his guard, as only then can accurate observations be made. Either inspiration or expiration may be unduly prolonged, the former being commonly associated with laryngeal or tracheal diseases, the latter with bronchial or pulmonary. A peculiar type, where successive respirations gradually get deeper and deeper till a maximum is attained, and then fall off again until a pause of complete apnoea occurs, to be followed by another wave of gradually deepening and then diminishing respiration, is known as *Cheyne-Stokes breathing*. The pause may last for fully half a minute, though it is often shorter, and the whole cycle is usually completed in less than two minutes. It is most conspicuous when the patient who exhibits it is asleep or unconscious, but may be overlooked if the patient is awake, and particularly if he is talking. Cheyne-Stokes breathing occurs most commonly in cardiac and renal failure, severe pneumonia, increased intracranial pressure and narcotic drug poisoning.

Note its amount of *movement*, whether it is expansile in character, and whether it is similar, or different, on the two sides and over corresponding areas. Movement and expansion are not interchangeable terms; in emphysema the chest may move considerably, but there is little expansion. Chest expansion in men can be measured with a tape measure round the chest just below the nipples. In a fit young man it may be 5–8 cm; in emphysema it may be 1 cm or less.

Diminished or absent expansion may be due to pleurisy with effusion, pneumothorax, consolidation, collapse, fibrosis or the presence of a neoplasm. It is also found in tuberculosis and lobar pneumonia, the former especially at the apices, the latter at the apex or base according to the situation of the disease.

PALPATION

Before making a systematic examination, it is well to lay the hand on any part of the chest which presents an obvious swelling, or where the patient complains of pain. Look at the face rather than the part under examination, so as to avoid causing unnecessary pain. Pain may be due to recent injury to the chest wall, or to inflammatory conditions; to intercostal muscular pain, where, as a rule, specially painful spots can be discovered on pressure; to a painful costochondral junction; to secondary malignant deposits in the ribs; to herpes zoster, before the appearance of the eruption; or to pleurisy. In the case of pleurisy, pressure may considerably increase the pain. Pain may also be due to cardiac causes, such as coronary thrombosis and pericarditis. At the same time the nature of any swelling should be investigated. Fluctuation occurs when an abscess has formed in the chest wall.

The positions of cardiac impulse and trachea should then be determined. Feel for the trachea in the suprasternal notch and decide whether it is placed centrally or deviated to one or other side, by its relation to the suprasternal notch and the insertion of the sternomastoids. Slight deviation of the trachea to the right may be found in healthy people. Displacement of the cardiac impulse alone may be due to scoliosis, the commoner form with its convexity to the right causing a displacement of the cardiac impulse to the left and vice versa, to funnel depression of the sternum or to enlargement of the left ventricle, particularly in aortic regurgitation and hypertension. In the absence of these conditions, a significant displacement of the cardiac impulse or trachea, or of both together, suggests that the position of the mediastinum has been altered by disease of the lungs or pleura. The main conditions which 'push' the mediastinum away from the affected side are pleural effusion and pneumothorax, and the main conditions which draw it towards the affected side are fibrosis of the lung in tuberculosis or after broncho-pneumonia, and collapse of one or more lobes. In fibrosis or collapse of the upper lobe of a lung, the trachea only is displaced.

The *nature of the respiratory movements* must next be studied. Make certain that the two sides of the chest move to approximately the same extent. This is done by fixing the fingertips of either hand at the patient's sides and making the tips of the thumbs just meet in the middle line in front of the chest. The patient is directed to take a full inspiration, when the distance of departure of the thumbs from the middle line indicates the extent of expansion of either half of the chest. The causes of diminished expansion have been mentioned under inspection.

Vibrations may be detected by palpation. For this purpose the palm of the hand should be applied flat on the chest. The patient is then told to repeat 'one, one, one', or 'ninety-nine', in a clear voice. The hand placed on the thorax detects distinct vibration whilst this is done and one must determine whether the vibrations in corresponding areas on the two sides of the chest are approximately equal in intensity; do not, however, forget that where the heart encroaches on the left lung the fremitus is much diminished. *Vocal fremitus is increased* when the lung is consolidated, or contains a large cavity near the surface. *Vocal fremitus is diminished* when the corresponding bronchi are obstructed or totally absent when the lung is separated from the chest wall by a pleural effusion. In this case the collapsed lung fails to convey the vibrations to the fluid; fluid itself is a good conductor of sound. In young persons and women, the vocal resonance is different both in character and intensity from that in male adults.

PERCUSSION

Method of percussion. The middle finger of the left hand is placed firmly on the part which is to be percussed. The back of its middle phalanx is then struck with the tip of the middle finger of the right hand. The stroke should be delivered from the wrist and finger joints, not from the elbow, and the percussing finger should be so bent that when the blow is delivered its terminal phalanx is at right angles to the metacarpal bones and strikes the pleximeter fingers perpendicularly. As soon as the blow has been given, the striking finger must be raised, just as the hammers of a piano fall back from the wires as soon as these have been struck. The blow should be no heavier than is necessary to elicit the resonance of the part being examined, and the wrist joint must move loosely. Repeated heavy blows cause much discomfort to sensitive patients.

The *character of the sound produced* varies quantitatively and qualitatively. When the air in a cavity of sufficient size and appropriate shape is set into vibrations which are not modified by excessive tension of the containing walls of the space, the sound heard has a tympanitic character; such a note is heard on percussion over an air-containing viscus, such as the stomach; but when the cavity is subdivided into a number of small loculi by numerous septa, more or less tense, a characteristic resonance, no longer tympanitic, is produced. Such conditions prevail in the healthy lung and the observer must learn by practice to recognize its distinctive quality. In general terms, this pulmonary resonance is low in pitch and clear in character.

Beginning in front, the examiner should tap lightly and directly (i.e. without pleximeter finger) on the most prominent point of each clavicle—being sure that the points examined correspond exactly with each other—and should observe the quality of the sound, and particularly whether the effects on the two sides are identical. Thereafter the other corresponding areas on either side should be carefully percussed in the manner already described. The presence of the heart will interfere, in parts of the left side, with the development of a sound resembling that from the corresponding point on the right. The back and axillary regions should then be examined in the same manner.

It is essential in all parts of the examination that the patient's attitude is a comfortable one and that his arms and shoulders are placed symmetrically, whether he is sitting up or lying down. When in the case of a very ill patient it is only possible to examine the back by rolling him on to his side, only gross differences in the note on the two sides are significant. If possible the patient should be examined lying first on one side and then on the other. Should the patient's chest by asymmetrical, from scoliosis or other cause, equal resonance on the two sides is not to be expected and again only gross differences between the two sides are significant.

The observer should have two objects in mind; first to make a comparison of the percussion note in comparable areas on the two sides; and second, to map out the limits of lung resonance particularly at the apices, the bases and the area of cardiac dullness.

The *normal degree of resonance* varies from individual to individual and in different parts of the chest in the same individual, being most resonant below the clavicles and scapulae where the muscles are relatively thin, and least resonant over the scapulae.

The lower limits of lung resonance should be determined by percussing from above downwards. The *lower border of the right lung* lies over the liver and is thin; therefore its exact situation is best made out by light percussion. Posteriorly, however, the muffling due to the thick muscles and fat of the back makes it necessary to percuss more firmly. When the patient is obese, very heavy percussion may be necessary. In quiet respiration and on light percussion the lower border is found to lie in the mammary line at the sixth rib, in the mid-axillary line at the eighth rib, in the scapular line at the tenth rib. On heavier percussion some loss of resonance, due to the underlying liver and diaphragm, is found at higher levels and in the mammary line can be detected from the fourth interspace downwards.

On the left side the lower border overlaps the stomach and so the transition is not from lung resonance to dullness, but to tympanitic stomach resonance. Posteriorly, however, the splenic dullness and the dullness of the various solid structures which lie below the lung near the spine are interposed, so that the conditions resemble those found on the right. The position of the lower border corresponds pretty closely with that on the right side; it may, however, be found a trifle further down.

Resonance is increased when the pleural cavity contains air and the lung is more or less collapsed towards the hilum. The note varies from one that is hyperresonant to one that is distinctly tympanitic, according to the amount of air in the pleural cavity.

A characteristic form of high-pitched tympanitic resonance, the *bruit d'airain* (*airain* = brass), 'bell-sound' or 'coin-sound', may also sometimes be heard in pneumothorax by percussion over the front of the chest with a couple of coins (one used as a plexor and the other as a pleximeter) whilst the observer listens with the stethoscope at the back of the patient. Failure to elicit the *bruit d'airain* does not mean, however, that a pneumothorax is not present.

Though a definite tympanitic or hyperresonant sound is regularly found in pneumothorax, it is not consistently found in any other pulmonary conditions. It may be found over some large cavities. It is often stated that resonance is increased in emphysema. In the diagnosis of emphysema it is more important to note the increased limits of resonance with loss of liver and cardiac dullness than the quality of the resonance.

Resonance is diminished when the pleura is thickened, when the underlying lung is more solid than usual for any reason and when the pleural cavity contains fluid. Thus, there may be slight impairment of resonance at one apex in a case of pulmonary tuberculosis due to local infiltration and fibrosis. Considerable impairment may be found over areas of lung affected by fibrosis or collapse. Percussion over a completely consolidated lobe produces a definitely dull note, whilst absolute dullness along with a peculiar sensation of resistance in the percussing finger, so-called 'stony dullness', is the characteristic finding over a pleural effusion of any size. In heart failure, impaired resonance or dullness may be found at the bases of both lungs, indicating oedema of the bases or bilateral effusions.

Myotatic irritability.   In certain conditions the muscles on the front of the thorax are unduly irritable, and a light tap over the sternum produces contractions, at some distance off, in the pectoral muscles. This phenomenon occurs in any wasting disease, and is known as myotatic irritability or myoidema.

AUSCULTATION

Three observations must be made at each point auscultated: first, the character of the breath sounds; second, the character of the vocal resonance; and third, the presence or absence of other sounds.

For good auscultation, a patient in bed should lean back against pillows, or lie on his back, and be completely relaxed. To examine the back, the patient should sit up, but if he is unable to do this he should be rolled round first to one side then to the other. In serious cases, the minimum necessary examination should be done. Take care that the chest-piece is accurately applied, that it is not allowed to move on the surface of the skin, and that no undue pressure is exerted. The patient should breathe with his mouth open, regularly and fairly deeply, but not noisily.

Character of respiratory sounds

There are two typical varieties of breath sounds, both of which are audible in health at certain parts of the chest. The first is known as vesicular breathing, the second as bronchial. Vesicular breath sounds are produced by the passage of air in and out of normal lung tissue, and are heard all over the chest under normal conditions. Bronchial breath sounds are produced by the passage of air through the trachea and large bronchi. Under normal conditions they can be heard by listening over the trachea, but they are not heard over normal lung tissue (except where they may modify the sounds heard over normal tissue situated near the trachea and large bronchi, as will be mentioned later). In disease, however, these sounds may be conducted from the bronchi to the chest wall, as, for instance, when a whole lobe is consolidated by pneumonia. Under these circumstances no air enters or leaves the alveoli and no vesicular breath sounds can be heard. Provided, however, that the bronchi are patent, so that bronchial sounds are produced and conducted through them, and provided that sufficient lung is consolidated to convey these sounds to the chest wall, bronchial breathing will be heard over the area affected by these changes.

In *vesicular breathing*, which can be heard typically in the axillary and infrascapular regions of a healthy individual, the inspiratory sound is fairly intense and is audible during the whole act. The pitch is low and the quality is characteristic, being somewhat rustling. The expiratory sound follows that of inspiration without a distinct pause. It only remains audible during the earlier part of the expiratory phase, and under normal conditions the inspiratory sound is heard for at least twice as long as the expiratory.

To learn to recognize *bronchial breathing* the student should listen over the trachea, though he must not expect to hear so intense a type of bronchial respiration when he subsequently examines a diseased lung. The inspiratory sound is moderately intense. It becomes inaudible shortly before the end of inspiration. Its quality is harsh and aspirate. The expiratory sound is generally more intense than the inspiratory; the pitch is often higher; the duration extends through the greater part of expiration, being as long as, or even longer than, the inspiratory sound. In quality it exactly resembles the inspiratory sound, being aspirate in character. Bronchial breathing can most readily be recognized by the quality of the expiratory sound and the definite gap between inspiration and expiration. Some prolongation of the expiratory sound is characteristic of asthma and emphysema and must not be mistaken for bronchial breathing. It is due to the fact that in these diseases the act of expiration is itself performed more slowly than in health.

When breath sounds in a superficial bronchus can be heard through normal lung, the sound of the breathing combines both vesicular and bronchial elements. This variety of breath sound is known as *bronchovesicular*, and it is usually the expiratory sound which has more of a bronchial character. It may occur in health near the roots of the lungs behind; in the upper portions near the middle line in front; and especially at the right apex for a few centimetres below the clavicle in front and above the level of the spine of the scapula near the midline behind. These findings, which sometimes lead to a mistaken diagnosis of disease at the right apex, are due to the fact that the trachea lies in immediate contact with the apex of the lung on the right side, whereas it is separated from it on the left by the aorta, the internal carotid artery and the oesophagus.

The breath sounds must be auscultated in the various regions that have already been examined by percussion, their character in each noted and similar regions on the two sides of the chest accurately compared.

If the student understands how vesicular and bronchial breath sounds are produced, he should have no difficulty in explaining the findings in disease. Vesicular breath sounds may be present but reduced in intensity in any condition in which the entry of air to that part of the lung is diminished, as, for instance, in bronchopneumonia, where some alveoli are affected and others not. Breath sounds of any kind may be diminished or absent where thickened pleura, pleural effusion or pneumothorax interferes with or prevents the conduction of these sounds to the chest wall. They may also be absent in any condition, such as collapse or fibrosis, in which no air enters or leaves alveoli, but at the same time the conditions necessary for the conduction of bronchial breath sounds to the chest wall are not fulfilled. Finally, bronchial breath sounds may be heard whenever patent bronchi are connected to the chest wall by a sufficiently uniform sound-conducting medium. This occurs classically over consolidated lung, occasionally in the presence of a large cavity, and very rarely over a pleural effusion.

Vocal resonance

The second series of observations is directed to *the intensity and character of the vocal resonance*. It varies in intensity even in health being more intense the nearer the stethoscope is to the larger bronchi. When the patient repeats the words 'one, one, one', or 'ninety-nine', the ear perceives, not the distinct syllables, but a resonant sound, the intensity of which depends on the loudness and depth of the patient's voice and on the conductivity of his lungs.

Each point examined on one side of the chest should be at once compared with the corresponding point on the other side. Vocal resonance of normal intensity generally conveys the impression of being produced just at the chest-piece of the stethoscope. If it seems to be nearer the ear than this, the resonance is increased. When it appears to be near the earpiece of the stethoscope the increase is marked and the condition is often described as *bronchophony*.

If the words become clear and seem to be spoken right into the auscultator's ear, it will generally be found that whispered words are distinctly heard. This condition is called *whispering pectoriloquy*. Increased resonance occurs when the lung substance conducts the sound waves set up by the voice more clearly than usual from the bronchi. Consolidation is the commonest cause. Bronchophony and whispering pectoriloquy occur when a moderately large bronchus is surrounded by layer of solid lung reaching to the chest wall, as in lobar pneumonia. Whispering pectoriloquy is also fairly characteristic of a cavity of some size communicating with a bronchus and may be heard above the level of pleural effusion. In some cases a certain degree of pectoriloquy is heard in health in the proximity of the trachea and large bronchi and particularly at the right apex.

Vocal resonance is either entirely abolished or much diminished where a layer of fluid separates the lung from the chest wall (except when bronchial breathing is heard, see above) and in pneumothorax. It is also diminished in cases of thickened pleura and of emphysema.

Above the level of a pleural effusion or in some cases over an area of consolidation, a nasal or bleating character may be imparted to the voice. It is known as *aegophony*.

Added sounds

Added sounds may arise in the lung or in the pleura. Sounds resembling pleural friction may be produced by movement of the stethoscope on the patient's skin, or of the observer's hands or clothes against the stethoscope. Sounds arising in the patient's muscles may resemble adventitious sounds and in particular the shivering of a cold patient makes any attempt at auscultation useless. The application of the stethoscope to hairy skins may produce sounds indistinguishable from crepitations. Sounds resembling coarse crepitations may also be heard over a broken rib.

The nomenclature of the added sounds arising in the lung has been confused since their original description by Laennec. He introduced the French word *râle* to describe any added sound heard in the chest and also used the Latin word *rhonchus* in the same connotation. As a result of confusion in translation, the terms are often used differently today. The least confusing classification of added sounds is to divide them into continuous wheezing sounds, or *rhonchi*, and interrupted bubbling or crackling sounds, or *crepitations*.

Rhonchi, which are prolonged uninterrupted noises, arise in the bronchi and are due to partial obstruction of their lumen, by swelling of the mucosa, by viscid secretion or by constriction of bronchial smooth muscle. They may be high or low pitched, depending on whether they arise in small or large bronchial tubes. High-pitched rhonchi are called *sibilant* and have a squeaky quality; low-pitched rhonchi are called *sonorous* and have a snoring quality. They may also be palpable. Rhonchi are characteristic of bronchitis and asthma, and in the latter are high-pitched and expiratory. When they are localized to one side of the chest, the possibility of a localized obstruction of a bronchial tube should be considered, as for example in bronchial carcinoma. The word 'bronchospasm' as a description of a physical sign should be avoided.

Crepitations are discontinuous crackling or bubbling sounds. They may be produced in the alveoli, bronchi or, occasionally, in cavities. There are several types of crepitation produced by different mechanisms. They may be heard at any time in the respiratory cycle but are most commonly heard at the beginning of inspiration.

Fine crepitations are thought to be due to the presence of fluid in the alveoli as occurs in heart failure or the early stages of pneumonia when there is exudate in the avleoli.

Course crepitations can be produced by two distinct mechanisms. They can occur as bubbling or clicking sounds due to secretion in the bronchi in bronchitis and bronchiectasis.

In fibrosing alveolitis a more crackling sound is characteristically heard, especially in early inspiration. This is thought to be due to the sudden 'snapping open' of the relatively stiff alveoli that are associated with fibrosis. Such crepitations are usually only present at the lung bases.

A few crepitations may be heard in health, particularly at the lower borders of the lungs. These are abolished if the patient is asked to cough and are of no significance. In other cases crepitations are intensified after a cough or may only then make their appearance; these are known as *post-tussive crepitations*. They are an important sign of tuberculous infiltration, and may also be heard over cavities.

A *friction sound* or *pleural rub* is characteristic of pleurisy at the stage when exudation is not abundant enough to separate the inflamed and roughened pleural surfaces. It has a creaking or rubbing character, often quite characteristic, but sometimes rather hard to distinguish from a crepitation. The friction sound may be fine or coarse. In some instances it is palpable, but since coarse crepitations may be so too, this does not distinguish them. The chief differences are that friction sounds occur during that part of inspiration when the roughened surfaces are rubbing against each other, to reappear at a corresponding period of expiration. They are, moreover, unchanged after the patient has coughed, whereas crepitations may alter under these conditions because of changes in disposition of the secretion which causes them.

Finally there are certain manifestations of pulmonary disease which should be looked for outside the chest itself. These include clubbing of the fingers and cyanosis (both mentioned in previous chapters), and enlargement of cervical or axillary lymph nodes or the liver from secondary carcinoma. Respiratory failure with carbon dioxide retention (p. 192) may be associated with certain neurological signs. These include a coarse flapping tremor of the hands (asterixis), generalized twitching movements and even convulsions. Such patients may become drowsy or stuporose and this is aggravated by sedatives or injudicious oxygen therapy. In some cases there is papilloedema.

THE SPUTUM

Sputum may be mucoid, purulent or frothy. Any of these varieties may contain blood, or the sputum may consist entirely of blood.

Mucoid sputum occurs characteristically in chronic bronchitis when secondary infection is not present. It is clear, tough and sticky and usually scanty. Particularly tenacious sputum may be found in asthma. This may block the bronchi by forming plugs, or else be coughed up as 'casts' of the bronchial tree—during or after an attack; alternatively, sticky particles like sago—the *perles* of Laennec—may be expectorated after an attack.

Mucopurulent sputum is seen in bronchitis (or other upper respiratory infections) when secondary bacterial infection has occurred: the sputum in bronchitis may also be frankly purulent.

Purulent sputum is thick and yellow (or green) and not sticky. It may occur in any condition in which infection is present and is characteristic of bronchiectasis, bronchopneumonia and lung abscess. In bronchiectasis and lung abscess it may be copious and its expectoration may be readily influenced by change of posture.

Frothy sputum, characteristic of pulmonary oedema, may be white or pink and is often copious.

Blood may be coughed up alone, or the sputum may be more or less blood-stained. It must be distinguished from blood brought into the mouth from epistaxis or haematemesis. Its brighter colour and its frothy appearance usually makes its origin obvious. Further, patients who have had a haemoptysis commonly bring up blood-stained sputum for a day or two, while bleeding from the upper intestinal tract is characteristically followed by melaena. Haemoptysis may be due to pulmonary causes, including tuberculosis, bronchiectasis, pulmonary embolus and carcinoma; to cardiac causes, including mitral stenosis; and very rarely to aneurysm of the aorta.

Several diseases cause a characteristic colouration of the sputum. In lobar pneumonia it may be rusty and so viscid that it often will not fall out of an inverted spittoon; it is bright yellow or green when a liver abscess has ruptured into the lung, and the latter colour also appears in some cases of pneumonia. When an amoebic hepatic abscess has discharged into the lung, the sputum has the appearance of anchovy sauce.

The quantity of sputum coughed up in 24 hours is important, especially whether change of position produces a large quantity. Bronchitic patients bring up most sputum during the first two hours after waking in the mornings.

The odour of the sputum is rarely important, but it may be putrid in bronchiectasis or lung abscess.

Microscopical examination of sputum

The principal value of microscopical examination of the sputum is in the detection of bacteria and in the recognition of malignant cells. Eosinophils may be found in the sputum in allergic conditions, e.g. some cases of asthma, and in pneumonia due to parasitic worms and in aspergillosis.

Malignant cells may be seen in the sputum, particularly in patients with squamous carcinomas of the main bronchi. Skill is required to differentiate them from epithelium and other cellular debris, but their appearance is sometimes unmistakable (Plate VII).

Less common constituents of the sputum include fungi, yeasts and golden yellow asbestos bodies in asbestosis (Plate VII)

X-RAY EXAMINATION

Radiological examination of the chest is most important, because many localized and even some widespread infiltrative lesions (e.g. sarcoidosis) may produce no abnormal physical signs. It is paramount, in the early diagnosis of tuberculosis and carcinoma. Serial X-rays form an integral part of the estimation of progress in many chest diseases. A brief outline of the standard methods will be given here.

Radiography

Posterior-anterior view.   The ordinary standard X-ray film of the chest is a postero-anterior view, that is to say one taken with the film against the front of the patient's chest and the X-ray tube 2 metres behind the patient. It is examined systematically on a viewing box. The following is a simple plan of examination.

1. *The bony skeleton.* Is the chest symmetrical? Is any scoliosis present? Are the ribs unduly crowded or widely spaced in any area? Are cervical ribs present? Are the ribs eroded or do they appear the site of malignant deposits?

2. *The position of the patient.* Is the patient straight or rotated? If straight, the inner ends of the clavicles will be disposed symmetrically with reference to the vertebral column.

3. *The position of the trachea.* This is seen as a dark column representing the air within the trachea. The cartilaginous rings are not visible. Is it centrally placed or deviated to one or other side?

4. *The outline of the heart and mediastinum.* Is this normal in size, shape and position?

5. *The diaphragm.* Can the outline of the diaphragm be seen on each side, and is it normal in shape and position? Are the cardiophrenic and costophrenic angles clearly seen?

6. *The lung fields.* For radiological purposes the lung fields are divided into three zones:

Zone 1 (upper zone)	extends from the apex to a line drawn through the lower borders of the anterior ends of the second costal cartilages.
Zone 2 (mid zone)	extends from this line to one drawn through the lower borders of the fourth costal cartilages and contains the hila of the lungs.
Zone 3 (lower zone)	extends from this line to the bases of the lungs.

Each zone is systematically examined on the two sides and any area which appears abnormal is carefully compared with the corresponding area on the opposite side. The minor interlobar fissure, which separates the right upper and middle lobes, may sometimes be seen running horizontally in the third and fourth interspace on the right side. The major interlobar fissure, which separates the lower lobes from the remainder of the lungs, is not seen in a normal postero-anterior film.

Lateral views. Lateral views are indispensable in the localization of lung lesions for the postero-anterior view does not show whether a shadow is situated in the anterior or posterior part of the chest, or (if in the mid zone) whether in the upper or lower lobe.

The following is a simple plan of examination.

1. *The bony skeleton*
2. *The position of the trachea*
3. *The diaphragm.* As the level of the diaphragm differs on the two sides, a double outline may be seen, that of the side nearer the film being the clearer.
4. *The lung fields* are obscured by two relatively opaque areas, one above and behind, due to the shoulder joint, and one below and in front, due to the heart, which rests on the anterior part of the diaphragm. There are thus left two relatively clear areas—one above and in front, behind the upper part of the sternum, and one below and behind, including the angle between the diaphragm and the spine.

In the lateral views, the interlobar fissures are more often seen. Their normal positions have already been described (p. 168). Their recognition is useful both in localizing lesions and in detecting shrinkage of a lobe from fibrosis or collapse.

Screening

Screening is used mainly to detect abnormalities of the heart and paralysis of the diaphragm. By standing the patient in different positions, it is possible to see enlargement of the various chambers of the heart and main vessels and paradoxical pulsation of the left atrium. Enlargement of the left atrium is detected by noting displacement of the barium-filled oesophagus. When a diaphragmatic paralysis is present *paradoxical* movement is seen when the patient coughs or sniffs, the diaphragm ascending when it should descend, and vice versa.

Bronchography

After local anaesthesia, a radiopaque iodized oil is introduced into the trachea and allowed to run into the bronchi. X-ray pictures are taken and the corresponding bronchi are clearly outlined. With suitable manipulations, the whole of the bronchial tree can be outlined, but more than one sitting may be required. Bronchography is rarely performed nowadays although it is sometimes a useful procedure. Its main use was to demonstrate bronchiectasis which is now much less common.

Tomography

An ordinary X-ray picture consists of shadows at all depths in the chest, superimposed on one another. It has the disadvantage that not more than some 40% of the lung tissue is shown without its being obscured by shadows of the bony thorax or of mediastinal contents. The tomograph is a device whereby a picture is obtained of a section of the thorax at any given depth. The tube and plate are moved in the arc of a circle as the exposure is made, in such a manner that the structures in one section only remain in focus and anything out of the plane of this section is blurred out. Sections can be taken at different depths in the chest, as desired, and so the appearances in chest X-rays can often be greatly simplified. It is mainly used to detect cavitation in apparently opaque shadows in the lung fields, and to give a clearer picture of hilar shadows. It may also indicate narrowing of a bronchus due to lesions such as carcinoma.

BRONCHOSCOPY, THORACOSCOPY AND MEDIASTINOSCOPY

By means of the bronchoscope, the main bronchi and their branches can be directly inspected, small portions of tissue can be removed for biopsy, and therapeutic procedures carried out. The main value of bronchoscopy is in the diagnosis of carcinoma of the bronchus and in deciding whether this is operable. With the aid of modern flexible fibreoptic bronchoscopes, very small bronchi can be visualized and washings for cytological examination taken from separate lung segments. The flexible bronchoscope enables examination of patients with severe cervical or skeletal deformities, and affords a good view of the upper lobe bronchi. After an artificial pneumothorax has been induced, the pleura can be inspected with the aid of a thoracoscope and further assistance in diagnosis may be obtained. Mediastinoscopy can be carried out by inserting an instrument behind the sternum. This enables the observer to inspect structures such as glands and to take specimens for biopsy. These are both specialized surgical procedures.

PLEURAL ASPIRATION AND BIOPSY

Pleural effusions may be drained by inserting a wide-bore needle into the fluid-filled pleural space through one of the rib spaces, under local anaesthesia. The needle is inserted perpendicular to the skin and pleura, just above a rib margin. Aspirations may be *therapeutic*, to relieve respiratory embarrassment due to a large effusion, or *diagnostic*, to remove fluid for examination.

Pleural fluid can be examined macroscopically and microscopically. Full details cannot be given here, but the colour, consistency and quantity should be noted. A *transudate* from the capillaries, as occurs in cardiac and renal disease, can be distinguished from an *exudate* resulting from pleural inflammation by its lower protein content (<3.0 g/100 ml) and specific gravity (usually <1.015). Frankly blood-stained effusions occur with carcinoma, pulmonary infarction or trauma. In tuberculosis effusions the fluid is straw-coloured and copious (often well over 1 litre) and may coagulate on standing; under the microscope many leucocytes are seen, lymphocytes often predominating. Tubercle bacilli are rarely seen, but can more commonly be cultured. In other inflammatory exudates, many polymorphs are seen. In *empyema* pus is aspirated which may be full of white cells and organisms.

Needle biopsy of the pleura may also be useful in establishing the diagnosis of the cause of a pleural effusion. In a high proportion of patients the presence of carcinoma or tuberculosis may be detected. Drill biopsy of lung can also be performed and is useful in establishing a histological diagnosis in diffuse lung diseases, such as fibrosing alveolitis.

LUNG FUNCTION TESTS

In recent years, tests of lung function of increasing complexity have been introduced, which are beyond the scope of this chapter, but some of the simple tests useful in clinical practice will be described. It must be stressed that lung function tests enable the clinician to make a *physiological* rather than a *pathological* diagnosis. That is to say, they will indicate that there is obstruction to air flow, but not that the patient has a bronchial carcinoma. Also, they are more likely to be abnormal if there is a diffuse process affecting the lung than if there is merely a localized lesion. They may be useful under the following circumstances:

1. To give an objective assessment of a patient's disability
2. To follow the progress of a disease and the effect of treatment
3. To try to differentiate possible causes of a patient's dyspnoea
4. To aid the management of cases of respiratory failure
5. To assess patients prior to anaesthetics and surgery, particularly thoracic surgery leading to lung resection.

Vital capacity and spirometry

The simplest and still perhaps the most valuable tests are the measurement of the patient's *vital capacity* and the recording of the *expiratory spirogram*. These can be measured by various types of *spirometer* and recorded graphically (Fig. 6.4). The patient inhales maximally and then breathes out as hard and as fast as he can. Measurements are then made of the amount of air he expels and the speed at which he does so. The amount of air expelled by maximal voluntary effort is the *vital capacity*. In normal subjects three-quarters of this air is expelled within the first second and all within about three seconds. Thus the normal curve is steep. In

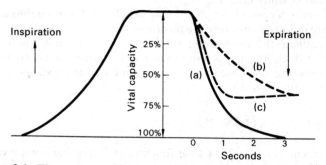

Fig. 6.4. The expiratory spirogram: (*a*) normal; (*b*) airway obstruction; (*c*) restriction.

diseases such as asthma, bronchitis and emphysema there is obstruction to the flow of air out of the lungs, owing to collapse or constriction of the airways, or intraluminal obstruction, owing to mucus or oedema, so that the curve is flattened (Fig. 6.4*b*). On scrutiny of the curves, this flattening is apparent, but a numerical value can be given to the degree of flattening by recording the volume expired in one second. This volume (*forced expiratory volume at one second*, or FEV1) is then expressed as a ratio of the *vital capacity* (VC). This ratio (FEV1/VC) is called the FEV% and should exceed 70% in healthy individuals under 60 years of age. If the percentage is below this figure, the patient may be described as suffering from *airways obstruction*. The test may be repeated after the use of a bronchodilator aerosol, and if the FEV1 improves, the *airways obstruction* is said to be *reversible*. In some patients, treatment for several days with oral bronchodilators or even steroids may be needed to demonstrate reversibility. Broadly speaking, in asthma and bronchitis the obstruction is partly reversible by bronchodilators, whereas in emphysema it is not. However, the distinction between these conditions is not as clear as might be supposed. Alternatively the maximum expiratory flow rate can be measured by means of a peak flow meter. This portable instrument (Fig. 6.5) measures directly the expiratory flow rate, which is reduced in airways obstruction. The other principal abnormality which can be recognized from the expiratory spirogram is pulmonary *restriction*. This may result from limitation of movement of the chest wall

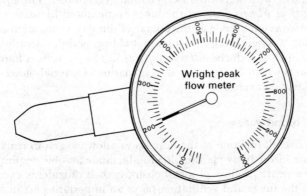

Fig. 6.5 A Wright peak flow meter.

(e.g. kyphoscoliosis) or diseases causing loss of lung volume (e.g. pulmonary fibrosis). In these conditions the vital capacity is reduced but the shape of the trace is similar to normal (Fig. 6.4c). The ratio FEV_1/VC remains normal (more than 70%) and the peak expiratory flow rate measured by the peak flow meter is also normal.

Diffusion and distribution

Having entered the lungs, air is normally fairly evenly distributed throughout them. Similarly the blood entering the lungs from the pulmonary arteries has a quite even distribution, although in health both ventilation and perfusion are greater at the bases compared with the apices of the lungs. Modern radio-isotope techniques can be used for looking at the pattern of perfusion or ventilation; some centres can perform simultaneous ventilation–perfusion scans. In disease both ventilation and perfusion can be quite uneven and may lead to abnormal gas exchange.

Oxygen and carbon dioxide must pass freely between alveoli and pulmonary capillaries. The passage of these gases occurs largely by diffusion. Carbon dioxide diffuses very readily and rarely presents a problem; but in certain conditions, notably the *interstitial fibroses*, and some pulmonary infiltrations, such as *sarcoidosis*, the diffusion of oxygen may be limited. Unequal *distribution* of inspired gas in relation to *perfusion* of the pulmonary capillaries may also cause abnormal oxygenation of the blood. The *diffusing capacity* or *transfer factor* of the lungs is measured by using *carbon monoxide* as a marker gas; the uptake of this gas is measured either during a single period of breath holding or by a steady-state technique. A reduced *diffusing capacity* or *transfer factor* is found in diseases which cause reduced oxygenation of arterial blood, particularly on exercise.

The blood gases

The overall function of the lungs is to allow oxygen to reach the tissues of the body via the blood to facilitate aerobic respiration; also a waste product of metabolism, carbon dioxide, is excreted from the lungs and ventilation plays an important part in acid–base regulation of the body. The effectiveness of gas exchange can be assessed by measuring the *partial pressure* of oxygen (PO_2) and carbon dioxide (PCO_2) in the arterial blood and acid–base status can be investigated by measuring arterial blood pH. All of these parameters can be measured by appropriate electrodes, and the apparatus is available in most hospitals. Also the arterial PCO_2 can be estimated indirectly by a simple rebreathing method.

Alveolar ventilation is the principal factor which determines arterial PCO_2. Alveolar hypoventilation with subsequent *respiratory failure* may result from drugs or diseases which impair ventilatory effort as well as from lung diseases. Normal arterial PCO_2 is in the range of 4·7–6·0 kPa (35–45 mmHg); a low PCO_2 may result from alveolar hyperventilation. Normal arterial PO_2 is 11·3–14·0 kPa (80–100 mmHg) and will be reduced in many lung diseases as well as in cardiac conditions which cause shunting of venous blood to the arterial circulation. The pH of arterial blood is normally kept within the tight limits of 7·38–7·42 but may be altered by renal failure and other metabolic disorders such as diabetic keto acidosis. Blood gas and pH measurements are widely used in clinical medicine and indeed to try to manage respiratory failure without them is analagous to treating diabetic coma without doing blood sugar measurements.

Other tests

Many other physiological tests of lung function are available including measurements of lung compliance, airway resistance and gas mixing in the lung. Exercise testing may be needed in some cases to fully assess every aspect of lung function.

IMMUNOLOGY

Skin tests can be valuable in the diagnosis of chest disease. Allergic asthma is associated with Type 1 hypersensitivity and immediate skin reactions to allergens such as grass pollen and house dust mite. Delayed hypersensitivity (Type 4) is shown by Mantoux tests used to detect the presence of tuberculous infection (previous or recent). The Kveim test is relatively specific for sarcoidosis. Here an intradermal injection of antigen is made and the site of the lesion is biopsied for histological examination six weeks later. Antibody levels in serum can now be measured and are of use in diagnosis of many conditions. Precipitating antibodies are present in patients with some fungal diseases, and specific reaginic antibodies (IgE) can now be accurately measured. IgE levels are often raised in asthma, particularly if this is due to allergy.

7

The cardiovascular system

ANATOMICAL LANDMARKS

The *praecordium* is a term used to indicate the anterior aspect of the chest which overlies the heart.

It is often necessary to define the exact situation of a point on the front of the chest, and certain landmarks, some natural and some artificial, are commonly used for this purpose.

The ribs and interspaces on either side form convenient horizontal landmarks. In order to count them, feel for the ridge which marks the junction of the manubrium with the body of the sternum, known as the angle of Louis, or sternal angle. When this has been found, run the finger outwards until it reaches the second costal cartilage, which articulates with the sternum at this level. The space immediately above this is the first intercostal space. The spaces should then be counted downwards well away from the sternum, where they are more easily felt.

The distance of any given point from the midline of the body may be referred to as a series of vertical lines. These are the *midclavicular line*, defined as the vertical line dropped from the centre of the clavicle, or, what amounts to the same thing, the line midway between the middle of the suprasternal notch and the tip of the acromion; and the *anterior*, *mid-*, and *posterior axillary lines*, descending respectively from the anterior border, the centre and the posterior border of the axilla.

Examination of the cardiovascular system should follow this sequence: the arterial pulses, the blood pressure, the venous pulse and finally the praecordium. The usual methods of inspection, palpation, percussion, and auscultation are used to examine the praecordium, although percussion gives only limited information. The order of examination of the cardiovascular system is important. The information obtained in earlier parts of the examination guides the clinician towards expected findings later on. This is especially helpful with regard to auscultation; here the experienced examiner anticipates the findings based on previously established clinical observations; in contrast the beginner arrives at auscultation with no expectation and so has less chance of a successful analysis. In selected patients a more detailed analysis of the peripheral vascular system, venous or arterial, may be required if insufficiency is suggested by the general examination.

ARTERIAL PULSES

The presence of the main peripheral pulses, the radial, brachial, carotid, femoral, popliteal, posterior tibial, and dorsalis pedis pulses, should be noted and the volume compared with the other side.

The following observations should then be made:

1. Rate of pulse
2. Rhythm
3. Character
4. Volume
5. Condition of vessel wall
6. The presence or absence of delay of the femoral pulses compared with the radials

To assess the rate and rhythm of the pulse the radial pulse at the wrist is usually used. It is best felt with the tips of the fingers, the patient's forearm being pronated and the wrist slightly flexed. A central pulse, in either the carotid or the brachial artery, is preferable for studying the character or wave-form of the pulse.

Estimates of the 'tension' of the pulse, that is of the blood pressure within the vessel, by palpation are quite unreliable. The blood pressure should be measured with the sphygmomanometer. The terms 'good', 'bad', 'strong' and 'weak' in relation to the pulse lack precision and should be avoided.

The *rate* of the pulse is stated as so many beats a minute. It is counted, not when the fingers are first laid upon the pulse, but when any quickening due to nervousness of the patient has subsided and the pulse has resumed its normal rate. Count the beats for not less than half a minute. In cases of atrial fibrillation, the pulse rate counted at the wrist may not indicate the true rate of ventricular contractions. In all such cases, the rate of the heart beat should be counted by auscultation at the apex, and the difference between this rate and the pulse rate at the wrist should be recorded. This difference is referred to as the *pulse deficit* which is due to some beats being of insufficient strength to reach the peripheral arteries, while the heart sounds indicate the true ventricular rate. The spontaneous resting rate shows marked variations (between 60 and 120 beats per minute) depending on the balance of activity between the vagal and sympathetic components of the autonomic nervous system. The pulse rate is increased during exercise, in fever and in thyrotoxicosis. It is also increased in rapid arrhythmias. It is slowed somewhat in myxoedema, and in complete heart block it beats at a steady 20–40 beats/minute.

Decide next whether the *rhythm* is regular or irregular. If it is irregular, decide if it is completely irregular, whether the irregularity has a recurring pattern, or whether an otherwise regular rhythm is occasionally interrupted by some slight irregularity. The pulse of atrial fibrillation is completely irregular. The irregularity is usually obvious when the rate is rapid, but becomes less easy to recognize when the rate has been slowed by digitalis. If the rhythm has a recurring pattern, or there are occasional irregularities, these are likely to be due to extrasystoles. An extrasystole is a beat which occurs prematurely, is small and is followed by an unduly long pause. Disorders of rhythm are described more fully under Electrocardiography (p. 229).

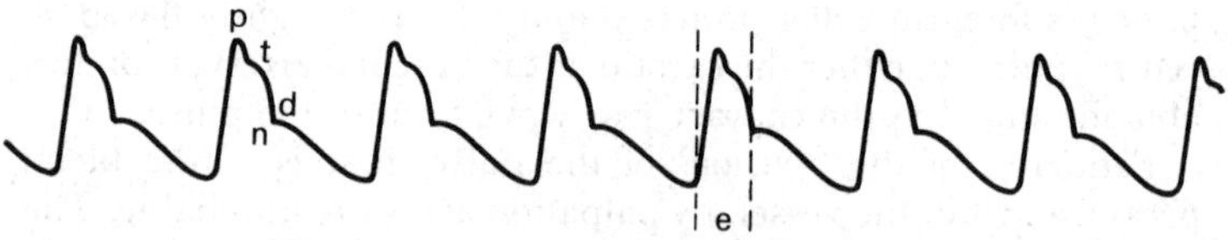

Fig. 7.1 A normal arterial pulse tracing.

p: percussion waves   d: dicrotic wave
t: tidal wave   e: period of ventricular
n: dicrotic notch   systole (aortic valve open)

Study the *character or form* of the individual pulse wave (Fig. 7.1). The character of the pulse becomes sharper in the more peripheral arteries and so in assessing the central wave form the carotid artery is most useful. It is best felt with the thumb, pressing backwards at the medial border of sterno-mastoid at the level of the thyroid cartilage. It is not usually possible to detect slight variations from the normal, but in certain diseases the character of the pulse is detectably abnormal. The most important of these are as follows:

Anacrotic pulse.   (The term anacrotic is a derivative of anadicrotic, meaning two up-beats.) Anacrotic pulse occurs in aortic stenosis, which gives rise to a slow ejection of blood from the left

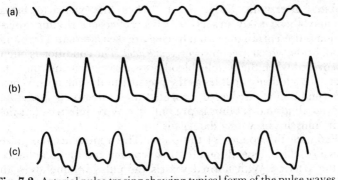

Fig. 7.2 Arterial pulse tracing showing typical form of the pulse waves in (*a*) aortic stenosis, (*b*) aortic incompetence and (*c*) pulsus alternans.

ventricle. The resulting pulse wave has a slow upstroke, an anacrotic wave on the upstroke, and the pulse is of small volume (Fig. 7.2a).

Collapsing (water-hammer) pulse. Collapsing pulse is characterized by a rapid upstroke and descent of the pulse wave. It occurs in aortic regurgitation. The abrupt upstroke is due to the greatly increased stroke volume, and the collapsing character results firstly from the diastolic leak back into the left ventricle as well as from the rapid run-off to the periphery because of the low systemic vascular resistance. Minor degrees of this type of pulse are seen with patent ductus arteriosus and other large arteriovenous connections and occasionally in thyrotoxicosis. (Fig. 7.2b).

Bisferiens pulse. Bisferiens pulse is a combination of the anacrotic and collapsing pulses occurring in combined aortic stenosis and incompetence. The anacrotic wave is of the same height as the percussion wave, and both can be felt distinctly.

Pulsus paradoxus. Normally with inspiration there is a slight fall in the peak arterial pressure (5–10 mmHg.) When ventricular filling is restricted during inspiration (as in constrictive pericarditis or cardiac tamponade) left ventricular stroke volume drops markedly so the arterial pulse becomes smaller, or in extreme cases becomes impalpable during inspiration. The degree of a paradox can be quantified using a sphygmomanometer. Pulsus paradoxus also occurs with severe airways obstruction.

Pulsus alternans. (Fig. 7.2c). When the ventricle beats strongly, then weakly, in successive beats of normal rhythm, alternation is present. In the radial tracing are seen alternate large and small beats, which are, however, *equidistant*. The condition is often discovered when the systolic blood pressure is taken, and the rate of sounds suddenly doubles as the pressure in the cuff falls. When this condition is discovered, provided the heart rate is moderate and no abnormal rhythm is present, it may be inferred that the heart muscle is severely damaged.

Estimate the volume of the pulse. This represents the pulse pressure which depends on the stroke volume and the compliance of the arteries. With normal vessels the pulse volume gives an indication of the stroke volume. In older subjects with normal stroke volume the rigid vessels cause the pulse pressure to widen.

Examine the *condition of the vessel wall*. Sufficient pressure should be exerted on the brachial artery to abolish pulsation in the radial vessel which should then be rolled beneath the fingers against the underlying bone. In young persons, the arteries cannot be felt or are soft. In older persons, they are more easily palpable. In arteriosclerosis they may feel hard like whipcord and may be tortuous.

Delay of the femoral compared with the right radial pulse is found in coarctation of the aorta.

The *typical pulse* of a healthy adult man should be described in the following terms. The rate is 70/minute. The beats are regular in rhythm and equal in volume. The pulse is of normal volume and the arterial wall is just palpable but is neither thickened nor tortuous.

The blood pressure

Certain details are important in the use of the *sphygmomanometer*. The patient should be sitting or lying at ease. The manometer is placed so as to be at the same level as the observer's eye. All clothing should be removed from the arm. The cuff should be applied closely to the upper arm, with the lower border not less than 2·5 cm from the cubital fossa.

The radial pulse is palpated while the cuff is inflated to a pressure of 30 mmHg above the level at which radial pulsation can no longer be felt. The stethoscope is then placed lightly over the brachial artery. The pressure in the cuff is lowered, 5 mmHg at a time, until the first sound is heard, which is the systolic pressure. Continue to lower the pressure in the cuff until the sounds become suddenly faint or inaudible: this is the diastolic pressure.

Arterial pressure shows temporary variations with change of posture, after meals, on exertion and notably on excitement. Hence it should be observed only after the patient has been reassured and when he is quietly resting, free from excitement and with the arm relaxed. In nervous patients the first reading is often too high and should be rejected; a second reading will more closely represent the true pressure. The pulse rate at the time should be noted, for blood pressure varies to some extent with the rate of the heart. It is essential to work as quickly as is compatible with accuracy, for compression of a limb itself induces a rise in blood pressure. To reduce this source of error when successive estimations are to be made, the air pressure in the armlet should always be allowed to fall to zero as soon as each reading has been taken. It is important to take the blood pressure of patients taking hypotensive drugs or otherwise suspected of postural hypotension in both the recumbent and the standing positions.

Occasionally the sounds disappear at a point below 200 mm for a period and then reappear, finally disappearing at the point of diastolic pressure. Thus the sounds may first appear when the mercury falls to 210 (systolic pressure), disappear from 180 to 160 (silent gap), reappear and finally disappear at 120 (diastolic pressure). This phenomenon of a *silent gap* is found in certain patients with hypertension; its significance is unknown, but its occurrence makes it important that the armlet pressure should always be well raised at the beginning of an estimation of blood pressure.

Check that the width of the cuff is correct. For an adult, the standard cuff width is 12·5 cm. If a narrower cuff is used, the recorded pressures will be falsely high.

For children, there is a variety of cuffs of different widths. Select the size which covers most of the upper arm but leaves a gap of 1 cm below the axilla and above the antecubital fossa.

Occasionally it becomes necessary to compare the systolic blood pressure in the arm with that in the leg. The patient lies face downwards and an 18 cm cuff is applied above the knee and auscultation carried out over the popliteal artery. In coarctation of the aorta, the blood pressure in the legs is lower than in the arms.

Normal blood pressure. The average systolic pressure in healthy adults is 100–140 mmHg, the average diastolic pressure, 60–90 mmHg. In children it approximates to the lower figure in each case, and in the elderly it reaches or even exceeds the higher figure. The difference between the systolic and the diastolic pressures—the pulse pressure—is 30–60 mmHg.

Abnormal blood pressure. Abnormal blood pressure must be considered in relation to the patient's age. A blood pressure of 140 over 90 would indicate quite severe hypertension in a child while much higher systolic pressure in an elderly patient is inevitable due to loss of elasticity resulting from degenerative arterial changes (arteriosclerosis). If a cause for hypertension cannot be found then a diagnosis of essential hypertension is made.

VENOUS PULSES

The neck veins

The neck veins communicate directly with the right atrium. Changes in the mean pressure within them, together with the pulsations that occur with each cardiac cycle, give direct information, therefore, about mean pressure in the right atrium and about pressure changes during the cardiac cycle.

The neck veins should be examined with the patient in a good light, and reclining at an angle of about 45° (Fig. 7.3). The neck should be supported so that the neck muscles are relaxed. The veins normally show slight pulsation, and two or three small waves can be distinguished in each cardiac cycle. There is, however, a mean level, and the perpendicular height of this level above the right atrium indicates the mean hydrostatic pressure within the right atrium. In health this level is the same as that of the sternal angle, whatever the position of the subject. The sternal angle is therefore a convenient reference point for measuring or estimating the right atrial pressure. This means that in a healthy person reclining at an angle of 45°, the mean level will be invisible, because it is below the clavicle, but some slight pulsation may appear above the clavicle.

Arterial pulsation may also be visible in the neck and has to be distinguished from venous pulsation. The venous pulse has a

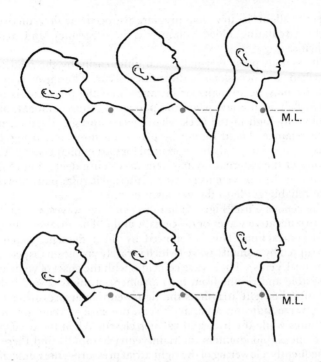

Fig. 7.3 In health the height of a column of blood in the jugular vein is about level with the manubrium sterni (ML) whatever the position of the patient. In heart failure, when the right atrial pressure is increased, the vertical height of this column is increased and is above the level of the manubrium sterni whatever the position of the patient.

definite upper level, though it may be necessary to sit the patient up higher or lay him lower to find it. This level falls during inspiration when blood is drawn into the heart. Venous pulsation is usually more sinuous and less sharp than arterial pulsation. Finally it is impalpable, or even when grossly abnormal, e.g. in tricuspid regurgitation, it is only just palpable, while arterial pulsation is easily palpable and thrusting in character.

A raised venous pressure is usually indicative of right heart failure. Occasionally it is due to obstruction of the superior vena cava, in which case the normal pulsations of the venous pulse are absent. A slight rise in venous pressure also occurs with an increase in the circulating blood volume, as in pregnancy and acute nephritis.

The venous pulse is usually seen quite easily by the methods described, but occasionally difficulties occur. The mean venous pressure may be so high, for instance, that the pulsation is obscured behind the jaw when the patient is semirecumbent, and visible only high in the neck when he sits upright. Further, too much reliance should be not be placed on the external jugular veins, as these may only be superficial for part of their course. Also kinking of the external jugular vein may cause distension of the vein above the true venous pressure. Internal jugular pulsation is a more reliable guide to the venous pressure.

The venous pulse (Fig. 7.4) has three positive waves, *a*, *c*, and *v*, and two negative waves or descents, *x* and *y*. The *a* wave is due to atrial contraction. This is followed by the *x* descent, which is interrupted by a small *c* wave (which is rarely visible on inspection of the neck veins). The *c* wave coincides with the onset of ventricular systole and results from the movement of the tricuspid valve ring into the right atrium as the right ventricular pressure rises. The *v* wave indicates a passive rise in pressure as venous return continues while the tricuspid valve is closed. When the tricuspid valve opens, blood enters the right ventricle rapidly and there is consequently a lowering of the right atrial pressure—the *y* descent.

The *a* wave is prominent when the resistance of the right ventricle to filling is increased, as in tricuspid stenosis, or from hypertrophy of the right ventricle due to increased pressure work, in pulmonary stenosis or pulmonary hypertension. In tricuspid regurgitation, the *v* wave is replaced by a large *systolic* wave due to regurgitation of blood into the right atrium during the right ventricular systole. This regurgitant wave has a surging expansile character.

Obviously *a* waves will disappear when there is no active atrial

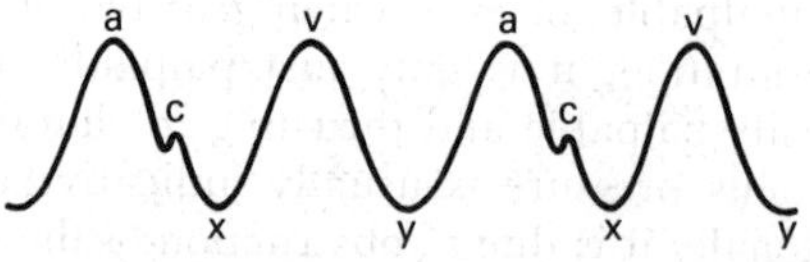

Fig. 7.4 The venous pulse.

Failure to detect the apex beat in the usual area is usually due to the fact that it is obscured by a rib. One should also remember that it is felt on the right side in congenital dextrocardia.

Other pulsations

In addition to the pulsations already described, movements should be looked for at the root of the neck, the front of the chest, and the epigastrium.

In the suprasternal notch the pulsation is usually systolic in time, and when well marked may be an indication of an unfolded aortic arch in hypertension or coarctation of the aorta or of aneurysm of the arch of the aorta.

In the neck various pulsations may be observed. These may be either arterial or venous. The carotids pulsate visibly on exertion, from mental excitement, in diseases which cause overaction of the heart, such as thyrotoxicosis, and in cases of aortic regurgitation, hypertension and aneurysm of the aorta. In hypertension, especially in women, and in association with a high aortic arch, the right carotid sometimes shows abnormal pulsation due to kinking, which must not be mistaken for aneurysm.

In the thorax, a rare source of pulsation in unusual parts is *aneurysm of the aorta*. Such aneurysmal pulsations always manifest themselves at first above the level of the fourth rib, though at a later period they may affect a considerable portion of the chest wall. The position of the impulse varies according to the part of the aorta which is diseased. If the *ascending aorta* is affected, the pulsation is chiefly to the right of the sternum, whilst the *transverse aorta* gives rise to less distinct pulsation under the manubrium sterni, and the *descending aorta* still more to the left. The time of this pulsation is systolic, following immediately on the apex beat, and it may be observed to be expansile in character.

In *coarctation of the aorta* a collateral arterial circulation develops, and pulsation may be detected in superficial arteries in the chest wall. This may best be seen over the back with the patient bending forward to touch his toes.

Pulsation *in the epigastrium* is most commonly due to nervousness or excitement in a thin person. Less commonly it is due to a hyperkinetic right ventricle, to thyrotoxicosis or to transmission of the aortic pulsation by a tumour, such as carcinoma of the stomach. Occasionally it is due to distensile pulsation of the liver in heart failure with tricuspid regurgitation; and very rarely to an aneurysm of the abdominal aorta, which may be palpable as an expansile swelling.

Thrills

Any sound or murmur which is loud will be palpable. A palpable murmur is called a thrill and transmits to the hand a sensation like the purring of a cat. The character, timing, and variation with respiration of thrills are the same as those of the corresponding murmurs and are discussed with murmurs. An abnormally loud sound is felt as a shock. A third sound or atrial sound is often easier to feel than to hear. The loud first sound of mitral stenosis is often palpable and the sounds of aortic and pulmonary valve closure are palpable in systemic and pulmonary hypertension respectively.

PERCUSSION

Where radiographs of the chest are readily available percussion of the cardiac dullness is hardly worth pursuing. Where radiographs are not so available percussion may assist in the diagnosis of large pericardial effusions and of aneurysms of the ascending aorta. In the former the whole area of dullness is increased; and in the latter an area of dullness to the right of the sternum at the level of the second interspace may be detected. In pulmonary emphysema the area of cardiac dullness may be diminished.

AUSCULTATION

Auscultation of the heart presents major difficulties to all students. As with other skills, such as driving a car or playing tennis, it requires a great deal of practice and constant repetition. The skilled examiner listens for specific findings, focusing attention on particular aspects of the cardiac cycle; a complete and detailed understanding of the events of the cardiac cycle (Fig. 7.5) is the basis of auscultation. The student must comprehend the sequence of events before any progress can be made. A common error is to

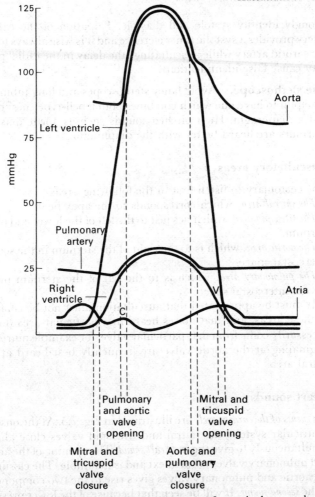

Fig. 7.5 The cardiac cycle. With the onset of ventricular systole the mitral and tricuspid valves close asynchronously. The ventricular pressure rises rapidly during isocolumic contraction and the semi-lunar valves open when the pressure in the ventricles exceeds the pressure in the great arteries. Towards the end of ejection the pressures in the great arteries fall and the aortic and pulmonary valves close. At the end of isovolumic relaxation the ventricular pressure falls below atrial pressure, the mitral and tricuspid valves open and ventricular filling occurs.

wrongly identify systole and diastole. Palpation of the carotid artery provides a systolic time reference and it is wise always to feel the carotid artery while auscultating (the delay in the radial pulse may cause false identification).

The stethoscope.   Avoid fancy stethoscopes and long tubing. It is helpful to have one which combines both a bell-type chest piece and a diaphragm. High pitched sounds such as aortic diastolic murmurs are heard better with the diaphragm.

Auscultatory areas

It is customary to listen first in the following areas:
  The mitral area, which corresponds to the apex beat.
  The tricuspid area, which lies just to the left of the lower end of the sternum.
  The aortic area, which is to the right of the sternum in the second intercostal space.
  The pulmonary area, which is to the left of the sternum in the second intercostal space.
  It must be appreciated that auscultation must not be confined to these areas, and that noises heard in a particular area do not necessarily come from that particular valve; for example murmurs originating at the aortic valve are frequently best heard at the mitral area.

Heart sounds

The events of the cardiac cycle are illustrated in Fig. 7.5. At the onset of ventricular systole, the mitral and tricuspid valves close almost simultaneously to give the *first heart sound*. The opening of the aortic and pulmonary valves occurs next and is inaudible. The closure of the aortic and pulmonary valves gives rise to the two components of the *second sound*. It will be seen that because of the lower pressure in the right ventricle compared with the left, closure of the pulmonary valve follows that of the aortic valve. After a brief period the mitral and tricuspid valves open inaudibly in the normal heart.

DEVIATIONS FROM THE NORMAL IN DISEASE

In disease the following deviations from the normal may occur:

1. The sounds may have a different intensity, both absolutely and relatively to each other, from that possessed in health.
2. The sounds may be abnormally split.
3. A triple rhythm may be present.
4. Adventitious sounds may be heard, either replacing or occurring along with the heart sounds.

Alterations in intensity

In patients with thick chest walls, and in those with a serious degree of emphysema, the heart sounds may scarcely be audible, though there is no heart disease. Conversely, in the presence of serious heart disease the sounds may appear quite normal. Thus alterations in the intensity of the heart sounds are significant only when considered in relation to all the other features of the case. The heart sounds are distant or inaudible in pericardial effusion. Accentuation of the first sound is often present in mitral stenosis and in tachycardia from any cause.

An absolute accentuation of the sound of aortic or pulmonary valve closure is found when there is systemic or pulmonary hypertension.

Splitting

The mitral valve closes slightly before the tricuspid valve, and this can give rise to splitting of the first sound. This splitting is difficult to detect by auscultation and even phonocardiography, because both components are very low-pitched and merge one into the other. When it is heard, splitting of the first sound is not a sign of heart disease and is of importance only because its two components may be confused with an atrial sound and a first sound, or with a first sound and a systolic ejection click.

Splitting of the second sound is much easier to hear because of the aortic and pulmonary valve closure sounds (A2 and P2) have high-pitched harmonics, and the two sounds can be separated, especially when the diaphragm is used for auscultation. Aortic valve closure (A2) is audible in all areas. Pulmonary valve closure (P2) is audible only in the pulmonary area and for a short distance down the left sternal edge, unless its intensity is greatly increased due to pulmonary hypertension. It follows that splitting of the second sound is usually heard only at and close to the pulmonary area. Splitting is most easily heard in children, and may not be audible in older adults, especially men, when muscle noise, a thick chest wall, and emphysema make P2 inaudible. Normally P2 always follows A2, and the splitting is widest during inspiration and narrowest in expiration, when the two components usually merge to give a single sound. Splitting of 0·06 second during inspiration and 0·02 second (a very close split or single sound) in expiration would be average for a child or young adult.

The mechanism of splitting of the second sound is as follows. During inspiration blood is drawn into the thorax, there is a relative rise in right atrial pressure, and the right ventricular stroke volume increases. The duration of right ventricular systole measured from the first sound to P2 is increased, and P2 is therefore slightly delayed. Conversely the left ventricular stroke volume falls during inspiration, because the greater negative pressure within the thorax enlarges the capacity of the left atrium and pulmonary veins and reduces left atrial pressure and hence left ventricular filling and stroke volume. Thus left ventricular systole is shortened and A2 is earlier. During inspiration, then, A2 occurs earlier and P2 later, so that splitting of the second sound widens. During expiration the changes are exactly opposite and the splitting narrows. Movement of P2 is considerably greater than that of A2. This concept of respiratory variation in right and left ventricular stroke volume is of the greatest importance.

Triple rhythm

Phonocardiography shows that in addition to the two heart sounds generally recognized, a third sound and an atrial sound are often present. When either of these additional sounds are prominent and audible, they give a cadence of sounds known as triple rhythm.

The third sound follows the aortic component of the second sound by about 0·15 second. It is usually best heard in the mitral area and is lower pitched than the second sound, which it follows. Triple rhythm from a third sound is common in healthy young persons. It is an important sign in heart failure from any cause, and may be heard shortly after cardiac infarction. The third sound is attributed to rapid ventricular filling and is found in the relatively hyperkinetic circulation of young persons and where the mitral diastolic flow is increased as in mitral regurgitation and ventricular septal defect. In heart failure the atrial pressure is increased and the early filling of the ventricle is rapid. A third sound is also heard in disease when the distensibility of the ventricular muscle is altered. The sound arises from vibrations in the atrioventricular valve structures and in the ventricular muscle. A third sound can arise on either side of the heart, but in fact usually arises in the left heart.

The atrial sound is a low-pitched sound occurring before the first sound. It is not heard in health. Triple rhythm from an atrial sound can originate in the right heart from pulmonary stenosis or pulmonary hypertension, and in the left heart from systemic hypertension. It is not always a sign of failure but does indicate that the heart is abnormal. Like the third sound, it used to be thought to be a 'filling sound', but now a valvular origin is suspected.

When the heart rate is rapid (100 or more), diastole tends to be relatively shortened compared with systole, and a third sound may come to overlie an atrial sound giving rise to a 'summation gallop'. Usually, when the heart slows, a loud third or atrial sound is audible.

Additional sounds

Systolic ejection sounds (clicks) arise from the semi-lunar valves, either aortic or pulmonary. Usually the valve is abnormal although this may be trivial, for example a bicuspid valve without stenosis. The systolic click coincides with the opening of the valve in early systole. When one of the great arteries is dilated, for example the pulmonary artery in pulmonary hypertension, a systolic ejection sound can frequently be heard without any valve abnormality.

Mid and late systolic sounds arise from the mitral valve. The valvar tissue is often found to be excessive, permitting prolapse of one or both cusps. The systolic sound is believed to arise from tension on the mitral valvar chordae by this bulging backwards of the cusp.

The opening of normal mitral and tricuspid valves is silent. An opening snap is always abnormal. When the mitral valve opens abruptly at the end of isometric relaxation, the rapid movement is arrested abruptly by fusion of valve commisures, producing an audible snap.

Murmurs

Murmurs have a blowing or musical quality. They are due to turbulence in the blood flow at or near a valve or an abnormal communication within the heart. Not all murmurs are due to organic damage in the heart; they may be due to such causes as an abnormally rapid flow of blood through a normal valve. Such murmurs are called flow murmurs. Murmurs also occur at the site of arterial stenoses. In examining a murmur the following points must be noted:

Time of occurrence.   Murmurs may be systolic, diastolic or continuous throughout systole and diastole. *Systolic murmurs* are either *pansystolic*, as in mitral or tricuspid regurgitation and ventricular septal defect, or *ejection*, when they arise either at the pulmonary or aortic outflow tracts. *Diastolic murmurs* are either *immediate* (or early), starting at the second heart sound and occurring as a result of aortic or pulmonary regurgitation, or *delayed* (or mid), when there is a short gap after the second heart sound and the beginning of the murmur. These murmurs arise at the mitral or tricuspid valve.

The behaviour of the murmur during respiration.   The stroke output of the right heart increases during inspiration, while that of the left heart is reduced. It follows that a murmur originating on the right side of the heart will become louder during inspiration. Any murmur which increases on inspiration can be attributed to the right heart and any murmur which increases on expiration can be attributed to the left heart. When the cardiac lesion is severe, however, the variation in stroke volume may not occur with respiration and the murmur is of constant intensity.

Point of maximum intensity and direction of selective propagation.   The maximum loudness of a murmur which has been produced at a given valve usually occurs at the point where the valve sound would be best heard in health. To this rule, however, there are some exceptions.

Murmurs are not equally well heard at all points on the chest wall which are equidistant from the point of their greatest intensity, but each is much more distinctly audible in some directions than in others, i.e. such murmurs have a direction of selective propagation.

The character of a murmur. The character of a murmur also helps to determine its origin. Obstructive murmurs, from obstruction to the onward flow of blood through a narrowed valve, are usually rough; regurgitant murmurs, from leakage backwards through a closed but incompetent valve, are softer and blowing. The loudness of a murmur has no relation to its importance. A very loud murmur may be less significant than one so soft as to be nearly inaudible.

It has already been stated that murmurs are due to turbulence in the flow of blood. The most important cause of turbulence within the heart is the rapid flow of blood through a relatively small orifice, and this means that there must be a considerable difference in pressure on the two sides of the orifice leading to a substantial gradient. In the normal adult heart, the pressure gradients across open valves are negligible because the valve orifices are fairly large in relation to the flow of blood through them. There are therefore no murmurs. If, however, a valve orifice should be narrowed by disease, a sufficient pressure gradient may build up at certain times during the cardiac cycle to produce a murmur.

In the next paragraphs the haemodynamics in some common forms of valvular disease are presented, in order to show how murmurs are produced and why they arise when they do.

MITRAL VALVE DISEASE

Mitral stenosis

Narrowing of the mitral valve orifice, mitral stenosis, is due to the fusion of the two valve cusps along their margins, extending from the valve ring at the periphery in towards the centre. The normal valve closed by the apposition of two mobile cusps over a length of 3·5 cm becomes a fibrotic diaphragm with a small central orifice closed by the apposition of 1 cm or less of cusp tissue.

The haemodynamics in a mild and a severe case of mitral stenosis are shown diagrammatically in Figs 7.6 and 7.7.

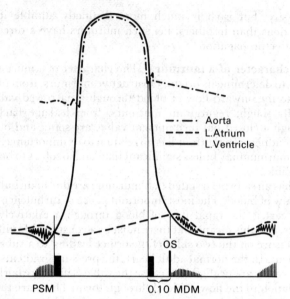

Fig. 7.6 The relationship of murmurs to haemodynamics in mild mitral stenosis. The left atrial pressure is only slightly raised so that mitral valve opening, the opening snap (OS), is not particularly early. During the early rapid phase of ventricular filling turbulence creates a diastolic murmur (MDM) and with atrial systole a further period of turbulent flow occurs across the mitral valve producing a pre-systolic murmur (PSM).

Loud first heart sound.   In normal subjects at the end of diastole the mitral valve is almost closed as ventricular filling is complete. In contrast, with mitral stenosis, the valve remains open at the end of diastole and is forcibly shut by the rise of pressure due to left ventricular systole. The mitral valve therefore closes very rapidly and a loud first heart sound results.

The opening snap of the mitral valve is a loud sound heard just after the second heart sound. It is a consequence of the high left atrial pressure, which forces the mitral valve to open rapidly when the ventricle relaxes. If the mitral valve is rigid and calcified, it follows that the first heart sound will not be accentuated and the opening snap will not be present.

The mitral diastolic murmur is a low-pitched rumbling murmur

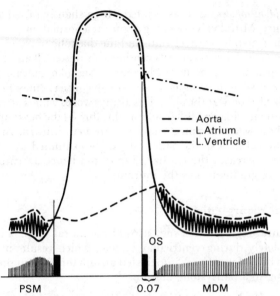

Fig. 7.7 The relationship of murmurs to haemodynamics in severe mitral stenosis. The elevated left atrial pressure opens the mitral valve prematurely causing an opening snap (OS), and turbulent flow throughout diastole produces a full-length diastolic murmur. PSM = presystolic murmur. MDM = diastolic murmur.

heard at the apex; it is due to blood passing through the narrowed mitral valve when there is a pressure gradient between the left atrium and left ventricle. (In the normal heart no such gradient exists and the pressures equalize rapidly when the mitral valve opens.)

The presystolic murmur results from atrial systole, and therefore immediately precedes the first heart sound. It is due to an increase in flow across the narrowed mitral valve during atrial contraction. It has been traditional teaching that when atrial fibrillation is present and there is no effective contraction of the atria, there cannot be a presystolic murmur; but a slight presystolic accentuation of the diastolic murmur may in fact be heard in the absence of atrial contraction, as the flow continues towards the end of diastole through a partially closed valve.

Mild mitral stenosis, is associated with a slightly raised left atrial pressure. Mitral valve opening occurs at a normal time, so that the opening snap is relatively late and the diastolic murmur is short.

Severe mitral stenosis causes a considerably raised left atrial pressure. The opening snap occurs early and the diastolic murmur is long.

The auscultatory signs in mitral valve disease may be sharply localized at or near the apex. It is always worth while listening with the patient lying on his left side, as this throws the heart up against the chest wall and apical murmurs are better heard. In cases of mild mitral stenosis the patient should be examined after exercise, for this increases the cardiac output and hence accentuates the pressure gradients and the murmurs.

Mitral regurgitation

In mitral regurgitation the cusps of the mitral valve fail to close completely during ventricular systole, which results in a jet of blood being forced back into the left atrium throughout the systole, leading to a pansystolic murmur.

The mitral pansystolic murmur. The mitral pansystolic murmur is due to blood leaking back through the mitral valve in ventricular systole. It starts therefore when the mitral valve normally closes, i.e. with the first heart sound, and continues throughout systole. It is best heard at the mitral area, and radiates into the axilla and increases in intensity with expiration.

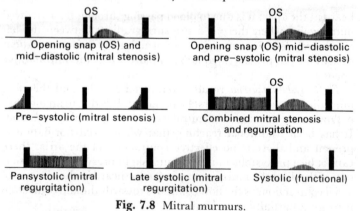

Opening snap (OS) and mid–diastolic (mitral stenosis)

Opening snap (OS) mid–diastolic and pre–systolic (mitral stenosis)

Pre–systolic (mitral stenosis)

Combined mitral stenosis and regurgitation

Pansystolic (mitral regurgitation)

Late systolic (mitral regurgitation)

Systolic (functional)

Fig. 7.8 Mitral murmurs.

The mitral late systolic murmur. The mitral late systolic murmur indicates mitral regurgitation and is usually associated with prolapse of floppy valvar cusps or disease of the chordae tendinae or papillary muscles of the mitral valve. Mid or late systolic clicks are frequently associated with late systolic murmurs.

The soft first heart sound. The bulk of the first heart sound is due to mitral valve closure, and if this closure is imperfect, the resulting heart sound will be softer than normal.

AORTIC VALVE DISEASE

Aortic stenosis

The haemodynamics in aortic stenosis are shown diagrammatically in Fig. 7.9. There is a considerable pressure gradient be-

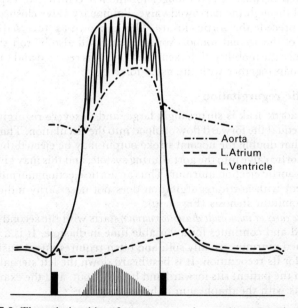

Fig. 7.9 The relationship of murmurs to haemodynamics in aortic stenosis. The slow ejection of blood into the aorta causes a slow rise to aortic pressure. The murmur follows the flow pattern rising to a peak in mid-systole then declining.

tween the left ventricle and aorta, and this gradient is greatest in the middle of systole, and is relatively small early and late in systole. The murmur of aortic stenosis is therefore midsystolic. All murmurs due to the ejection of blood through abnormal semilunar valves, or to abnormally high blood flow through normal semilunar valves, have this same pattern and are called 'ejection' systolic murmurs.

The aortic ejection murmur is heard in the aortic area and radiates into the neck although it is frequently well heard at the mitral area. It increases on expiration.

The aortic ejection click is due to opening of the aortic valve in aortic stenosis. It is therefore heard just after the first heart sound at the beginning of the ejection murmur. When the valve is rigid from fibrosis or calcification, no click is heard.

Delayed and soft closure of the aortic valve are much less easily detectable signs of aortic stenosis. The aortic valve closure is delayed because it takes longer for the left ventricle to expel its blood through the narrowed valve. Pulmonary valve closure may then precede the aortic closure. This is known as 'reversed splitting' of the second sound. Aortic closure will also be soft simply because the mobility of the semilunar cusps is reduced and they do not snap together with the usual force.

Aortic regurgitation

The aortic leak is surprisingly large, and in severe regurgitation may equal the forward flow of blood into the circulation. That is to say that double the normal stroke output may be ejected through the aortic valve into the aorta during systole, and this may give rise to an aortic ejection murmur. Thus an aortic ejection murmur in a patient with aortic regurgitation does not necessarily indicate a concomitant stenosis (Fig. 7.10).

The early or immediate diastolic murmur starts with the second heart sound and continues for a variable time in diastole. It is a high-pitched murmur, usually soft, and often requires intent auscultation for its recognition. It is best heard down the left sternal edge when the patient sits forward and breathes out, and the examiner listens with the diaphragm of his stethoscope.

TRICUSPID VALVE DISEASE

Organic tricuspid valve disease is almost always of rheumatic aetiology and is almost always accompanied by rheumatic mitral

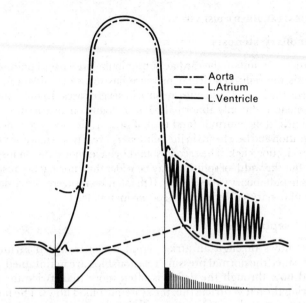

Fig. 7.10 The relationship of murmurs to haemodynamics in aortic regurgitation. The greatly increased stroke volume causes an ejection systolic murmur even without stenosis. The regurgitation commences as soon as the left ventricular pressure is lower than aortic pressure, i.e. immediately after the aortic valve closure. The murmur tails off as the diastolic pressure and so the gradient across the valve diminishes and the left ventricle fills.

and aortic valve disease. The diagnosis can often be made from inspection of the neck veins (p. 202). The murmurs of tricuspid stenosis and tricuspid regurgitation have the same timing and character as the corresponding mitral lesions, but are best heard at or near the lower end of the sternum and may be louder in inspiration. Tricuspid opening snaps are rare.

Functional tricuspid regurgitation is often found with congestive failure from any cause. It is due to dilation of the tricuspid valve ring, consequent on dilation of the right ventricle, and the characteristic changes in the venous pulse disappear or diminish when the heart failure is controlled.

CONGENITAL HEART DISEASE

Pulmonary stenosis

In order to maintain the cardiac output in the presence of pulmonary stenosis the right ventricular pressure has to rise considerably and exceeds the level of systemic pressure in severe cases. In mild pulmonary stenosis the only abnormal signs are found on auscultation. The ejection systolic murmur (and thrill if present) is most prominent in inspiration and best heard in the pulmonary area. It is usually preceded by an ejection click. The second sound behaves normally on inspiration, but the width of splitting may be wider than normal because of a delay in pulmonary valve closure. If the stenosis is severe, the closure of the pulmonary valve becomes soft or inaudible.

Atrial septal defect

Blood flows through an atrial septal defect from left atrium to right, since the normal pressure relationships are maintained. The blood flow through the defect is often more than twice the flow entering the left ventricle (i.e. the systemic blood flow). The flow of blood entering the right atrium will then be the systemic flow plus the flow from the left atrium through the atrial septal defect, i.e. three times the systemic flow. This torrential flow passes from the right atrium to the right ventricle, pulmonary artery, lung vessels and so back to the left atrium.

Because the defect is very large and the pressure gradient very small (about 1 mmHg), there is little turbulence and no murmur from blood flowing through the defect. The characteristic auscultatory sign is the relatively wide splitting of the second heart sound, uninfluenced by respiration as the large right ventricular stroke volume does not vary with respiration. The torrential blood flow through a normal pulmonary valve produces a functional ejection pulmonary systolic murmur which is moderately loud. A functional tricuspid flow murmur is often present. It is mid-diastolic, soft and best heard at the lower end of the sternum during deep inspiration.

Ventricular septal defect

Ventricular septal defects are rarely as large as atrial septal defects and usually less than 1 cm in diameter. The right ventricular systolic pressure is normally about one-fifth of that in the left ventricle, so that there is a pressure gradient from left ventricle to right throughout systole.

In mild cases where the defect has the cross sectional area of a pencil lead, the only abnormal sign is a pansystolic murmur, loudest in expiration, usually accompanied by a thrill, and best heard at the lower end of the sternum.

In more severe cases there is evidence of increased blood flow through the left heart and blood vessels of the lung. In addition to the pansystolic murmur and thrill there may be a soft short mid-diastolic murmur due to the rapid flow of blood through a normal mitral valve. Splitting of the second sound is normal, though A2 may be difficult to hear as it tends to be obscured in the loud pansystolic murmur in small and moderate sized defects. Where there is pulmonary hypertension the second sound becomes single.

Patent ductus arteriosus

The communication has the same size range as in ventricular septal defect, but its length also tends to limit flow. The pressure gradient from aorta to pulmonary artery is present throughout the cardiac cycle and is greatest towards the end of systole. The increased flow affects the left heart and pulmonary circulation exclusively.

Again, if the communication is small, a murmur is the only abnormal sign. It is best heard at the pulmonary area in expiration, and is called continuous. The accentuation of the continuous murmur about the time of the second sound gives it a particular character, and it is sometimes described as a machinery murmur. In addition to the continuous murmur, a short soft functional mitral diastolic murmur may be present.

A continuous murmur is not specific for patent ductus arteriosus, but can be produced by an arteriovenous communication or the rapid flow of blood through any narrowed vessel. Patent ductus arteriosus is the commonest of several such possible conditions within the thorax. Particular care should always be taken not to confuse it with a venous hum.

Fallot's tetralogy

Fallot's tetralogy consists of pulmonary stenosis, ventricular septal defect, right ventricular enlargement and overriding of the aorta, i.e. the aorta arises astride the ventricular septal defect. The essential features are pulmonary stenosis of at least moderate severity and a large ventricular septal defect, so that the pressure in the two ventricles is equalized. The right ventricular output is ejected partly into the pulmonary artery through the pulmonary stenosis, and partly into the aorta through the ventricular septal defect. The admixture of deoxygenated blood with the left ventricular output makes the patient cyanosed.

The auscultatory signs are a pulmonary ejection murmur and a single second sound. P2 is inaudible because of the low blood flow and low pressure in the pulmonary artery.

Coarctation of the aorta

In coarctation of the aorta there is a stricture of the aorta at or near the insertion of the ligamentum arteriosum. In order to maintain a satisfactory distal circulation, the arterial pressure proximal to the coarctation rises considerably and leads to elongation of the ascending aorta. Prominent arterial pulsation behind the manubrium sterni in a young person strongly suggests this diagnosis, and the radial and femoral pulses should be felt simultaneously. Normally the timing of the pulse wave is identical. In coarctation the femoral pulse is both delayed and diminished, or it is absent. The arterial pressure is considerably raised; the left ventricle is readily palpable and hypertrophied; there is often an ejection click and an aortic ejection systolic murmur from a congenital bicuspid aortic valve which is often associated. Collateral vessels linking the subclavian arteries which arise above the stricture with intercostal arteries arising below the stricture can usually be felt above the scapulae, and are well seen with the patient bending forwards in a good light (Plate XII).

PULMONARY HYPERTENSION

A rise in pulmonary artery pressure to systemic or near-systemic levels is always associated with narrowing of the pulmonary arterioles either from vasoconstriction or thrombosis and embolism. Pulmonary hypertension may be found in some cases of pulmonary heart disease, in some cases of septal defect, with mitral stenosis, or without apparent cause—primary pulmonary hypertension.

There is usually a prominent *a* wave in the neck, the pulse is often very small from the severe obstructive lesion in the pulmonary arterioles, and pulsation over the right ventricle may be palpable. On auscultation there is a loud ejection click, close splitting of the second sound with a very loud and palpable pulmonary valve closure and sometimes a pulmonary diastolic murmur due to functional pulmonary regurgitation.

FLOW MURMURS

Systolic flow murmurs are due to an abnormally high flow of blood through a normal valve, which causes turbulence of the blood stream. They are common and in themselves of no serious significance; yet many people have been labelled as having heart disease, simply because they had a systolic flow murmur. By contrast *diastolic murmurs are always significant*.

Systolic flow murmurs are common in infants and young children, and in the elderly. They also occur in any condition such as anaemia, thyrotoxicosis or hypertension which cause an increased blood flow.

In the adult most flow murmurs are aortic. They are loudest in expiration, heard best in the mitral or aortic area, soft, and never accompanied by a thrill. The other findings in the cardiovascular system are normal, except where the cardiac output is raised. The distinction between trivial aortic stenosis and an aortic flow murmur is difficult.

EXOCARDIAL SOUNDS AND MURMURS

Venous hum

Sometimes in children a continuous murmur can be heard in the neck and upper chest which is due to kinking and partial obstruction of one of the larger veins in the neck, and interference with continous flow of blood through the vein. The origin of the murmur should be suspected because of the youth of the patient, and the loudness of the murmur in the neck. The hum can be obliterated by pressure on the neck, which produces complete obstruction of the vein, or by altering the position of the neck so as to relieve the venous obstruction. It is particularly important to exclude a venous hum if a diagnosis of patent ductus is being considered.

Cardiorespiratory murmurs

Cardiorespiratory murmurs are systolic and due to the rhythmic compression of a lobule of lung by the beating heart. Characteristically these murmurs are loudest at a particular point in the respiratory cycle, disappearing as the patient breathes in a little more or out a little more. They also vary markedly with a change in posture.

Pericardial friction rubs

Pericardial friction rubs have a superficial 'leathery' quality and have a to-and-fro character, being present both in systole and diastole. The sounds may be sharply localized and vary in position from day to day. Effusion into the pericardium, by separating the pericardial surfaces, may eliminate the rub. Pleural rubs from pleurisy of a portion of lung near the heart may have a similar quality but are much reduced in intensity by having the patient hold his breath.

PERIPHERAL VASCULAR SYSTEM

Examination of the peripheral vascular system, including both the arterial and venous system, is often carried out as part of the general examination. It is particularly important, however, in patients with symptoms of arterial or venous disease of the limbs, and in those with cerebral or coronary arterial disease. Further, many patients with hypertension or diabetes mellitus have associated arterial disease, and degenerative vascular disease is common in the elderly. Special attention must therefore be paid to the arterial system in those patients.

Peripheral arterial system

Intermittent claudication is the term used to describe the cramp-like aching pain felt in the calf muscles during exercise. The pain only occurs during exercise, often after walking a certain distance, and it gradually ceases when the patient stops walking. It is ischaemic pain due to failure of the peripheral arterial system to allow a sufficiently increased blood flow to the legs to match the metabolic demands of muscular work. In certain forms of inflammatory arterial disease, e.g. polyarteritis nodosa or temporal arteritis, similar ischaemic pain may occur in other muscles. Intermittent claudication of the legs is not associated with numbness or tingling in the feet or legs unless the blood supply of the cauda equina or of the spinal cord is affected.

Impaired blood supply to a limb can be assessed by its lowered skin temperature and by its impaired nutritional status. Temperature differences can only be reliably assessed when the limbs have been exposed to a constant room temperature for 10–20 minutes. In an ischaemic leg the skin of the foot will be cold and pale or cyanosed, and capillary filling after blanching with light finger pressure is delayed. *Reactive hyperaemia* is also delayed. This can be demonstrated with the patient lying down. The leg is elevated for several minutes to allow the venous pool of blood in the leg to drain into the circulation, and then the patient sits up and allows the leg to hang over the edge of the bed. Normally the foot will flush pink in about 10 seconds; the flush takes a longer time to appear if blood flow is inadequate. When there has been chronic arterial insufficiency the skin becomes thin and shiny, often losing its hair, and the nails become brittle. Late severe manifestations of arterial insufficiency are chronic ulceration and even gangrene, especially of the distal parts of the toes or feet, the dead area becoming shrivelled, blackened and often demarcated from neighbouring healthy tissue by a thin red zone of inflamed tissue. In *acute interruption of arterial flow* to a limb, as in embolic or thrombotic occlusion of a femoral artery, the affected leg becomes colder than the normal limb, peripheral pulses below the level of the obstruction disappear, and the skin, which is at first white, becomes blue and, later, gangrenous.

Diminished or absent pulsation of vessels is of great value in localizing arterial lesions, both acute and chronic. In the legs the femoral, popliteal, posterior tibial and dorsalis pedis pulses should be carefully palpated with the fingers, not with the thumb, and their pulsation compared with that in the contralateral vessels. In addition, the thickness and hardness of the walls of the femoral and politeal vessels should be assessed and any tortuosity noted. Using the bell of the stethoscope a careful search for the hissing systolic sound (arterial bruit), associated with partial obstruction, should be made in both femoral arteries, in the abdomen (aortic bruits) and in the loins (renal artery bruits). Sometimes a thrill may be palpable in these larger vessels.

In patients with claudication the distal pulses should also be examined after exercise since the diversion of blood flow to exercised muscle may cause previously detectable pulses to disappear, indicating restriction of flow in the affected limb.

In the arms the subclavian, axillary, brachial and radial pulses should be similarly assessed and bruits listened for in the subclavian and brachial vessels. The carotid arteries should similarly be examined; it is particularly common to find systolic bruits in these vessels, and to recognize tortuosity and thickening of their walls since they are relatively accessible to examination. Arterial pulsation in the limbs can be assessed quantitatively with a Döppler ultrasonic flow meter or by oscillometry.

In coarctation of the aorta, a cause of hypertension in the young, the femoral pulses are diminished and delayed. The delay can be measured roughly by comparing the timing of the femoral pulse with that of the radial artery; the femoral and radial pulses are normally synchronous since they are equidistant from the heart.

Spasm of arterioles may occur in the presence of normal peripheral pulses. This is usually seen in the hands; the digital arteries go into spasm in response to cold or to emotional stimuli so that the fingers become white and then cyanosed. When the spasm passes off the fingers become hyperaemic and pink. This sequence of changes is termed *Raynaud's phenomenon*. Very rarely it may lead to superficial necrosis of the skin of the fingers.

In patients with arterial disease it is important to remember that the arterioles, capillary bed and small veins can be inspected directly in the retina by ophthalmoscopy (see p. 378). Some patients with arterial disease associated with hyperlipidaemia show deposition of cholesterol lipid in the margin of the cornea, the arcus senilis, and in the skin of the eyelids and elbows (xanthelasma).

Peripheral venous system

Varicose veins should be looked for with the patient standing. Superficial varicosities are then obvious. The efficiency of the valves of the long saphenous vein should be detected by Trendelenberg's test. With the patient lying the saphenous vein is emptied by elevating the leg. The upper end of the vein is then occluded by finger pressure on the saphenous opening. While the examiner maintains this pressure, the patient stands. If the valves are incompetent the vein will fill from above when the pressure is released.

Venous thrombosis is rare in healthy mobile subjects but may be seen in women taking contraceptive steroids. However, it is a frequent complication of enforced bed rest particularly after surgery. Congestive cardiac failure also leads to venous stasis and thrombosis. The affected limb is swollen, tender and warmer than normal. Dilated superficial veins may be seen which do not collapse when the leg is elevated. Forceful dorsiflexion of the foot will cause pain in the calf (Homan's sign), but this manoeuvre is not recommended as it may dislodge a clot. Sometimes extension of deep venous thrombosis upwards to the thigh may cause secondary arterial spasm, the whole leg becoming white, painful and swollen.

Studies with radioactive fibrinogen, which is taken up by the forming thrombus, and venography have shown that quite extensive venous thrombosis can occur without significant physical findings. Pulmonary embolism may thus be the first sign of a deep vein thrombosis in the leg.

ELECTROCARDIOGRAPHY

The action of the excitable tissues of the body is associated with electrical activity. Changes in electrical potential associated with the contraction of the heart can be recorded from the body surface.

There must be two points of contact with the body to lead the electrical activity of the heart to the galvanometer. These connections are termed electrocardiographic leads. The leads in common use are:

The standard limb leads (bipolar limb leads).

> Lead I   right arm–left arm
> Lead II   right arm–left leg
> Lead III left arm–left leg

The unipolar or V leads. The two connections in these leads are (*a*) an exploring electrode (Fig. 7.11) and (*b*) an indifferent electrode which is produced by joining the limb leads together and thence through a resistance—for all practical purposes it is neutral.

The deflections or waves of the electrocardiogram are designated by the letters PQRST as shown (Fig. 7.12). The P wave is associated with atrial excitation, the QRS with ventricular excitation (depolarization), and the T wave with ventricular recovery

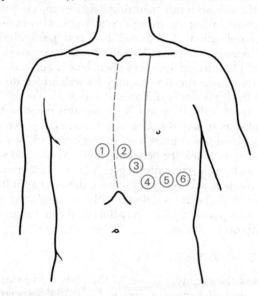

Fig. 7.11 The position of the exploring electrode for chest leads.

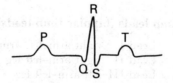

Fig. 7.12 The terminology of the electrocardiogram.

(repolarization). The Q wave is an initial downward deflection in the QRS complex.

The PR interval (measured from the beginning of the P wave to the beginning of QRS complex) is normally less than 0·2 second. The duration of the QRS complex is normally less than 0·12 second. The appearance of a normal electrocardiogram is shown in Fig. 7.21.

READING AND INTERPRETATION OF THE ELECTROCARDIOGRAM

An electrocardiogram must be examined systematically. A convenient method is as follows:

1. Determine the cardiac rate and rhythm (see below).
2. Assess the PR interval and the width of the QRS complex.
3. Examine the P wave (atrial contraction) and the QRS complex (ventricular depolarization).
4. Examine the ST segment and T wave (ventricular repolarization).

It is not possible in this text to do more than give some examples of the kind of abnormalities that can be demonstrated in electrocardiograms. Those who wish to understand this subject must refer to specialized textbooks. Considerable experience is required even to be familiar with the limits of the normal tracing. One should also notice that, since many electrocardiographic abnormalities can arise from a variety of causes, they cannot be finally interpreted unless they are considered in relation to the clinical findings.

THE ELECTROCARDIOGRAM IN DISORDERS OF CARDIAC RHYTHM

By providing together a record of atrial excitation (P waves) and ventricular excitation (QRS complexes) the electrocardiogram has advanced our understanding of the cardiac dysrhythmias. P waves are ususally best seen in Lead II or in the right-sided chest leads (V1) and these leads are therefore most valuable in the disorders of cardiac rhythm.

In health the heart beat is initiated in the sinoatrial node (pace-maker) which lies near the entry of the superior vena cava into the right atrium. The impulse spreads through both atria and thence to the atrioventricular node. The AV (atrioventricular) node is continuous with the bundle of His and its branches. The commonest disorders are listed below.

Sinus tachycardia

The cardiac impulse arises normally, and the electrocardiogram is normal in form. The pulse rate is increased above 90 or 100 (adults). Sinus tachycardia may result from emotion, exercise, fever, hyperthyroidism and anaemia.

Sinus bradycardia

Again the electrocardiogram is normal in form, but the heart rate is less than 60/minute. Sinus bradycardia occurs in athletes, and in patients with increased intracranial pressure, myxoedema and jaundice.

Sinus arrhythmia (Fig. 7.13)

The cardiac impulse arises normally in the sinoatrial node, the rhythmicity of which varies; the heart rate increases with inspiration and diminishes with expiration. The electrocardiogram is normal apart from variation in the R–R intervals. This arrhythmia is a normal finding in young people; it is increased by deep breathing and abolished by exercise.

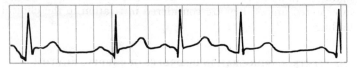

Fig. 7.13 Sinus arrhythmia.

Extrasystoles or ectopic beats (Figs 7.14 and 7.15)

Ectopic beats arise from foci in the atria or ventricles which stimulate the heart before the next sinus beat is due. In ventricular extrasystoles P waves are absent and the QRS complexes are broad, the T wave pointing in the opposite direction to the major deflection of the QRS. The extrasystole comes prematurely and is followed by a pause (the compensatory pause).

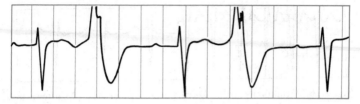

Fig. 7.14 Ventricular extrasystoles. Note that there is no P wave before the second extrasystole, and there is an abortive P wave just before the first extrasystole.

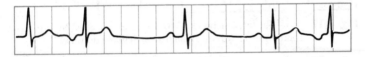

Fig. 7.15 Atrial extrasystoles. Note the abnormal (inverted) P wave. The R–R interval is longer after the extrasystole than in the normal cycle.

The electrocardiogram of an atrial extrasystole shows the P wave to be abnormal in form, but the QRS which follows it is normal. The pause which follows the extrasystole is longer than normal.

Extrasystoles are thus premature beats followed by an abnormally long pause and can be recognized by auscultation or from palpation. Extrasystoles occur both in health and in patients with heart disease. If an extrasystole follows after each normal beat as in Fig 7.14 the pulse is said to be coupled (pulsus bigeminus). Digitalis often causes coupling.

Atrial tachycardia and atrial flutter (Figs 7.16 and 7.17)

Atrial tachycardia and atrial flutter are due to the presence of an ectopic focus in the atrium which beats regularly at a rapid rate. The P waves are abnormal in shape, but the QRS complexes are usually normal, although at faster rates a bundle branch block pattern (p. 237) may develop. As a rule not all atrial impulses are conducted to the ventricles. Often alternate beats are conducted

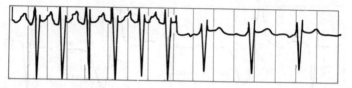

Fig. 7.16 Atrial tachycardia. During attack, pulse rate 225; after attack, sinus tachycardia, pulse rate 130.

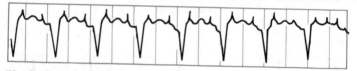

Fig. 7.17 Atrial flutter, 2:1 block. Atrial rate about 300. Note the two spiked flutter waves to each ventricular complex.

when 2 : 1 atrioventricular block is said to be present. Occasionally 3 : 1 or 4 : 1 block is present and sometimes the block varies.

Atrial flutter and tachycardia may occur in hearts which are otherwise normal, in thyrotoxicosis and in rheumatic or ischaemic heart disease.

Atrial fibrillation (Fig. 7.18)

There is no coordinated atrial activity (either electrical or mechanical) in atrial fibrillation. The electrocardiogram shows *f* (fibrillation) waves representing the atrial activity instead of P waves, especially in lead V1. The QRS complexes are normal, but irregularly spaced.

Atrial fibrillation is recognized clinically by complete irregularity of the pulse both in rate and volume. Mitral valve disease, ischaemic heart disease and thyrotoxicosis are the commonest causes of fibrillation.

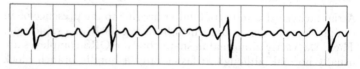

Fig. 7.18 Atrial fibrillation. Note the f waves and irregular ventricular rhythm.

Heart block (Figs 7.19 and 7.20)

In first degree atrioventricular block the P–R interval exceeds 0·2 second and all the impulses reach the ventricles. When some impulses fail to reach the ventricle but others do reach it, then there is second degree heart block. In complete heart block (third degree) the atria and ventricles beat independently, i.e. they are dissociated, and the ventricular rate is usually slow, 20–40 beats/minute.

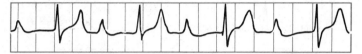

Fig. 7.19 First degree heart block. P–R interval = 0·42 second.

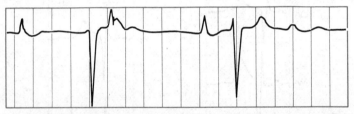

Fig. 7.20 Complete heart block. Atrial rate 55; ventricular rate 39.

Ventricular fibrillation

A similar mechanism operates in the ventricles as in the atria with atrial fibrillation. There are no distinct QRS complexes, but bizarre undulations of the tracing of irregular height and rate.

THE ELECTROCARDIOGRAM IN SOME OTHER CONDITIONS

Ventricular hypertrophy

Ventricular hypertrophy is diagnosed principally from the chest leads and in particular V_1 and V_6. Fig. 7.22 shows the appearance

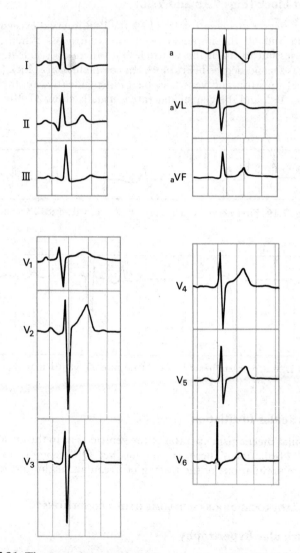

Fig. 7.21 The normal electrocardiogram. Standard leads (I, II, III), V (unipolar) limb leads, V (unipolar) chest leads V1–V6.

of the QRS complexes in V₁ (over the right ventricle) and V₆ (over the left ventricle). It must be appreciated that the QRS complex from any lead represents the algebraic sum of the electrical activity of both ventricles. At any point in time the ECG will show an R wave if the resultant is directed towards the electrode and an S wave if the resultant is going away from the electrode. Ventricular hypertrophy is associated with an increase in the electrical activity of depolarization. As a result there is an increase in the magnitude of the QRS deflections best seen in the chest leads.

Left ventricular hypertrophy.   (Fig. 7.22a). As the left ventricle lies to the left and posteriorly there is an increase in the size of the R wave in the left chest leads (V₅–V₆) and lead I and an increase in the S wave in the right chest leads (V₁ or V₂).

Right ventricular hypertrophy.   (Fig. 7.22b). The R wave in the right chest leads is increased and there is a deeper S wave in the left chest leads and in lead I as the increased electrical activity is associated with the anteriorly placed right ventricle.

Both types of ventricular hypertrophy may in addition show a *ventricular strain pattern*. This is an abnormality of ventricular repolarization associated with hypertrophy. It causes the T wave to point away from the affected ventricle giving ST depression and T wave inversion in leads I, aVL and the left chest leads in left ventricular hypertrophy, and in leads V₁, V₂, II and III in right ventricular hypertrophy. Other causes of T wave changes are mentioned on p. 242.

Bundle branch block (Fig. 7.23)

In bundle branch block (Fig. 7.23) owing to an interruption of a branch of the bundle of His, conduction to one ventricle is delayed. The QRS duration is greater than 0·12 second. For example, if the left bundle is interrupted, conduction to the left ventricle is delayed and it becomes activated at a time when it is no longer opposed by the right ventricle, and therefore produces large deflections, as in hypertrophy of the left ventricle.

Cardiac infarction

Cardiac infarction alters the electrocardiogram by the production of abnormal Q waves or abnormalities in the S–T segments and T

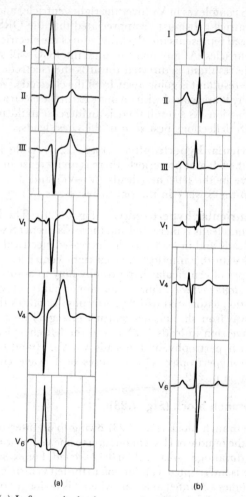

(a)   (b)

Fig. 7.22 (a) Left ventricular hypertrophy. Note the deep S wave in V₁; the tall R wave in V₆; and S–T depression and T wave inversion in lead I and V₆. (b) Right ventricular hypertrophy. Note the tall R wave in V₁; deep S wave in V₆; and T wave inversion in lead III and V₁. In this tracing the T wave is normal in lead II, though it is usually flat or inverted in right ventricular hypertrophy. The P wave in V₁ is sharp and peaked, suggesting right atrial hypertrophy.

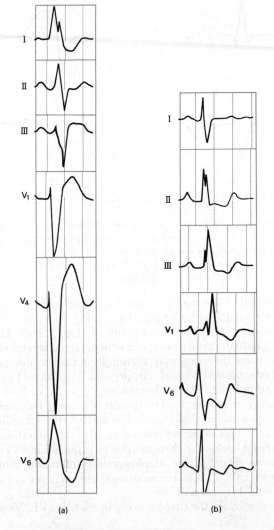

Fig. 7.23 (a) Left bundle branch block. Note the wide QRS complexes (0·15 seconds) and deep wide slurred R wave in V6. (b) Right bundle branch block. Note the wide QRS complexes (0·15 seconds), RSR pattern in V1 and deep wide S wave in V6.

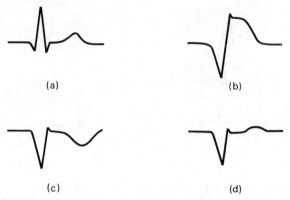

Fig. 7.24 The evolution of the changes in the QRS complex, S–T segment and T wave after cardiac infarction. (*a*) Normal pattern. (*b*) A few hours after infarction: a Q wave is present and the S–T segment is elevated (Pardee's sign). (*c*) After a time the S–T segment returns to the base line and the T wave becomes steeply inverted. (*d*) After a further period the T wave becomes inverted, flat and finally upright. Note that the Q wave persists.

waves, or both. Within a few hours of infarction the S–T segments become elevated (Pardee's sign) (Fig. 7.24b). In a few days the T waves become inverted, often steeply so (Fig. 7.24c). The S–T segment gradually returns to the base line, taking several weeks to do so. T wave inversion may eventually return to normal (Fig. 7.24d), but some inversion usually persists. Abnormal Q waves are usually permanent. The leads showing Q waves or S–T and T wave change are determined by the site of infarct. The electrocardiograms illustrating classical anterior and inferior infarction (Fig. 7.25) are tracings taken several weeks after the infarction.

In *anterior infarction* the changes are seen in leads I and V1 to V4.

In *inferior infarction* (or diaphragmatic infarction sometimes erroneously called posterior infarction) the changes are seen in leads II and III and aVF.

In *lateral infarction* the changes occur in leads I, aVL, V5 and V6.

P wave changes

In right atrial hypertrophy, due for example to chronic cor pulmonale or pulmonary stenosis, the P wave is tall and sharp. In left

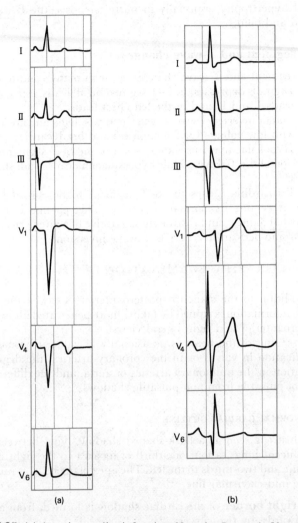

Fig. 7.25 (*a*) Anterior cardiac infarction. Note the Q wave in V₁ and V₄. The T wave is low in lead I and inverted in V₄. (*b*) Inferior cardiac infarction. Note the Q waves in leads II and III. The T wave is slightly inverted in lead II and inverted in lead III. V₆ also shows a Q wave and a low T wave, so that this is really inferolateral infarction.

atrial hypertrophy, especially in mitral stenosis, the P wave is broad and bifid.

S–T segment and T wave changes

S–T segment and T wave changes occur in many conditions:

1. Digitalis depresses the S–T segment in all leads, especially in limb leads I and II and in the left chest leads.

2. Flat or inverted T waves occur in myxoedema and are associated with low voltage QRS complexes and bradycardia.

3. Hypokalaemia causes depression of the S–T segments and inversion of the T waves, while hyperkalaemia causes tall sharp T waves.

4. Pericarditis causes the S–T segment to be elevated. The segment retains its normal concavity. This change is due to epicardial damage and is strongly suggestive of acute pericarditis. In chronic pericarditis there is T wave inversion.

RADIOGRAPHIC EXAMINATION OF THE HEART

In addition to the standard posteroanterior X-ray of the chest much information is gained by taking more penetrated films of the posteroanterior and right lateral views.

Screening of the heart is occasionally of value in visualizing calcification in valves or in the coronary arteries, the degree of pulsation in the pulmonary arteries or aorta, and the differentiation of pulsatile from non-pulsatile shadows.

THE NORMAL CARDIAC OUTLINE

The heart is seen as a flask-shaped shadow, lying between the translucent lungs, about one-third of its area to the right of the midline and two-thirds to the left. The apex of the heart is internal to the mid-clavicular line.

The right border of the cardiac shadow is formed, from above downwards, by two curves:

1. A slightly curved portion, the outer edge of the superior vena cava with the ascending arch of the aorta.

2. A more convex portion, the outer border of the right atrium, which ends at the diaphragm.

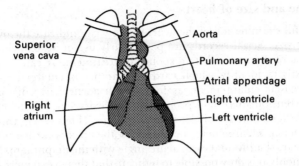

Fig. 7.26 The cardiac silhouette in the anteroposterior position. This is particularly useful in studying the outflow from the left ventricle, the pulmonary artery and the aortic knuckle.

The left border is made up from above downwards by:

1. The prominent knuckle produced by the arch of the aorta as it passes backwards, slightly to the left, then downwards.

2. The straighter line of the pulmonary artery.

3. The wide sweep of the left ventricle, ending at the apex, where it rests on the diaphragm.

In the overpenetrated posteroanterior film the left atrium can be seen, especially if enlarged, and the aorta is particularly well shown. Calcification in the pericardium or valves is usually apparent. The right lateral film is also of value in showing calcification and in addition is helpful in right ventricular hypertrophy when the cardiac shadow comes closer to and higher up the sternum than usual.

COMMON ALTERATIONS IN DISEASE

Position of the heart in the chest

Displacement of the heart as a whole is seen in pleural effusion, pneumothorax and fibrosis of the lung. In distension of the stomach and obesity, the heart is raised with the diaphragm and the apex tilted upwards. The common type of scoliosis (convexity of the curve to the right) is a frequent cause of displacement of the heart to the left. In narrow chests the heart often lies centrally and seems small and slender.

Shape and size of heart

Careful examination of the heart shadow can indicate the overall heart size. Serial records are particularly useful in following the course of disease and its response to treatment. It can be more difficult to identify which cardiac chamber is enlarged. In left ventricular enlargement, as found with aortic valve disease or hypertension there is a prominent convexity curving below the diaphragm and forming an obtuse angle (Fig. 7.27). In right ventricular enlargement the outline of the apex is turned up and the heart shadow makes an acute angle with the diaphragm. More commonly it is only possible to indicate that there is an increase in ventricular mass without being able to accurately predict which chamber is responsible.

The left atrium is enlarged in mitral stenosis and mitral regurgitation. The left atrial appendix (Fig. 7.28) shows in chest X-rays as a straightening or convexity of the normally concave left border of the heart below the pulmonary artery.

The overpenetrated grid film is particularly useful in detecting left atrial enlargement. The outline of the enlarged left atrium can usually be seen through the right atrial shadow on the right border. On the left, the dark shadow of the left main bronchus is displaced upwards by the enlarged left atrium and lies more horizontally.

Left atrial enlargement can also be assessed by giving the patient barium paste to swallow and screening him in the right oblique position. The oesophagus is displaced backwards and to the right by the enlarged left atrium.

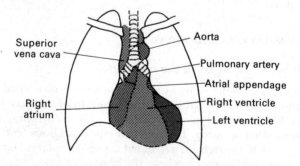

Fig. 7.27 Diagram of cardiac outline in left ventricular enlargement.

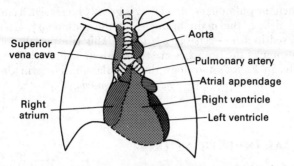

Fig. 7.28 Diagram of cardiac outline in mitral stenosis showing prominence of left atrial appendage at left heart border.

Shape and size of the aorta and superior vena cava

Enlargement of the ascending aorta occurs in syphilitic aortitis with aneurysm, in aortic stenosis (post-stenotic dilatation) and in aortic regurgitation.

Unfolding of the aorta is seen in atheroma, especially when hypertension is associated. The shadow of the superior vena cava is widened in congestive heart failure.

Pulsation of the heart and aorta

An abnormal degree of aortic pulsation is a feature in the cardio-scopic examination of cases of aortic regurgitation. In mitral re-gurgitation, the shadow of an enlarged left atrium is seen in the anteroposterior view to expand markedly during ventricular systole. A saccular aneurysm of the aorta appears as a rounded outgrowth from some part of the aorta, which itself will often be dilated. Its relation to the course of the aorta and its pulsation help to distinguish it from an intrathoracic tumour.

The hilar shadows and lung fields

In mitral stenosis, where the left atrial pressure is significantly raised, horizontal lines (Kerley B lines) due to engorged sub-pleural lymphatics are seen at the lung bases. The hilar shadows are heavy and rather ill-defined. Similar changes are found in left ventricular failure.

When the pulmonary blood flow is greatly increased, as in atrial septal defect, the main branches of the pulmonary artery are increased in size—*'pulmonary plethora'*. This is especially obvious when some of the branches are seen end-on near the hilum. Conversely, in Fallot's tetralogy the vascular markings in the lung fields are inconspicuous—*'pulmonary oligaemia'*.

SPECIAL INVESTIGATIONS

Electrocardiography and chest radiography are essential in the proper assessment of the cardiovascular system and so are considered as part of the routine examination. The need to establish precisely the diagnosis and functional status of patients, frequently as a preliminary to cardiac surgery, has required the development of special techniques.

External pulse recording and phonocardiography

Using suitable transducers, carotid and venous pulsation can be displayed along with the cardiac impulse (apex cardiography) and the recordings of heart sounds and murmurs. This is useful in confirming the time relationships of the physical signs and should be considered an adjunct to the physical examination. However useful in assisting interpretation, these techniques cannot be used to elicit new information; phonocardiography will not reveal significant heart murmurs that cannot be heard by auscultation.

Echocardiography.   The use of ultrasound to obtain images of cardiac structures has become especially useful when applied to valvar disease and congenital heart disease. The identification of pericardial effusion is quite precise using echocardiography, and it is the optimal method of identifying atrial myxomas. It can also give some information on the dimensions of cardiac chambers and from the pattern of movement of the myocardium functional assessment can be attempted. Conventional echocardiography is restricted by the fact that it can only visualize events in one dimension. The development of real-time two dimensional techniques promises to expand the usefulness of the method.

Cardiac catheterization and angiography

Catheterization of the heart is performed to obtain detailed haemodynamic information and to assist in the diagnosis or assessment of heart disease. Right heart catheterization is performed by passing a flexible radiopaque catheter via a vein into the right atrium, right ventricle and pulmonary artery under fluoroscopic control. The left heart can be entered by the retrograde passage of a catheter from an artery to the aorta and thence to the left ventricle; or by puncturing the atrial septum with a needle passed through the venous catheter and subsequently advancing the catheter over the needle into the left atrium and left ventricle. Information can be obtained in several ways:

1. The pressure within the cardiac chambers and vessels can be measured. Abnormal pressure gradients across valves may be demonstrated.

2. The cardiac output can be measured using either the Fick principle or dilution techniques.

3. Septal defects may be demonstrated by passing the catheter through the defect and by measuring the oxygen saturation of blood samples taken from different chambers. For example if the oxygen saturation in the pulmonary artery and right ventricle is 80% and in the right atrium is 65% this would indicate a shunt of blood through a ventricular septal defect from the left ventricle, and the amount of the shunt can be calculated.

Angiocardiography consists of the injection of contrast material into the chambers of the heart, the great vessels (aorta and pulmonary artery) or the coronary arteries, while serial X-ray films are exposed. Usually high speed cine-angiography using 35 mm film is used in one or two planes. Occasionally a larger format 100 or 105 mm or, less commonly now, full sized X-ray films are exposed serially when detailed anatomy is to be demonstrated.

These two techniques are used together to identify cardiac lesions and assess their severity; and to indicate patients suitable for cardiac surgery.

PLATE I

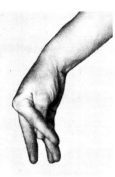

Tetany

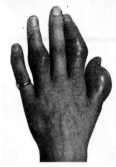

Gout

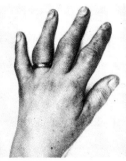

Rheumatoid arthritis

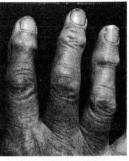

Heberden's nodes

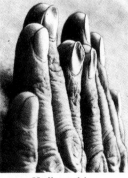

Koilonychia

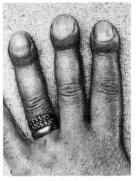

Clubbing

THE HAND

PLATE II

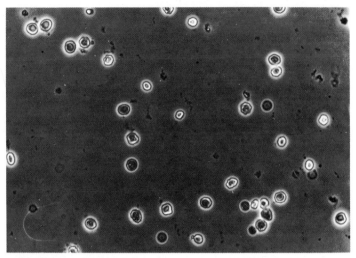

Erythrocytes in urinary sediment

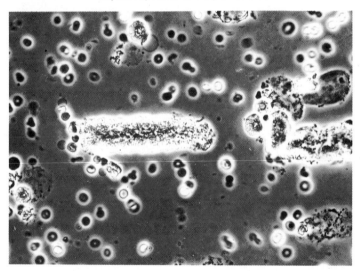

Granular casts in urinary sediment

Plates II and III illustrate the urinary sediment as seen by phase contrast microscopy. Readers using ordinary microscopy must not expect to see casts and cells so clearly defined.

PLATE III

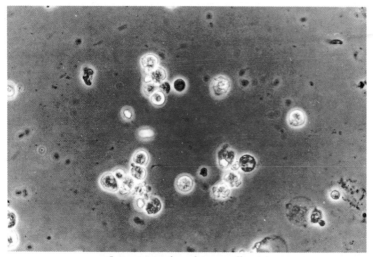

Leucocytes in urinary sediment

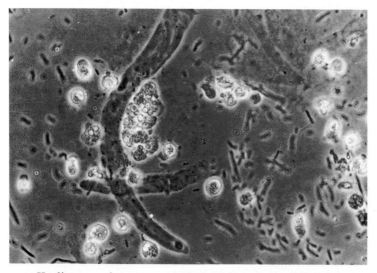

Hyaline casts, leucocytes and bacteria in urinary sediment

Plates II and III reproduced, by kind permission of the publishers, from: Edwin S. Spencer and Ib Pederson (1971) Hand Atlas of the Urinary Sediment. Copenhagen: Munksgaard.

PLATE IV

INTESTINAL PARASITES

1   *Entamoeba histolytica.* Fully developed four-nucleated cyst, containing chromatid bodies, as seen in saline preparations. × 1500

2   *Entamoeba histolytica.* Four-nucleated cyst as seen in iodine preparation. ×1500

3   *Entamoeba histolytica.* Active form, containing included red blood cells, as seen in saline preparations. × 1500

4   *Iodamoeba bütschlii.* Cyst, as seen in saline preparations. Note the unstained glycogen vacuole. × 1500

5   *Entamoeba coli.* Fully developed eight-nucleated cyst, as seen in saline preparations. × 1500

6   *Entamoeba coli.* Eight-nucleated cyst stained by Lugol's iodine solution. × 1500

7   *Entamoeba coli.* Active form, as seen in saline preparations. × 1500

8   *Iodamoeba bütschlii.* Cyst stained by Lugol's iodine solution. × 1500

9   *Giardia lamblia.* Cyst form, stained by Heidenhain's haematoxylin. × 1500

10   *Giardia lamblia.* Active form, stained by Heidenhain's haematoxylin. × 1500

11   *Trichomonas hominis.* Stained by Giemsa's method. × 1500

12   *Isospora belli* (*I. hominis*). Undeveloped oocyst as passed in human faeces. × 500

13   *Balantidium coli.* Active form stained by Heidenhain's haematoxylin. × 350

14   Ova of *Ankylostoma duodenale* (hookworm). × 500

15   Ova of *Enterobius vermicularis* (threadworm). × 500

16   Ova of *Taenia solium* and *T. saginata* (tapeworms). × 500

17   Ova of *Trichuris trichura* (whipworm). × 500

18   Ova of *Ascaris lumbricoides* (roundworm). × 500

19   Ova of *Schistosoma haematobium.* × 300

20   Ova of *Schistosoma japonicum.* × 300

21   Ova of *Schistosoma mansoni.* × 300

All magnifications approximate

Drawings by W. Cooper

PLATE IV

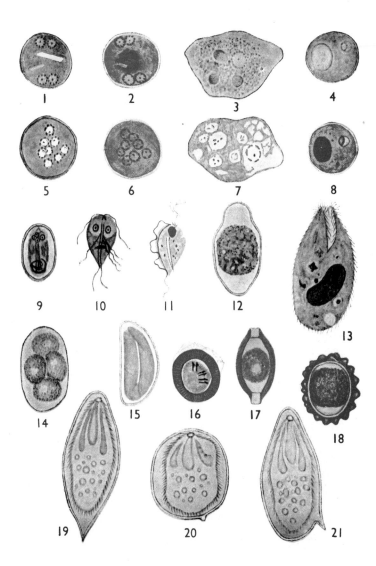

INTESTINAL PARASITES

PLATE V

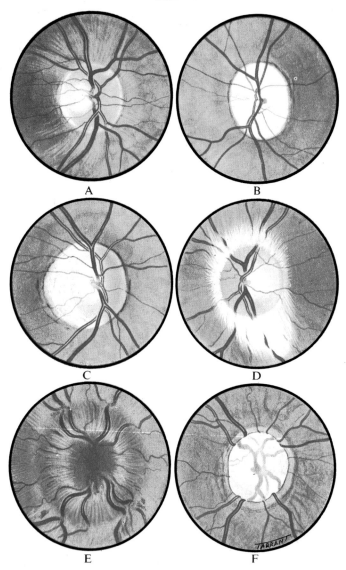

FUNDUS OF THE EYE

CAPTIONS ON FACING PAGE

PLATE VI

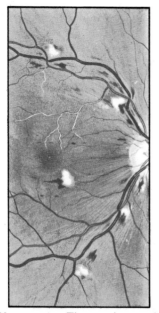

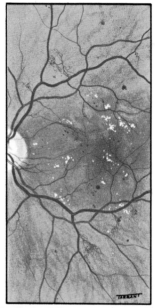

Hypertensive. The arteries are irregular in calibre and show 'silver-wiring'. Arteriovenous nipping is present. Characteristic 'flame-shaped' haemorrhages and 'cotton wool' exudates can be seen

Diabetic. Micro-aneurysms (tiny red dots), round haemorrhages, waxy exudates and areas of new vessel formation are characteristic of this condition. In many patients hypertensive retinopathy is also present

RETINOPATHY

A   *Normal optic disc*

B   *Optic atrophy.* The disc is white and the number of small vessels crossing its edge is reduced

C   *Myopic crescent.* A crescent or ring of exposed white sclera, seen particularly in high myopia

D   *Opaque nerve fibres.* The characteristic appearance of medullated nerve fibres

E   *Papilloedema.* A red swollen optic disc with dilated veins. The retinal vessels bend sharply as they dip down from swollen disc to surrounding retina. A similar appearance occurs in papillitis

F   *Glaucomatous cupping.* A form of optic atrophy due to raised intraocular pressure. The floor of the cup is depressed below the level of the surrounding retina

PLATE VII

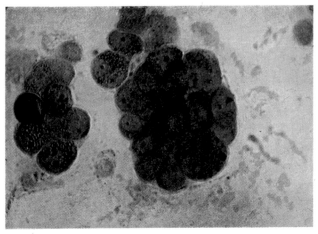

Carcinoma cells

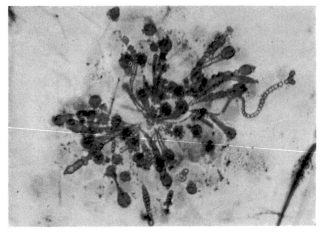

Asbestos bodies

SPUTUM

PLATE VIII

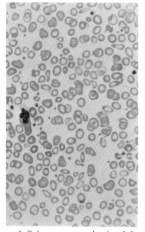

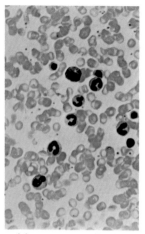

Iron deficiency anaemia (peripheral blood) Hypochromia, microcytosis, anisocytosis and target cells are shown

Normal bone marrow cells Nucleated red cells and granulocyte precursors are visible

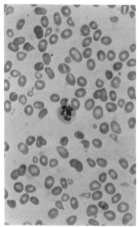

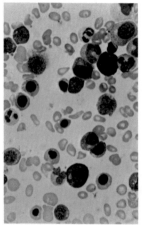

Macrocytic anaemia (peripheral blood) Macrocytosis, anisocytosis poikilocytosis and a hypersegmented neutrophil polymorph are shown

Megaloblastic anaemia (bone marrow) Early, intermediate and late megaloblasts visible; granulocyte precursors larger than normal with abnormal nuclear morphology

PLATE IX

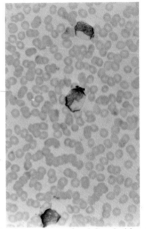

Glandular fever (peripheral blood). Atypical mononuclear cells are visible

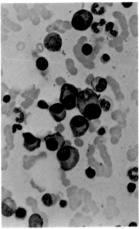

Myelomatosis (bone marrow). The marrow is infiltrated with plasma cells

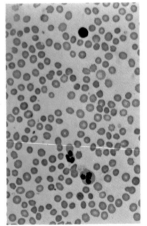

Spherocytosis (peripheral blood). Microspherocytes are small dense red cells which are characteristic of hereditary spherocytosis and auto-immune haemolytic anaemia

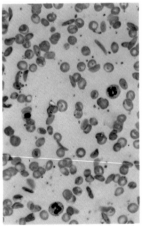

Sickle haemoglobin disease (peripheral blood). In the homozygous form, sickle cells and target cells are visible together with nucleated red cells and polychromatic cells

PLATE X

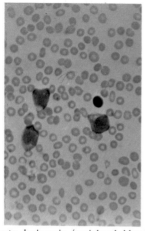

Acute leukaemia (peripheral blood). Large primitive blast cells are found in the peripheral blood and bone marrow

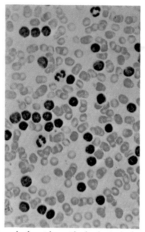

Chronic lymphocytic leukaemia (peripheral blood). Increased white cell count; cells are small mature lymphocytes

Chronic granulocytic (myeloid) leukaemia (peripheral blood). There is an increased number of granulocytes; most are mature neutrophils. A few more primitive cells are also found

Thrombocytopenic purpura of the skin

PLATE XI

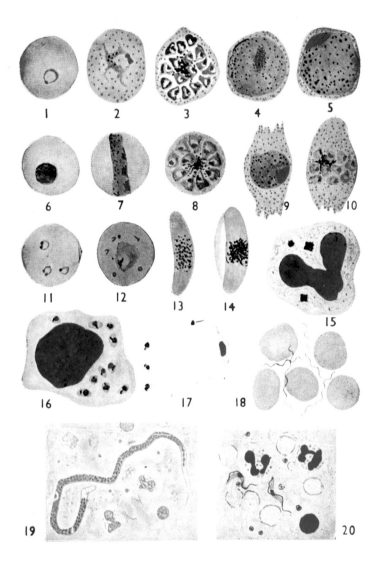

PARASITES OF THE BLOOD

PLATE XI

PARASITES OF THE BLOOD

1   *Plasmodium vivax*. Ring stage. × 2000
2   *Plasmodium vivax*. Amoeboid form. × 2000
3   *Plasmodium vivax*. Fully developed schizont. × 2000
4   *Plasmodium vivax*. Male gametocyte. × 2000
5   *Plasmodium vivax*. Female gametocyte. × 2000
6   *Plasmodium malariae*. 'Compact' form. × 2000
7   *Plasmodium malariae*. 'Band' form. × 2000
8   *Plasmodium malariae*. Fully developed schizont. × 2000
9   *Plasmodium ovale*. Female gametocyte. × 2000
10   *Plasmodium ovale*. Fully developed schizont. × 2000
11   *Plasmodium falciparum*. Red blood corpuscles containing various types of young rings. × 2000
12   *Plasmodium falciparum*. 'Old' ring, showing altered staining reaction and Maurer's dots. × 2000
13   *Plasmodium falciparum*. Male gametocyte or crescent. × 2000
14   *Plasmodium falciparum*. Female gametocyte or crescent. × 2000
15   *Plasmodium falciparum*. Pigment in polymorphonuclear leucocyte. × 2000
16   *Leishmania donovani* from a spleen smear. Some lying free and others within the cytoplasm of an endothelial cell. × 2000
17   *Trypanosoma cruzi*. Adult form as seen occasionally in the blood of patients suffering from Chagas's disease. × 2000
18   *Borrelia recurrentis*. × 2000
19   *Microfilaria loa loa*. × 600
20   *Trypanosoma rhodesiense* as seen in a thick blood film of patients suffering from trypanosomiasis. × 1000

Drawings by W. Cooper

PLATE XII

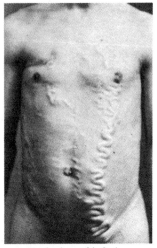

Occlusion of inferior
vena cava

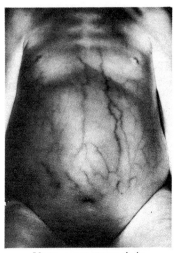

Venous anastomosis in
portal obstruction

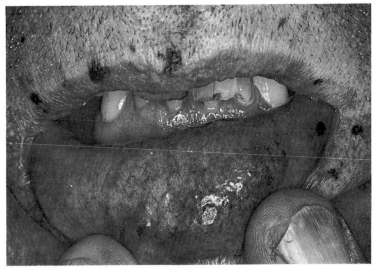

Hereditary telangiectasia The telangiectasia can be seen at
the margins of the lips and on the lower lip

PLATE XIII

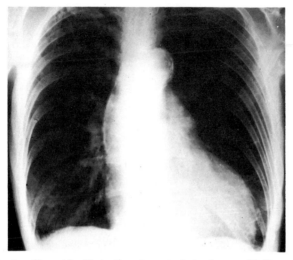

Chest radiography Note the characteristic shape of left ventricular enlargment in this patient with syphilitic aortic regurgitation. This egg-shell calcification is seen in the aortic wall.

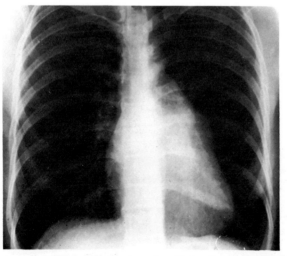

Chest radiography Mitral stenosis. Note the characteristic bulging of the left heart border associated with left arterial enlargement

PLATE XIV

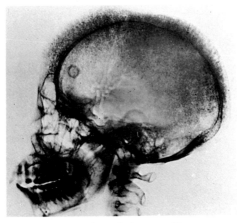

Skull radiograph showing 'hair-on-end' appearance in the calvarium in thalassaemia

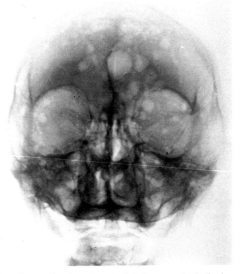

Skull radiograph showing multiple osteolytic lesions in myelomatosis

8

The nervous system

The aim of a neurological examination is to determine the site and nature of disease of the nervous system. In simplified form it is also an essential part of any routine clinical examination. Clinical examination of the nervous system should be thought of as a technique for precisely delineating the patient's disability in physiological and anatomical terms. It gives information about the condition at the time of the examination but gives no clue as to the natural history nor, therefore, to the pathogenesis of the disorder. For the latter, precise history taking is of particular importance since it alone enables the evolution of the disease to be studied.

A detailed neurological examination is an ordeal for ill patients and a test of concentration and co-operation for those in good general health. Care should be taken not to fatigue the patient unduly. Overlong examination may defeat its own ends, especially when sensation is being investigated, by leading to variable and incongruous findings. It may therefore be necessary to conduct the examination in more than one session.

The order of examination outlined in this chapter need not be rigidly adhered to. For example, if a patient is complaining of sciatic pain, it is appropriate to begin with the examination of the lower limbs and lumbar spine. An abbreviated scheme for routine use is set out at the end of the chapter. Observation of the patient's ordinary activity, for example the way he walks into the room and undresses for examination, is often helpful in deciding how to begin the examination.

ANATOMY AND PHYSIOLOGY

The dominant hemisphere is that which plays the major part in control of a person's abstract activities, especially of language. The left hemisphere is dominant in almost all right-handed people and in most left-handed people.

THE MOTOR SYSTEM

The lower motor neurones

Muscular movement depends ultimately on the integrity of the lower motor neurones, which connect striped muscles with the central nervous system. The lower motor neurones consist of the anterior horn cells, homologous cells in the brain stem and their efferent nerve fibres, which pass via the anterior spinal nerve roots and peripheral nerves to the muscles.

If this final common pathway is interrupted at any point, *weakness, fasciculation, muscle wasting, loss of tendon reflexes* and *hypotonia* occur. These are the cardinal signs of a *lower motor neurone lesion*.

Although various reflex movements operate at a spinal level, the initiation of voluntary movements and the maintenance of posture and muscle tone depend on impulses arising from higher centres. These impulses can only reach the muscles if the final common path is intact. These higher centres consist of the corticospinal and extrapyramidal systems and the cerebellum.

The corticospinal (pyramidal) system

The corticospinal system consists of the pathways which directly link the pyramidal cells in the fifth layer of the motor cortex with the lower motor neurones in the brain stem and spinal cord. The fibres concerned are gathered together in the corticospinal tracts. The corticospinal tracts, however, also contain fibres which arise from the postcentral cortex and subcortical structures. The motor area of the cortex occupies the anterior wall of the central sulcus (Rolandic fissure) and the adjacent parts of the precentral gyrus. There is localization of function in the motor cortex, different parts of the opposite side of the body being separately represented. Those parts of the body which carry out the most skilled movements, for example the fingers and thumb, have the largest areas of representation. The areas for tongue, jaw and facial movements lie lowest in the motor cortex, those for the arm, trunk and leg following successively as the motor area ascends on to the medial aspect of the hemisphere (Fig. 8.1).

The fibres of the corticospinal tracts pass downward from their cells of origin into the internal capsule, occupying the anterior two-thirds of the posterior limb. Here the order of representation of the body is face, shoulder, elbow, hand, trunk and lower limb from before backwards. The corticospinal fibres then descend to occupy the middle three-fifths of the peduncles of the mid-brain in the same order. Passing through the pons, the tract becomes broken into scattered bundles by the transverse pontine fibres and nuclei

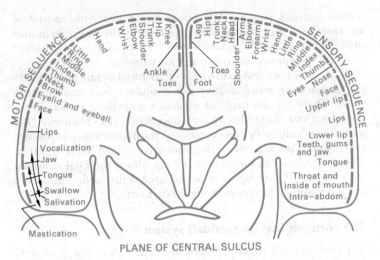

Fig. 8.1 Rasmussen and Penfield's diagram of localization in the motor (left) and sensory (right) cortex.

pontis. In the upper part of the medulla the fibres join to form the pyramids, which appear as well marked protuberances on the anterior aspect of the brain stem. In the lower part of the medulla the majority of the corticospinal fibres decussate with those of the opposite side and pass posteriorly to run down the spinal cord in the lateral columns as the crossed corticospinal tracts. A smaller number of fibres do not decussate, but continue downwards in the anterior columns as the direct corticospinal tracts, which decussate at segmental levels in the anterior commissure. A few uncrossed fibres descend in the crossed corticospinal tract of the same side, ending in the ipsilateral anterior horns. At different levels the corticospinal fibres terminate in the grey matter of the brain stem motor nuclei or in the anterior horns of the spinal cord.

The corticospinal system is concerned with the initiation of voluntary and skilled motor acts, particularly of fine distal movements. Contrary to former teaching the paralysis resulting from lesions affecting corticospinal fibres alone is limited to impairment of fine and rapid distal movements of the digits, as in picking up a small object. The more familiar occurrence of widespread paralysis of one side of the body (*hemiplegia*) or of a single limb (*mono-*

plegia) is usually the result of a more extensive lesion affecting extrapyramidal or other subcortical structures in addition to the corticospinal fibres themselves. Even in cases of dense hemiplegia movements of the head and trunk (axial movements) usually escape altogether. The nervous pathways for such postural movements are predominantly under subcortical control and are represented bilaterally.

Since, in clinical practice, most lesions of the corticospinal system also damage neighbouring extrapyramidal nuclei and pathways, the distinctions drawn above are rarely of clinical importance. All such cases are loosely grouped as 'corticospinal lesions'. The classical signs of such a lesion (an *upper motor neurone lesion*) are *weakness*, which predominantly affects fine, distal movements, hip flexion and shoulder abduction, *spasticity*, *increased tendon reflexes*, and an *extensor plantar response* (p. 315).

When the corticospinal system is suddenly damaged or destroyed, as by haemorrhage or injury, there is a temporary depressant effect on the anterior horn cells (neuronal shock). Paralysis is accompanied at first by loss of muscle tone and absent or reduced tendon reflexes. The characteristic hypertonia and increased reflexes of a corticospinal lesion appear after a few hours or days.

The extrapyramidal system

The term extrapyramidal system is applied to those parts of the nervous system, excluding the motor cortex and corticospinal pathways, which are concerned with movement and posture. The system includes the basal ganglia, the subthalamic nuclei, the substantia nigra, the red nuclei and other structures in the brain stem. The connections of these extrapyramidal centres are complex and include fibres from the cerebral cortex and the thalamus. There are no direct pathways from the basal ganglia to the spinal cord; the connections with the lower motor neurones are indirect, via several paths arising in the brain stem. These include the dentatorubrospinal, reticulospinal, vestibulospinal and olivospinal tracts.

The extrapyramidal system, which must clearly be considered in close relation with the corticospinal system, is important in the control of posture and in the initiation of movement, especially those movements which affect postural mechanisms such as sitting, standing, turning over in the lying position, walking and running. Complex volitional movements, such as reaching for an object, require both postural adjustments and fine distal movements, which are themselves broadly speaking under corticospinal control.

Diseases affecting the extrapyramidal system are characterized by difficulty in initiating voluntary movement, by impairment of orienting and balancing reflexes, by alterations in muscle tone and by the appearance of involuntary movements. Muscle power is rarely weakened.

The cerebellum

The cerebellum receives afferent fibres from the spinal cord, vestibular system, basal ganglia and cerebral cortex. It influences the lower motor neurone mainly through its connections, via the thalamus, with the basal ganglia and cerebral cortex.

Lesions of the cerebellum cause muscular hypotonia and incoordination (ataxia). Paralysis is not a feature of cerebellar disease. Lesions of the cerebellar vermis cause a characteristic ataxia of the trunk, so that the patient has difficulty sitting up or standing. In such patients there may be little or no incoordination of the limbs.

THE SENSORY SYSTEM

Sensory input reaches the nervous system from specialized receptors and free nerve endings in the skin and superficial tissues; from other receptors, such as muscle spindles, Golgi tendon organs, Pacinian corpuscles and free nerve endings in muscles; and from other specialized receptors in the joints. All afferent fibres enter the central nervous system through the posterior root ganglia and the posterior roots. Disease of these 'first sensory neurones' may thus affect all modalities of sensation. It must be remembered, however, that much sensory input is concerned with the reflex control of posture and movement and as such does not reach consciousness or is not consciously perceived. Thus the conscious recognition of posture and position of a limb is dependent on input from cutaneous and joint receptors. Muscle spindles and tendon organs also seem to play some part in this sensation (kinaesthesis) although clearly their major role is in the control of voluntary and reflex movements.

After they have entered the spinal cord, the various sensory fibres are rearranged and grouped into other systems. The majority of these afferent fibres terminate in the grey matter of the posterior horn at or near the level at which they enter. The secondary sensory fibres arise from these cells in the posterior horn. Some of these cross immediately, or within a few segments, to the opposite lateral and anterior columns of the cord and so ascend to the brain stem as the anterior and lateral spinothalamic tracts. Impulses from which the sensations of pain and temperature are derived ascend in the *lateral spinothalamic tract*, the fibres from the lower part of the body being placed laterally. Other peripheral fibres do not synapse in the grey matter of the posterior horns of the spinal cord, but ascend in the ipsilateral posterior columns: these posterior column fibres carry impulses upon which depend the appreciation of position, movement, size, shape, discrimination and texture, and vibration (which should be regarded only as touch rapidly applied). The medial of the two posterior columns, the *fasciculus gracilis*, contains fibres originating in the lower part of the body, whereas the lateral, the *fasciculus cuneatus*, carries fibres predominantly from the upper limbs. It should be noted, therefore, that somatotopic lamination of fibres in the posterior columns is the converse of that in the lateral spinothalamic tracts.

At any level of the spinal cord, therefore, there are two major groups of sensory fibres conveying sensory information towards the brain: one in the anterior and lateral columns carrying pain and temperature from the opposite half of the body, and a second in the posterior column, conveying the appreciation of posture, weight, size, shape and other qualities of sensation from the same side of the body. A unilateral lesion of the spinal cord, therefore, results in loss of pain and thermal sensibility below the level of the lesion on the opposite side of the body, while on the side of the lesion there is, in addition to spastic paralysis, disturbance of the sense of position and of movement and loss of recognition of weight, size, shape, touch and vibration. This group of clinical signs is called the *Brown-Séquard syndrome*.

At the upper end of the spinal cord the posterior column fibres terminate in the gracile and cuneate nuclei. The fibres of the secondary sensory neurone originate in these nuclei and immediately cross to the opposite side of the medulla in the sensory decussation. In the medulla, therefore, *all* sensory impulses are carried in sensory tracts situated on the opposite side to that from which they arise. But even here all do not run in a single pathway: spinothalamic fibres pass through the lateral part of the medulla, while those afferent impulses carried by the posterior columns enter the medial lemniscus. Higher in the brain stem the two sensory pathways are joined by the secondary sensory fibres from sensory cranial nerve nuclei. Finally the fibres of the medial lemniscus and spinothalamic tract terminate in the thalamus. All secondary sensory fibres synapse in the thalamus. From this level a third system of sensory fibres conveys sensory impressions through the internal capsule to the cerebral cortex.

The description of the major sensory pathways given above is sufficient for the practical work of diagnosis but it is a gross oversimplification of a complex subject. There are, for example, many afferent pathways other than the two described. These two pathways themselves are not modality specific in the sense that certain fibres 'carry' vibration sense or other forms of sensation: but rather the interaction of different patterns of impulses in different sized fibres of differing conduction velocity determines the sensation perceived at the highest levels of the nervous system. The importance of spinal mechanisms in the control of the flow of afferent information has recently been emphasized in the 'gate control' theory of sensation. This work has emphasized, furthermore, the pre-eminent role of the dorsal columns in exploratory, movement-directed behaviour, rather than in the passive reception of sensory input.

THE SPINAL CORD

The spinal cord extends caudally to the interspace between the 12th thoracic and 1st lumbar spines; the thecal membranes are continued down as far as the body of the 2nd sacral vertebra. The cervical enlargement reaches to the 7th cervical spine. Its largest part is at the level of the 5th and 6th cervical vertebrae. The lumbar segments lie opposite the 10th and 11th thoracic spines and the next interspinous space.

Since the cord ends at the level of the lower border of the first lumbar vertebra, spinal segments do not correspond with the vertebrae overlying them. To determine which spinal segment is related to a given vertebral body:

For the cervical vertebrae, add 1.

For thoracic 1–6, add 2.

For thoracic 7–9, add 3.

The 10th thoracic arch overlies lumbar 1 and 2 segments.

The 11th thoracic arch overlies lumbar 3 and 4 segments.

The 12th thoracic arch overlies lumbar 5.

The 1st lumbar arch overlies the sacral and coccygeal segments. In the lower dorsal region the tip of a spinous process is on a level with the body of the vertebra below.

The spinal cord is made up of segments from each of which a pair of anterior (motor) and posterior (sensory) nerve roots arises. The *myotomes* and *dermatomes* supplied by the pairs of nerve roots are shown in Tables 8.1 and 8.2 and in Fig. 8.2. It is important to remember these, since accurate knowledge of them enables quick and easy separation of nerve root and peripheral nerve lesions to be made by simple clinical examination. The sensory loss found after some common peripheral nerve lesions is shown in Figs 8.3 and 8.4. They should be carefully compared with the patterns of sensory loss shown in Fig. 8.2. Note that C8 and C6 sensory loss extends to the elbow on both ventral and dorsal surfaces of the forearm, but that ulnar and median nerve sensory loss predominantly affects the palmar surface of the hand and extends no further proximally than the wrist.

Vascular supply of the brain and spinal cord

The *brain* is supplied by the internal carotid and vertebral arteries (Fig. 8.4). Owing to the position of origin of the left common carotid, an embolus can enter it more easily than it can the artery of the opposite side. Embolic lesions are therefore more frequent in the left than in the right cerebral hemisphere.

The two *vertebral arteries* unite at the lower border of the pons to form the basilar, which runs up the middle of the anterior surface of the pons, dividing into the two posterior cerebrals. It gives off the paramedian and short and long circumferential branches which supply the pons and parts of the mid-brain and cerebellum.

The *posterior cerebral* supplies the occipital lobe, the lower part of

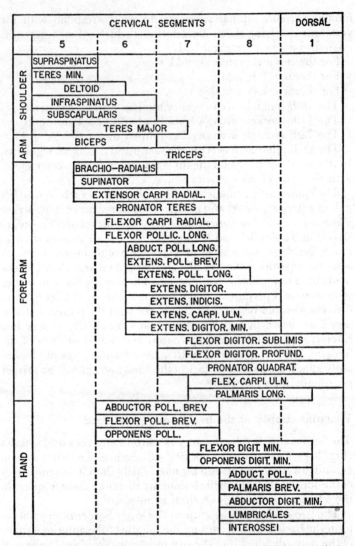

Table 8.1 Segmental innervation of the muscles of the upper limb.

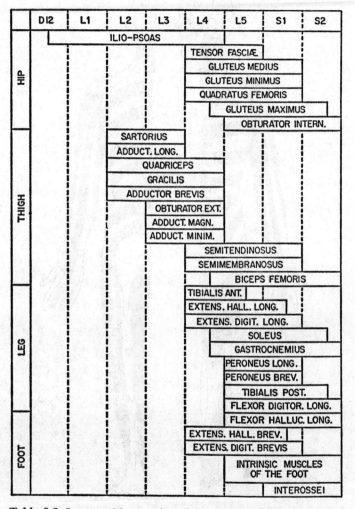

Table 8.2 Segmental innervation of the muscles of the lower limb.

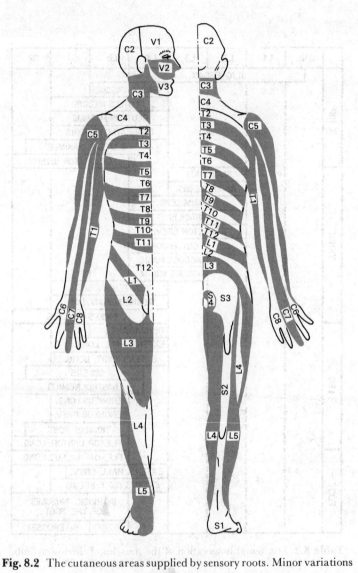

Fig. 8.2 The cutaneous areas supplied by sensory roots. Minor variations are common.

the temporal lobe and the uncus, the inner part of the crus and the corpus quadrigeminus, and the posterior part of the posterior limb of the internal capsule. Occlusion of this artery at its origin will therefore involve the visual cortex and the sensory fibres, but thrombosis often involves the calcarine branch and hence the visual cortex alone.

The *internal carotid* gives off the *anterior cerebral* artery, which curves round the anterior end of the corpus callosum, and is chiefly distributed to the inner surface of the cerebral hemisphere as far back as the parieto-occipital fissure. It also supplies the superior frontal gyrus, and gives a branch to the anterior part of the internal capsule and to the basal ganglia.

The internal carotid is predominantly directed into the *middle cerebral artery*, which lies in the lateral sulcus (Sylvian fissure). An embolus which has found its way into the internal carotid, therefore, usually ends in the middle cerebral or one of its branches. The

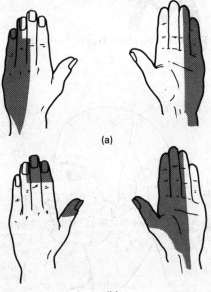

(a)

(b)

Fig. 8.3 Cutaneous sensory loss. (*a*) After division of the ulnar nerve above the elbow. (*b*) After division of the median nerve in the arm. These areas are subject to considerable variation.

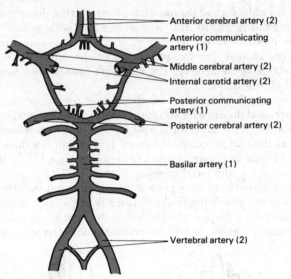

Anterior cerebral artery (2)

Anterior communicating artery (1)

Middle cerebral artery (2)

Internal carotid artery (2)

Posterior communicating artery (1)

Posterior cerebral artery (2)

Basilar artery (1)

Vertebral artery (2)

Fig. 8.4 The blood supply to the brain.

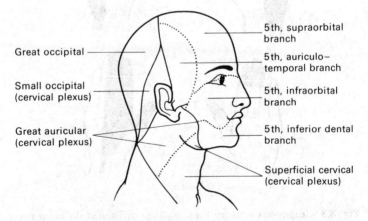

Great occipital

Small occipital (cervical plexus)

Great auricular (cervical plexus)

5th, supraorbital branch

5th, auriculo–temporal branch

5th, infraorbital branch

5th, inferior dental branch

Superficial cervical (cervical plexus)

Fig. 8.5 The distribution of the sensory nerves of the head. Compare with the sensory distribution shown in Fig. 8.2.

middle cerebral gives off cortical branches, which supply the motor area and the upper part of the parietal and temporal lobes. These branches anastomose freely with those of adjoining arteries so that occlusion of one of them may be largely compensated by the establishment of a collateral circulation. It also gives off *central branches* which penetrate into the brain substance and supply the white matter and the basal ganglia. There are two chief groups of these central arteries—an anterior group called the *lenticulostriate*, and a posterior group, the *lenticulo-optic*. The lenticulostriate are the source of hypertensive cerebral haemorrhage more often than are the lenticulo-optic. These central arteries also anastomose with one another.

Venous blood leaves the brain in the *venous sinuses*. Blood from the interior of the brain is chiefly returned by the cerebral veins, which end in the straight sinus.

Spinal arteries

The anterior and posterior spinal arteries arise from the vertebrals and travel downwards in the pia mater, the former in the anteromedian fissure and the two latter alongside the posterior nerve roots. Although they have a long and tortuous course, they do not diminish in size, being reinforced by radicular tributaries from the intercostal and lumbar arteries. The anterior spinal artery supplies most of the spinal cord, only the posterior parts of the posterior horns and columns being supplied by the posterior spinal arteries. Both anterior and posterior spinal arteries function as anastomotic vessels linking the radicular feeding vessels. Flow does not therefore occur in any particular direction in these vessels but varies, or may even reverse, in response to local factors such as changes in posture and variations in intra-abdominal and intrathoracic pressure.

The chief *veins of the spinal cord* are situated dorsally and ventrally in the middle line. Like the arteries, they communicate by radicular branches with the lumbar and intercostal veins, and empty into the vertebral veins. The blood in them flows upwards; hence in compression of the spinal cord, as by tumour or tuberculous abscess, there is venous engorgement below the level of pressure. This may very rarely result in a secondary, haemorrhagic, venous infarction of the spinal cord with paralysis and loss of sensibility below the level of the lesion. *However, if spinal compression is treated promptly, before cord infarction has occurred, recovery may occur.*

MENTAL FUNCTIONS

It is important to analyse the patient's intellectual state early in the examination, even if the analysis is limited to a subjective opinion of personality, memory, education and abstractional ability formed during the process of history taking, since this opinion is helpful in the subsequent investigation of symptoms. For example, if the patient's memory is deficient, only a limited value can be attached to his account of his illness or the state of his previous health. Or if he is comatose or unable to understand speech, any attempt to investigate the state of his sensory functions is likely to be frustrated. If for any reason the patient's own history is incomplete, it is essential to obtain a history from the relatives or friends.

Appearance and behaviour

The patient's bearing or his actions when lying in bed are important. Note whether there is any disturbance of consciousness such as confusion, stupor or coma. Is he unduly disturbed or apathetic, or in a state of agitation or terror? Is his attention easily held or fleeting? Does he show a reasonable degree of interest in his surroundings? How does he react to your approach and greeting? Is he well-groomed or unkempt? What is the condition of his hair, and hands? Any other features which strike one as unusual about his behaviour (e.g. facial tics or any inappropriate behaviour) should be noted.

Note whether his conversation flows easily or not: whether he is mute, answers only by monosyllables or is over-talkative. Do his remarks hold together as replies to questions? Do they show looseness of association? Do they show *flight of ideas* (a rushing stream of ideas with some connection) or the '*Knight's move*' in association (when one remark follows another with only indirect connection)? This name derives from chess, in which all pieces move on straight or diagonal lines, except the knight, whose move involves a change of direction. Do his replies to questions suggest *thought blockage*, or does he keep on repeating your question or his own remarks (*perseveration*)? He may use strange words (*neologisms*) or normal words strung together oddly (*word salad*).

Emotional state

It is important to note his mood. Is he happy or distressed? Is he happier than his condition would warrant (*elation* or *euphoria*) or filled with despair or dismay (*depression*)? Does his conversation lead you to feel that there is flattening of emotion, e.g. he speaks of family or financial success without pleasure or in an incongruous manner (he laughs after relating a misfortune or breaks into tears when given some pleasant news)? Is he able to enjoy anything? Does he feel that nothing is worth while? Does he feel fed up with life, or so fed up that he might as well end it (so that there is a risk of suicide)? Does the play of his features suggest that he enjoys a private world of his own, such as smiling or grimacing at odd times? Does he appear perplexed? Ask him whether persons or things seem as real as they once were, or whether they seem changed in some mysterious way (*depersonalization*). It is, however, unwise to ask leading questions about depersonalization, as neurotic patients will often respond affirmatively. Note whether the patient seems irritable or resentful, or whether he receives your words with suspicion.

Inquiries should be made about the patient's *sleep*. Does he sleep too much or too little? If too much, is any particular action likely to precipitate the hypersomnia? If too little, is the difficulty that of falling off to sleep, or of waking frequently, or waking early in the morning and being unable to go to sleep again? Where there is no physical cause for the insomnia, such as pain, cough, asthma or the wearing of some uncomfortable plaster, the insomnia is likely to be due to some psychological disorder, e.g. the restlessness of mania, the early waking of depression, or the turmoil of the mind with difficulty in getting off to sleep in the anxiety states.

Inquire about *dreams*. These are frequent and sleep-disturbing in the anxiety states, whether the source of the anxiety is apparent or not. In these conditions sleep is not refreshing and the patient may complain of being as tired in the morning as at night.

Delusions and hallucinations

Delusions are false beliefs which continue to be held despite evidence to the contrary. Hallucinations are false impressions referred to the organs of special sense (hearing, seeing, smelling, etc.) for which no cause can be found and which the patient knows to be imagined or unreal events. The patient's conversation may have already indicated that these are present. Note their content and the patient's attitude when you express doubt about what seems so real to him.

Neither delusions nor hallucinations may be voiced spontaneously. They have then to be inquired for and the introduction of the subject may call for considerable tact. Is his mind or his body interfered with by others or by some physical agency, e.g. electricity, radio or TV, or poison? Has he felt that others talk about him or shun him? Are his relatives, neighbours and colleagues at work kind to him or difficult to get on with? Has he ideas of supernatural power or inordinate wealth or, conversely, does he feel that he is weakened physically, morally or financially? Has he feelings of guilt? Does he think that he caused his own illness?

Hallucinatory experiences may be carefully hidden. Auditory and visual hallucinations are commonest. Of these visual hallucinations are usually organic and, except in temporal lobe epilepsy, auditory hallucinations are usually due to non-organic psychoses such as schizophrenia. Does he hear or see anything unusual? Does he taste or smell what he has not expected? Hallucinations may only occur at certain times of the day or in certain places and this should be noted. Delusions which are secondary to the hallucinatory experiences must be noted, e.g. that 'the neighbours are against him, because his bedroom is filled with gas, which he assumes the neighbours have engineered'. Notes should be made of any unusual actions upon the patient's part which have been prompted by delusions or hallucinatory ideas, e.g. ideas that his wife is in the pay of his enemies, or his clutching at small animals which he 'sees' crawling over his bedclothes.

Orientation in place and time

Does the patient appreciate his surroundings and know where he is, or is he wholly ignorant, and does he try to explain his ignorance in some way such as *confabulation*? Can he tell the date approximately, if not correctly? Can he tell the approximate time without looking at a watch or clock? Does he know why he is in hospital?

Clouding of consciousness

It is important to recognize states of clouded consciousness and to be able to describe and define them to others, particularly in the context of patients with head injury or raised intracranial pressure who may gradually deteriorate during a period of clinical observation. *Coma* is a state in which the patient makes no psychologically meaningful response to external stimulus or to inner need. In *stupor* the patient, although inaccessible, does show some response, for instance, to painful stimuli. Above these deep levels lie various degrees of altered consciousness and lethargy, which may be accompanied by confusion. The questioner must be alert to observe any minor defects in the patient's capacity to grasp what is required of him and what has happened to him. Such defects will usually be manifest in the responses to tests for orientation, recent memory and appreciation of environment.

Memory

Inability to grasp and retain images and ideas is a marked feature in acute toxic–delirious reactions and in the subacute and chronic organic psychoses. In these cases recent events may have been registered but cannot be recalled, although later when recovered, the patient may be able to remember them. It is more often correct that, in such patients, events have not been registered.

The degree to which recent memory is lost is an index of the severity of organic brain disorder (not necessarily permanent). Inquire about the day of the week and of the month and the names of prominent public figures. Ask the patient to recall what he has read in the paper or seen on television. In formulating questions on these lines, regard should be paid to the patient's educational background and his likely personal interests. More subtle changes are discovered by seeing whether the patient can repeat seven digits forwards or five digits backwards. Bring up a subject discussed three minutes previously or give the patient a simple story or address to remember and note how much is remembered after a short interval.

General intelligence

It is usually necessary to ascertain the patient's general intelligence or how it has been affected by brain injury or disease. The standard which he reached before leaving school, the character of his work and his work record give a rough-and-ready approximation. Frequent changes of job may indicate mental defect or personality disorder. Frequent changes after an accident or a serious illness with a previously good work record is suggestive of mental impairment.

Tests of memory as given above will indicate the more serious defects and these can be further exposed by tests of reasoning, more particularly where the tests show inability to criticize. Ask the patient to take sevens from a hundred (i.e. 100, 93, 86, 79 . . .), or to reverse in his mind's eye the hands of a clock. The absurdities test (e.g. 'What would be absurd if I told you I had three brothers, John, Fred and myself?') indicates grosser disability. A man with relatively low intelligence can give the months of the year parrot-fashion but is unable to say which months precedes May and which October, etc.

Tests in which the patient is asked the meaning of rare words or to interpret common proverbs or sayings are commonly used as an index of abstractional abilities. Judgement may similarly be assessed: 'What would you do if you saw a house on fire or a stamped addressed envelope lying in the road?' These questions often provoke concrete answers or a confused reply in the demented patient. Constructional and drawing tests may also be useful. These are briefly described on p. 275.

Released reflexes in dementia

In the demented patient and in other organic confusional states, a number of reflexes, released from the control of higher centres, may be elicited. Some may also be found in patients with large focal lesions; for example, the grasp reflex is characteristically released in patients with contralateral frontal lobe disease. In infancy the pressure or absence of three reflexes is used as part of the developmental assessment (p. 430). The most important of these higher level reflexes are the *grasping* and *avoiding responses*, the *palmo-mental reflex*, the *glabellar tap reflex* and released oral responses such as the *snout response* and tactilely and visually evoked *sucking reflexes*.

Grasping and avoiding responses. *Grasping* is elicited by stroking the palmar surface of the patient's hand on its radial aspect, preferably using a firm, distally moving stimulus between the patient's thumb and forefinger. The patient's hand grasps the examiner's and this grasp is not easily inhibited even if the patient is distracted by being asked his address. If traction is applied by simply pulling against the patient's flexed fingers the patient tends to oppose with an equivalent force. Grasping is typically associated with contralateral frontal lobe disease.

The avoiding response consists of a tendency for the patient's hand to move away from palmar or dorsal stroking or touch. It is usually evoked by stimuli on the ulnar surface of the hand. It is found in patients with contralateral parietal lobe disease, or lesions in its connections.

The palmo-mental reflex consists of a brief contraction of the ipsilateral mentalis muscle, causing puckering of the chin, in response to scratching the skin near the thenar eminence with a key or pin.

Glabellar tap reflex. A series of sharp finger taps to the glabella normally elicits only two or three blinks before this response is inhibited but in patients with diffuse degenerative disorders, especially senile dementia, and also in Parkinson's disease, the response is disinhibited and a blink follows each of a train of stimuli.

Snout reflex. Firm pressure of the examiner's knuckle against the patient's lips causes reflex puckering of the orbicular oris. This is usually associated with similar contraction of the facial musculature evoked by very light taps to the lips with a tendon hammer, or with the fingers.

Sucking reflexes. Anticipatory opening of the mouth as part of released sucking may be elicited by approaching visual stimuli, e.g. the shining metal end of a tuning fork, or by light contact with the cheeks near the corners of the mouth.

SPEECH

In considering speech disorders, it is essential to distinguish between defects of articulation and enunciation of speech (*dysarthria*) and disturbances of the structure and organization of language itself, *aphasia*.

DYSARTHRIA

Supposing that the patient is able to speak, one should note whether there is any abnormality in *articulation* apart from the variability inherent in various regional and other accents. The following are the chief abnormalities which may be present:

Stammering. This is a developmental disorder, more common in boys than girls. It is only very rarely due to organic brain disease.

Lalling or baby speech. Ask the patient to read something aloud. In lalling all the difficult consonants are dropped; he speaks like a baby. Lalling is usually the result of congenital or infantile deafness: very rarely it may be due to a congenital defect in the appreciation of the meaning of sounds—congenital auditory imperception. Speech is usually louder than normal in this disorder.

Scanning or staccato speech (cerebellar dysarthria). The patient speaks slowly and deliberately, syllable by syllable, as if scanning a line of poetry. The normal prosodic rhythm of syllable, word and sentence production is lost and in extreme forms each syllable is given equal emphasis. Ask him to say 'artillery': he will pronounce it 'ar-til-ler-y'. This is the classical form of severe *cerebellar dysarthria*. It is important to recognize it in minor, less obvious forms since its presence indicates bilateral disease of the cerebellum or its brain stem connections.

Spastic dysarthria. The syllables are slurred together as in a state of intoxication. Thus 'British Constitution' becomes 'Brizh Conshishushon'. This form of dysarthria is due to bilateral lesions in the corticospinal fibres supplying the muscles of the face, larynx, tongue and respiration concerned with speech, i.e. the lesion is supranuclear to, or above the level of, these brain stem nuclei. It is therefore a manifestation of *pseudobulbar palsy*: the jaw jerk is invariably brisk.

Bulbar palsy, due to lower motor neurone lesions affecting the speech musculature, results in some non-specific slurring of speech which can usually be readily separated from other forms of dysarthria.

Cortical dysarthria. An apractic hesitancy in word production, associated with difficulties in abstract, volitional movements of the lips and tongue is commonly associated with aphasia due to left frontal and temporal lesions. It never occurs as an isolated abnormality and the term should therefore be used with care, since it leads to confusion.

ASPHASIA

If the patient's defect consists not so much in a disturbance of articulation as in an inability to use language, whether speaking, writing or comprehending it, then he is suffering from *aphasia*.

Aphasia may be classified or described in a number of different ways. From the clinical viewpoint it is necessary to ascertain, first, where the responsible lesion is likely to be and, second, what is the significance of the functional defect in language in relation to the patient's disabilities: how does it affect him?

Everyday use of language includes:

1. The ability to *use words* in spoken speech. This includes *articulation, fluency* (the ability to put words together into phrases and sentences of varying complexity, in various grammatical constructions, without hesitations and errors), *naming* and ready accurate *repetition* of complex statements and concepts.

2. The ability to *comprehend* spoken speech.

3. The ability to *read* to oneself (not aloud).

4. The ability to *write*.

5. The ability to comprehend *other symbols*, e.g. mathematical or musical symbols.

Speech defects may readily be analysed in these terms as disturbances of *articulation, fluency, verbal comprehension, naming, repetition, reading* and *writing*. If a simple rough score is given to each of these categories (Fig. 8.6), a broad analysis of speech function which has some localizing value can be built up. It can be seen for example, that disturbances of fluency, verbal comprehension, repetition and writing, are all prominent in left anterior temporal lobe lesions (amnestic or Wernicke's aphasia). Frontal lesions affect articulation and fluency more than the other categories of language.

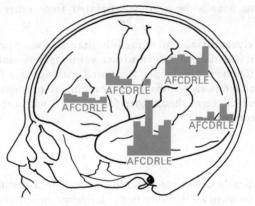

Fig. 8.6 The average degree of disturbance of various language modalities which occurs when there is an isolated lesion of various lobes (frontal, rolandic, parietal, temporal and occipital). A, articulatory disturbances; F, disturbances in the fluency of speech; C, disturbances of verbal comprehension; D, disturbances of naming; R, disturbances of repetition; L, disturbances of reading; E, disturbances of writing.
(*After H. Hecaen and R. Angelergues* (1964) *in Ciba Foundation Symposium on Disorders of Language. London: Churchill.*)

Parieto-occipital lesions impair reading (visual language functions) and parietal lesions impair several associative functions, but particularly writing.

Spoken speech

It will be noted that assessment of articulation and fluency, on the one hand, and reading and writing on the other, enables separation of lesions in front of and behind the central sulcus (Rolandic fissure): this is a useful clinical concept which may be referred to as the 'anterior' and 'posterior' aphasic syndromes. Use of the terms 'receptive' and 'expressive' aphasia is to be discouraged because, not only does this classification not allow insight into the nature of the patient's functional defect (since it ignores the equally important functions of reading, writing, repetition, articulation and fluency), but it provides little information of localizing value. Similarly, an excessive concern with 'pure' varieties of aphasia and the establishment of theoretical centres for various aspects of language leads to great complexity and confusion, with little practical benefit.

A simple scheme for the practical examination of the aphasic patient follows:

First find out whether the patient's hearing is good. Roughly assess his speech disorder in the context of an ordinary conversation about everyday things. Note the presence of hesitations, the searching for a forgotten word, the compensation by the use of a descriptive phrase, replacing that which was forgotten (*paraphasia*), neologisms (invented or nonsense words), inappropriate words or phrases, syntactical and semantic errors. Note also any articulatory disturbances, particularly clumsiness and difficulty in coordinating movements of lips and tongue (*orofacial apraxia*). This is usually very pronounced when the patient is commanded to put out his tongue or close his eyes and these movements should not, therefore, be used to establish comprehension of speech or the patient's cooperation. Disturbances of fluency may also be noted in this way.

Formal tests of the ability to comprehend and carry out complex commands may then be useful. Inability to comprehend spoken words may be regarded as a special form of *auditory agnosia* (word deafness).

Spontaneous speech production.   If the patient can use only a few words, make a note of what these are. If he repeats any word or phrase again and again (*perseveration* or *repetitive utterance*), note what it is.

If he has a considerable vocabulary, first make a note of any examples of lalling, slurring, etc., as an indication of *articulation*. Test him with such words and phrases as 'British Constitution', 'West Register Street', 'biblical criticism', 'artillery'. Then show him common objects—a knife, a pen, a matchbox, ect.—and ask him to *name* them or, if he is speechless, to indicate with his fingers the number of syllables in the name of each. Sometimes the patient has a general idea of the word he wants to use, but forgets exactly how to pronounce it; he omits some syllables or substitutes others for them, so that the listener may hardly be able to make out what word he wishes to use. These are signs of *amnestic* or *nominal* aphasia.

If he makes mistakes in his use of words, calling the knife a pen, he is suffering from *word substitution*. In that case, one should note whether or not the patient shows that he is aware of his error by trying to correct himself, or whether he continues with similar errors or even uses nonsense words without realizing that they are not real words (neologisms). This is called *jargon aphasia* and indicates a lesion situated posteriorly in the temporal lobe.

Speech repetition.   Ask him to repeat words after you. If necessary try to make clear your request by the aid of pantomime, repeating the word or phrase slowly and clearly several times. Remember never to shout at an aphasic patient: his hearing is normal. If he is able to repeat what you say, endeavour to find out whether or not he understands what he is saying.

Written speech

Speech comprehension.   Ascertain whether or not his sight is good. If so, write on a piece of paper such questions or commands as: How old are you? Put out your tongue. If he does not respond satisfactorily, there is some word blindness present. Inability to read is called *alexia*.

Production.   Ask him to write his name. (This can often be done when all other power of writing is lost.) If he is able to do so, ask him some simple question—How many do two and two make?—and get him to write a reply. If he has poor verbal comprehension put your question in writing. If his right hand is paralysed, make him write or print with his left. If he writes well, get him to write an account of his illness and note whether he makes use of the wrong word at times or whether there is repeated use of any particular word.

Can he write to dictation or copy words and sentences? Try, using a newspaper. If he succeeds, does he understand the meaning of what he writes?

Comprehension of other symbols.   Write down certain numerals:

$$\frac{\begin{array}{r}2\\+2\end{array}}{4} \qquad \frac{\begin{array}{r}2\\+2\end{array}}{5} \qquad \frac{\begin{array}{r}2\\+2\end{array}}{6}$$

and ask him to point out which is correct. Inability to understand amd manipulate mathematical symbols, termed *acalculia*, may occur in posterior parietal lesions affecting the dominant hemisphere. If he can read music, test him with musical notes.

Gesture. Many aphasic patients make attempts to use gesture to communicate, but this too is usually defective. Furthermore these patients do not readily understand complex gestural instructions.

Use of common objects. Occasionally a patient who has neither motor nor sensory paralysis, nor ataxia, cannot perform certain acts, though he can easily execute their component movements. He is consequently unable to make use of objects, though he can recognize their use. This is known as *apraxia*. It results from damage to the parietal cortex or white matter of the left or of both hemispheres, or from disease of the connections between the two hemispheres through the corpus callosum, and of the left parietal lobe. It affects only the left limbs, i.e. the right hemisphere, when the callosal fibres only are injured, but it is more commonly a bilateral disorder. It may be tested for by asking the patient to use certain objects, or make or imitate certain movements. For instance he may be given a box of matches and a cigarette and asked to light the latter. If there is apraxia, he may fail to open the box, or to take a match from it, or to strike the match, or even to light the cigarette with the match if he has succeeded in striking it. It is, of course, important to make sure that the patient understands the request.

THE CRANIAL NERVES

In this section a brief *résumé* of the essential points in the anatomy of each cranial nerve will be given indicating its function and, in some cases, the symptoms resulting from lesions affecting it. The method for clinical examination of each cranial nerve will be described.

FIRST OR OLFACTORY NERVE

Anatomy. The central processes of the bipolar sensory cells in the olfactory epithelium pass through the cribriform plate to the olfactory bulb, where the cells of the second olfactory neurones lie. Nerve fibres pass thence to the olfactory area of the cerebral cortex, the uncus of the parahippocampal gyrus.

Test

Have three small bottles containing some oil of cloves, some oil of peppermint and some tincture of asafoetida. Apply these to each nostril separately and ask the patient if he recognizes them. In testing, avoid the use of such irritating substances as ammonia, for these act partially through the 5th nerve. The sense of smell may be abolished. This is known as *anosmia*. Before concluding that this is due to neurological disease exclude local changes in the nose itself, e.g. catarrh. *Parosmia* is the name applied to that condition in which the sense of smell is perverted, so that, for instance, offensive substances seem to have a pleasant odour and vice versa.

Inquire also regarding *hallucinations of smell*. These sometimes constitute the aura of an epileptic fit.

SECOND OR OPTIC NERVE

Anatomy. From the retina, the fibres of the optic nerve pass back to the optic chiasma. Here the fibres from the inner half of each retina decussate, whilst those from the outer half remain on the same side. Each optic tract, therefore, consists of fibres from the outer half of the retina on the same side and the inner half of the retina on the opposite side. Each tract passes back to the superior colliculus, the lateral geniculate body and the pulvinar of the thalamus of the same side. In these most of the fibres of the optic tracts terminate. A further system of fibres, which is known as the optic radiation, takes origin in the lateral geniculate body and passes through the posterior limb of the internal capsule and then backwards to the cortex around the calcarine sulcus. Those subserving the upper visual fields pass down through the substance of the temporal lobe, whilst those mediating impulses from the lower field pass up into the parietal lobe. The occipital cortex around the calcarine fissure constitutes the chief visual centre, and represents the opposite half of the field of vision, the left half of the field of vision being represented in the cortex of the right hemisphere and vice versa (Fig. 8.7).

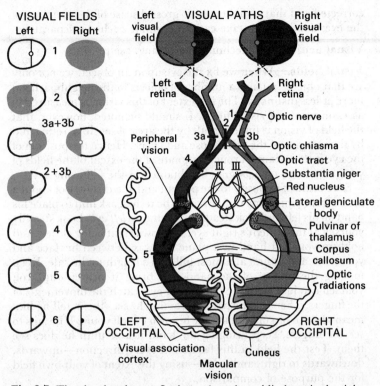

Fig. 8.7 The visual pathways. Lesion at 1 produces blindness in the right eye with loss of direct right reflex. Lesion at 2 produces bitemporal hemianopia. Lesion at 3a and 3b produce binasal hemianopia. Lesion at 2 and 3b produce blindness of the right eye with temporal hemianopia of the left visual field. Lesion at 4 produces right homonymous hemianopia with hemianopic pupillary response. Lesion at 5 produces right homonymous hemianopia with normal pupillary reaction to light. Lesion at 6 produces right homonymous central hemiscotoma.

Test

In testing the optic nerve, one has to investigate three functions: (*a*) visual acuity; (*b*) visual fields; and (*c*) colour sense.

Certain preliminaries must always be conducted. One of these is to see that any error of refraction in the patient's eye is first corrected and that also there is no gross disease of the structure of the eye; another is to take care to examine each eye separately.

Visual acuity.   For technique of testing, see p. 374.

Visual fields.   When we fix the eye upon an object, we not only see that object, but also a number of objects in the neighbourhood more or less distinctly. The full extent of this vision is measured in assessment of the visual fields. It should be noted, however, that the field of vision is limited both by the area of sensitive retina and by the margins of the orbit, nose and cheek. Hence the position of the eye is important. A rough estimate of the extent of the fields of vision for large objects may be obtained in the following way.

Seat yourself opposite to the patient and at a distance of about a metre from him. If his right eye is to be tested, ask him to place his hand on his left and look steadily at your own *left* eye. Look steadily yourself at the patient's right eye, your own right being closed, and hold up your left hand in a plane midway between his face and your own, and at first at almost full arm's length to the side. Keep moving the fingers of the hand and bring it nearer until you yourself can just 'with the tail of your eye' catch the movements of the fingers. Then ask the patient whether he sees them, telling him meanwhile to be sure not to take his own eye off yours. If he fails to see the fingers, keep bringing the hand nearer until he does see them. Test the field in this fashion in every direction—upwards, downwards to right, and to left—using the extent of your own field for the purpose of comparison.

This gives the outline of his field for appreciation of a moving object, which may, however, be relatively intact when the fields for other forms of stimulation are seriously constricted. The field for smaller objects must also be tested, therefore, when disease of the visual pathways is suspected. This can conveniently be done using a red pin-head held up in the patient's field in the manner described above. This method allows the patient's field, including the size of his *blind spot* (see below), to be compared with the examiner's field very exactly. Further central areas of impaired vision (central scotoma) can be recognized by this method either because the red pin-head cannot be perceived in the scotoma or, in less severe examples, because the intensity of the red colour is lower in this part of the field. A good rough test in preliminary assessment is to ask the patient to compare the contour and colour of the examiner's palm held up in the right, left and central fields of each eye separately.

Considering the field of vision in more detail, whereas images falling on the central part of the retina (the macula) are seen in minute detail and bright colouring, objects seen farther and farther from the point of fixation are perceived with less and less distinction and colour, until at the periphery of the field we can only appreciate the presence of an object of considerable size without being able to judge its form. To the temporal side of the central point of vision is the *blind spot* which represents the optic nerve head area in which there are no light receptors. Perimetry surveys the field of vision and the limits of perception are charted. The centre point of the chart corresponds to the visual axis; the point of fixation is therefore the point of more distinct vision. Around this point are arranged a series of more or less concentric lines, each of which denotes equal visual acuity, and is called an *isopter*. For purposes of investigation we divide the visual field into three parts:

1. An area surrounding the point of fixation to 20°.
2. An intermediate area between 20° and 50°.
3. An outer area from 50° to the periphery.

The fixation point is not exactly central so that the outer and inner part of the field is unequally divided. Further, the boundary is delimited inwards and upwards by the nose and brow. Testing with a 5 mm object we find the extent of the average field of vision is 100° outwards, 60° upwards and inwards and 75° downwards. The field charted with a 20 mm object is shown in Fig. 8.8; note the restriction of the lower nasal field by the bridge of the nose.

The binocular field extends 200° or more laterally and about 140° vertically, in the middle of which is a circular portion common to each eye with a diameter of about 120°. On each side of this paired area is a lateral semilunar area which is unpaired (monocular) and which accounts for the remainder of the field.

Perimetry is concerned with an investigation of the uniocular field of vision. As visual acuity is much lower at the periphery than at the point of fixation this acuity may be tested with objects of different size, as a very small object visible at and near the fixation point fades from view as it is withdrawn towards the periphery. By using a graduated series of objects, it is possible to plot out a series of isopters each of which corresponds to a known size of object used at a known distance from the eye.

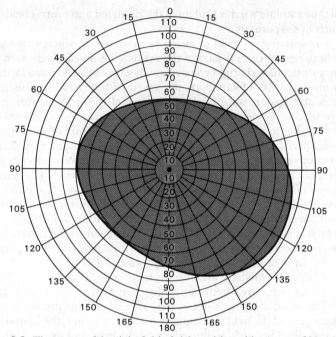

Fig. 8.8 The extent of the right field of vision with a white target of 20 mm diameter mapped on a perimeter at a distance of 330 mm.

That part of the field between the periphery and the 30° circle is investigated by means of a perimeter. A 3 mm white test object is usually used, but when visual acuity is impaired, a larger diameter may be required. Thus the fraction of diameter of object/distance (usually 3/330 mm) is a measure of the visual acuity at the particular point on the field which is being tested.

The area within the 30° circle is examined by means of test objects upon a black screen—*Bjerrum's screen*—at a distance from the patient of 1000 or 2000 mm.

The patient is seated comfortably at this distance with the head steadied by a chin and head rest, and a grey object 1 cm in diameter with a black centre is fixed to the screen on a level with the patient's eye.

The blind spot is first of all mapped out with a white object 20–30 mm in diameter. The peripheral field is then mapped with a

10 mm object: at a distance of 2000 mm it should be circular and extend to about 25°, that is to the edge of the 2 m² screen. With the small object areas of blindness or defective perception should be sought around the blind spot, especially between this area and the macula, the centrocaecal area, and in the horizontal meridian on the nasal side of the fixation spot. The findings are marked upon the screen with black pins, and subsequently transferred to a chart.

Changes in the field of vision.   The field of vision may be contracted all round its periphery. This is spoken of as *concentric constriction* of the field of vision. This occurs in long-standing papill-oedema, some forms of optic atrophy, bilateral lesions of the anterior part of the striate (visual) cortex, retinal disorders and hysteria.

Sometimes the loss of vision is confined to the centre of the field, a *central scotoma*. Sometimes it is due to local disease of the choroid or of the retina in the neighbourhood of the macula. In that case it may affect only one eye. A unilateral central scotoma is commonly produced by retrobulbar neuritis, which in most cases in Britain is a symptom of multiple sclerosis. More rarely, it may be due to toxic causes or vitamin deficiency, when it is generally bilateral. Pressure on the optic nerve is another cause. It may also result from a lesion of the posterior part of the cortical visual centres and is then bilateral, but this is very rare.

Hemianopia means loss of sight in one-half of a visual field. When the same half of both fields of vision is lost, the hemianopia is described as homonymous, e.g. right homonymous hemianopia when the blindness occupies the right half of the field of both eyes. (Fig. 8.8). Hemianopia limited to one quadrant of the field is termed a quadrantanopia.

Superior and *inferior hemianopia* means loss of the upper and lower halves of the visual field respectively. This *altitudinal hemianopia* is rare; it is usually due to occipital lesions.

Bitemporal hemianopia means loss of vision in the temporal or outer halves of both fields, and is due, therefore, to loss of function of the nasal half of each retina. It can only be produced by a lesion of the optic chiasma, involving those fibres of the optic nerves which decussate. It can be due to a tumour of the pituitary gland or sella turcica but may also be produced by inflammatory or traumatic lesions of the optic chiasma (Fig. 8.9).

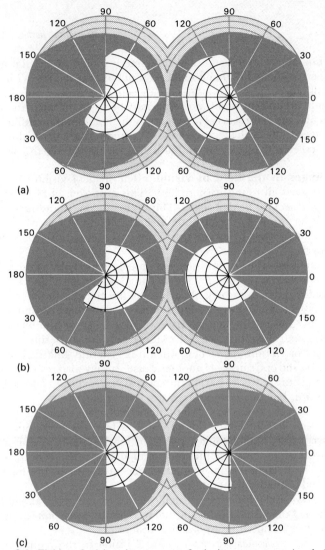

Fig. 8.9 Fields of vision in a case of pituitary tumour (probably chromophobe adenoma) showing the development of bitemporal hemianopia. (*a*) May: VA Lt 6/12 Rt 6/18. (*b*) August: VA Lt 6/12 Rt 6/12. (*c*) October: VA Lt 6/12 Lt 6/12. The fields were plotted on a Bjerrum's screen at a distance of 20 m from the eye to the point of fixation at the centre of the screen, using a 10 mm white object. The tan areas show the average normal field of vision and the white areas the patient's fields.

Binasal hemianopia signifies a loss of the nasal or inner half of each field and indicates a diminution of visual function of the temporal half of each retina. It is very rare but can result from bilateral lesions confined to the uncrossed optic fibres on each side of the chiasma, and it may also occur in open-angle glaucoma.

Temporal and nasal hemianopia are sometimes described as heteronymous, in contradistinction to the homonymous variety.

Colour sense. For method of testing see p. 375.

Subjective visual sensations

Among the commonest subjective visual sensations is the occurrence of what are known as *muscae volitantes*—little specks seen floating before the eyes, especially on looking at a white surface or up to the sky. They commonly occur in normal subjects and are frequently complaints in anaemic and debilitated persons. In migraine, peculiar zigzag lines, known as 'fortification figures' or *teichopsia*, are often seen at the beginning of the attack and in the investigation of such a case they should always be inquired for. Visual hallucinations occur in a number of neurological diseases, notably in delirium tremens and in temporal and occipital lobe disorder; they may also form part of the aura in epilepsy. *Photopsias*, tiny white flashes seen in the visual field, often particularly during ocular movement, may occur in acute retrobulbar neuritis.

THIRD, FOURTH AND SIXTH NERVES

It is convenient to consider these together, as together they innervate the muscles which move the eye.

Anatomy. The fibres of these nerves take their origin from a series of nuclei which begin in the floor of the cerebral aqueduct below the superior corpora quadrigemina, and extend down as far as the eminentia teres in the floor of the 4th ventricle. The nucleus for the 3rd nerve is farthest forward; its most rostral nerve cells supply the ciliary muscle and iris (Edinger-Westphal nucleus), those for the ocular muscles being more caudally situated. Caudal to this is the nucleus of the 4th, and, most caudal of all, that of the 6th. The 3rd nerve emerges on the inner aspect of the crus, and is therefore likely to be involved in lesions of that part of the brain.

The trochlear nerves emerge on the anterior part of the roof of the 4th ventricle. They are peculiar in that they are the only cranial nerves which decussate between their nuclei and their point of emergence and that they emerge dorsally.

The 6th nerve merges between the medulla and pons. Its long intracranial course renders it particularly liable to the effects of pressure.

Functions

The 6th nerve supplies the external rectus, the 4th supplies the superior oblique. All the other extraocular muscles, the sphincter pupillae, the muscle of accommodation, and the levator palpebrae superioris, are supplied by the 3rd.

Ocular movements

Horizontal movement outwards is described as abduction, inwards as adduction; vertical movement upwards as elevation and downwards as depression. The eye is also capable of diagonal movements at any intermediate angle. Rotatory movements, the eye rolling like a wheel towards the nose (internal rotation) or away from the nose (external rotation), do not occur normally but may be seen in some varieties of ocular palsy. Note that the *recti act as elevators and depressors alone when the eye is in abduction, and the obliques act similarly when the eye is in adduction* (Fig. 8.10). Their function may therefore be assessed by testing the movements of elevation and of depression in both full abduction and full adduction. This is more important than simply testing elevation and depression in the

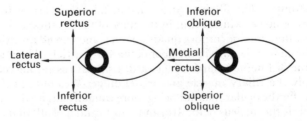

Fig. 8.10 The action of the external ocular muscles.

mid-position of gaze, with lateral gaze the so-called *cardinal directions* of gaze. The internal and external recti always act directly in a single plane, but all movements require the coordinated activity of the whole group of extra-ocular muscles. The eyes normally move 50° laterally, 50° medially, 33° upwards and 50° downwards.

Normally the movements of the two eyes are symmetrical, so that the visual axes meet at the point at which the eyes are looking. This is spoken of as conjugate movement of the eyes. *Infranuclear* (lower motor neurone) lesions of the 3rd, 4th and 6th nerves lead to paralysis of individual eye muscles or groups of muscles. *Supranuclear* (upper motor neurone) lesions lead to paralysis of conjugate movements of the eyes.

Lower motor neurone (infranuclear) lesions

Sixth nerve. Inability to move the eye outwards and diplopia on looking in that direction. Possibly internal squint.

Fourth nerve. Impaired downward movement, and on attempting to look downwards in the mid-position of gaze the eyeball is rotated inwards by the unopposed action of the inferior rectus (Fig. 8.10). Diplopia only below the horizontal plane, with the images uncrossed, but the false one tilted. There is rarely a visible squint.

Third nerve. Ptosis. The eye is displaced downwards and outwards and further movement is only possible outwards and a little downwards. Pupil usually dilated and fixed. Loss of power of accommodation.

Paralysis of the 3rd nerve is not infrequently partial—only one or a few of these functions being lost.

It must be remembered that smooth muscle in the upper lid is innervated by the cervical sympathetic and exerts a tonic elevating action. Slight ptosis therefore occurs after a lesion of the cervical sympathetic but the pupil is then small, rather than large (Horner's syndrome) (p. 293).

Thus the signs of a lesion involving one or more of these nerves may be: (*a*) defective movement of the eye; (*b*) the presence of a squint; (*c*) the presence of diplopia; and (*d*) pupillary abnormalities. Of these signs diplopia and pupillary abnormalities are the most reliable.

Strabismus

By *squint* or *strabismus* is meant a condition in which the visual axes do not meet at the point of fixation. Of this there are two varieties, *paralytic* and *concomitant*.

Paralytic strabismus.   The following are the characters of a paralytic squint:

1. *Limitation of movement*. Paralytic strabismus is due to weakness in one or more of the extra-ocular muscles; a prominent feature, therefore, is lack of ability to move the eye in the direction of the physiological action of the muscle affected. Although this weakness is usually apparent, it is sometimes so slight, or the unaffected muscles mask it so much, that the defective movement of the eye is hardly visible.

If an eye fails to move at all, or fails to move throughout the normal angular excursion, the deviation of the eye in a direction opposite to the physiological action of the muscle is called the *primary deviation* or *squint*, and it is measured by the angle which a line from the object to the nodal point of the eye makes with the visual axis. If now we cover the unaffected eye and so cause the patient to take on fixation with the affected eye, we shall find that the eye that is covered will deviate still more than the primary deviation of the affected eye. This deviation of the healthy eye is the so-called *secondary deviation* or *squint*, and this difference in amount between the primary and secondary deviation is the most important distinguishing feature between paralytic and concomitant strabismus.

2. *False orientation of the field of vision* is an erroneous judgement by the patient of the position of an object in that portion of the field of vision towards which the paralysed muscle should normally move the eye. Take the case of a patient who has paralysis of the right external rectus muscle. If such a patient closes the left eye and is asked to touch suddenly an object held in the horizontal direction on his right side, he may fail and strike wide of the object on his right-hand side.

3. *Dizziness* is occasionally a symptom of paralytic stabismus when both eyes are opened. It is due partly to the confusion of double vision and partly to false orientation.

4. *Double vision (diplopia)*. In order to overcome double vision, the patient turns his head in the direction of the action of the

paralysed muscle. The way in which the head is held gives information as to which muscle is involved.

Patients with paralytic squint complain of double vision. This occurs because defective movement of one eye results in the images found by the two eyes falling upon non-identical points of the two retinae. Binocular fusion cannot therefore occur in the visual cortex and two separate or overlapping images are perceived. Further, in paralytic strabismus, the image of the object fixed falls upon the macula of the healthy eye and is seen with distinctness and detail, and is called the *true image*, whereas in the affected eye the image falls upon the retina outside the macula, and as in consequence it is indistinct and blurred, it is called the *false image*. Most patients can therefore clearly recognize which of the two images they perceive is the true image and which the false. This false image is therefore projected into that part of the field of vision into which the paralysed muscle should move the eye if it were normal; it is perceived *in the direction of action of the weak muscle*. Doubt as to which is the false image can usually be resolved by covering one eye with a red glass and asking the patient whether the red or the normally coloured image is the real one.

The investigation of a case of paralytic strabismus and the diagnostic value of diplopia. First make certain that the diplopia is *binocular*, since certain conditions, for example lens opacities and astigmatism, may produce monocular diplopia.

Diplopia should always be assessed in the *cardinal* horizontal and vertical planes only, greatly simplifying its analysis and interpretation.

When the images in diplopia are separated laterally, so that the right image belongs to the right eye and the left to the left eye, the condition is called *homonymous* or *uncrossed diplopia*. If, however, the left image belongs to the right eye and the right to the left, it is called *heteronymous* or *crossed diplopia*. The real image always belongs to the healthy eye, and the false image to the paralysed eye.

The production of homonymous diplopia. If, as the result of paralysis of an abductor muscle (external rectus muscle), there is deviation of the eye inwards (convergent strabismus), the image in this eye will fall upon a point of the retina internal to the macula. Two things will result: (*a*) the image will not be so sharp as the image in the healthy eye, proving that the *false* image belongs to the affected eye; and (*b*) since images that fall upon the retina on the nasal side of the macula are projected in space to the temporal side of the eye, it follows that *paralysis of an abductor producing convergent strabismus causes homonymous or uncrossed diplopia*.

The production of heteronymous or crossed diplopia. If, as the result of paralysis of an adductor muscle (internal rectus), there is a deviation of the eye outwards (divergent strabismus), the image in this eye will fall upon a point of the retina external to the macula. The false image is produced in the affected eye, and since images that fall upon the retina to the temporal side of the macula are projected into space to the nasal side of the eye, it follows that *paralysis of an adductor producing divergent strabismus causes heteronymous or crossed diplopia*.

In a similar way it may be shown that in paralysis of an elevator muscle the false image (which belongs to the affected eye) lies on a higher level than the true image, and in paralysis of a depressor muscle the false image lies below the true image.

If a rotator muscle is weak, the false image is tilted. This often results in a compensatory head tilt.

Method of finding the direction of maximum diplopia. The patient is seated with the head fixed in position (preferably in a head rest) with a red glass before the right eye, and a green glass before the left. At a distance of about 5 metres the observer moves a light in the direction indicated in Table 8.3, each of the lateral squares corresponding to a pair of true associated muscles; thus a maximum vertical diplopia produced when the patient looks up and to

Table 8.3. CHARTING THE FIELD OF DIPLOPIA IN A CASE OF PARALYTIC STRABISMUS

	The patient looks	
Upwards to the left	Upwards	Upwards to the right
Left superior	*Superior median*	*Right superior*
area	*area*	*area*
To the left	Straight ahead	To the right
Left external	*Primary*	*Right external*
area	*area*	*area*
Downwards to the right	Downwards	Downwards to the left
Left inferior	*Inferior median*	*Right inferior*
area	*area*	*area*

the right into the right superior square shows that either the right superior rectus or the left inferior oblique muscle is the one affected. It is only necessary to find to which eye the false image belongs to decide which muscle is paralysed. The higher of the two images indicates the affected eye.

Note that in using this chart the area of greatest vertical diplopia is the namesake of the affected muscle or its true associate in the other eye; further, the true associates always bear names which are the most contrary possible, thus *left inferior oblique* is in every term opposite to *right superior rectus*.

Concomitant strabismus. It has been explained when dealing with paralytic squint that the amount of angular deviation of the two visual axes varies with different positions of the two eyes, and also that secondary deviation is always greater than primary deviation.

In concomitant strabismus, as its name implies, the angular deviation of the visual axes is the same in whatever position the eyes may be; in other words, the primary and secondary deviation are always equal.

The *cover test* is performed as follows. Ask the patient to look at an object immediately in front of him. Suddenly cover the apparently fixing eye and ask the patient to fix the object with the uncovered eye. If this eye makes any movement in taking up fixation, it must have been previously deviating. If now the eye behind the screen (which was previously fixing) is observed it will be seen to deviate in the same relative direction as was the other eye, and *to the same angular amount*, that is the primary and secondary deviation are equal.

The *clinical features* of concomitant strabismus are:
1. It always begins in early childhood, over 70% before the fifth year and the great majority before 3 years of age.
2. The movements of the eyes are good in all directions.
3. Diplopia is practically never a symptom.
4. The primary and secondary deviation are equal.
5. The deviating eye usually has defective vision.

A squint may be *intermittent* or *constant*, and if constant, *monocular* when the same eye deviates whilst the other usually fixes, or *alternating* when either eye fixes indifferently.

Upper motor neuron (supranuclear) lesions
In addition to the defects of movement due to paralysis of the individual ocular muscles, weakness or paralysis of the movement

of both eyes in one direction sometimes occurs. Thus the patient may be unable to look to either side, or upwards or downwards; or the power of convergence alone may be lost. Weakness of conjugate lateral movement may occur in hemiplegia due to cerebral lesions, especially in the acute stage. Palsy of this movement occurs with lesions in the pontine gaze centre, near the vestibular nucleus; the pontine paramedian reticular formation (PPRF); the lesion is on the side to which lateral gaze is weak. Bilateral paralysis of lateral conjugate gaze may occur in centrally placed pontine lesions above the level of the 6th nerve nuclei. Palsies of conjugate upward gaze are always associated with disease of the central parts of the mid brain or inferior thalamic region, or in the neighbourhood of the oculomotor nuclei. Impaired downward gaze is very rare, but occurs with brain stem lesions at a lower level.

If both eyes are kept persistently turned in one direction, the condition is spoken of as tonic or maintained conjugate deviation of the eyes. It is usually either to the right or to the left. It may be due either to a lesion which produces paralysis or to one which causes irritation or spasm. In the former, the eyes (and usually also the head) are turned towards the side of the lesion, provided the lesion is in the cerebral hemisphere. The patient 'looks towards his lesion'. An irritative lesion in a similar situation causes deviation towards the healthy side. If, however, the lesion is in the pons, these rules are reversed, the deviation being towards the sound side in a paralytic lesion and towards the affected side in one which is irritative. Irritative lesions in the brain stem, it should be remembered, are very rare. Assessment of saccadic (rapid, programmed, conjugate, fixation movements) and pursuit (following) movements can be performed separately but localization of abnormalities of these two systems of ocular movement is not yet well understood.

Skew deviation of the eyes—in which, for example, one is directed upwards and the other downwards—occurs in lesions of the labyrinth and in cerebellar disease. Other abnormal ocular movements, such as *ocular bobbing*, *opsoclonus* and *ocular dysmetria* are rare. Abnormal *saccadic* (cogwheel) jerky movements of the eye during voluntary following movements occur in certain diseases of the basal ganglia; they are especially characteristic of *Parkinson's disease*.

Internuclear ophthalmoplegia is due to a lesion which destroys one medial longitudinal fasciculus in the midbrain or upper pons. On attempted lateral gaze there is pronounced rhythmic nystagmus of the abducting eye and impaired medial deviation of the adducting eye. In addition the adducting eye moves more slowly than the contralateral abducting eye. All other gaze movements and the pupils are normal. The lesion is on the side of the impaired adduction, not on the side of the nystagmus. This sign is important because it is common in multiple sclerosis.

The term *nystagmus* is applied to a disturbance of ocular movement characterized by involuntary, often rhythmical oscillations of the eyes. These movements may be horizontal, vertical or rotary. The speed of the movements may be the same in both directions, or quicker in one direction than another; in the latter case the quicker movement indicates the direction of the nystagmus. To examine for nystagmus, ask the patient to look straight in front of him and observe whether the eyes remain steady. Then ask him to look or to follow your finger to his extreme right, then to the left, and then upwards and downwards. Observe the rate, amplitude and rhythm of the movements in each direction. Some forms of nystagmus, particularly that associated with benign epidemic vertigo, and with posterior fossa neoplasms, may be induced only by certain movements of the head (*positional nystagmus*).

A few irregular jerks of the eyes are often seen in full lateral deviation in normal subjects. The brief duration and irregularity of these movements distinguish them from true nystagmus.

Nystagmus is most commonly due to disorders of the vestibular system (either centrally or peripherally), lesions affecting the central pathways concerned in ocular movements, e.g. the medial longitudinal fasciculus, or to weakness of the ocular muscles. Nystagmus may also be induced by certain drugs. Nystagmus of visual origin is pendular and often rotary on central fixation of the eyes. Congenital nystagmus also shows this pendular quality.

Examination of the pupils

The following points must be noted about the pupils in every patient:

Size. Compare the size of the two pupils, first in a bright light and then in a dim light. Note whether the pupils are large or small and whether any irregularity is present. The size of the pupil in health is very variable. As a rule, the pupils are larger in dark eyes than in light and they tend to be small in elderly subjects. Slight inequality of the pupils may also be present in perfectly healthy subjects.

If one pupil is larger than the other, one must decide which is the normal. This is not always very easily answered, but the pupil which is less mobile is usually the abnormal one.

Shape.   Note whether the pupil is circular in outline, as it should be, or whether its contour is irregular. Such irregularities may be due to adhesion of the iris to the lens, as a result of an old iritis, or to neurosyphilis.

Mobility.   The *reaction to light* is a reflex. The afferent fibres involved are contained in the optic nerve, travelling to the oculomotor nuclei whence the efferent fibres pass by the 3rd nerve, through the ciliary ganglion, to the pupillary sphincter.

Examine each eye separately. Place the patient opposite a bright light, be sure his accommodation is relaxed and cover the eye with the hand. Leave it covered until the pupil dilates, then withdraw the hand and watch the pupil closely. It should contract almost immediately, then dilate again a little, and, after undergoing slight oscillations, settle down to its normal size. The test may also be carried out by shining a bright light into one eye and then the other.

Owing to the decussation of some of the fibres in the optic nerves at the optic chiasm, light shone into one eye stimulates the brain stem nuclei (3rd nerve) concerned with pupillary constriction bilaterally. This pathway is pregeniculate. As a consequence, if light is shut off from one eye both pupils dilate, and if bright light is made to enter one eye both pupils contract. This is known as the *consensual reaction* of the pupils. It should be tested by keeping one eye in the shade while the other is tested. The effect on the pupil of the shaded eye is then observed.

Reaction to accommodation. The pupils become smaller on accommodating for a near object (*miosis*). Convergence of the eyes, accommodation and miosis are due to closely related reflexes.

Hold up one finger close to the patient's nose. Ask him to look away at a distant object. Then ask him to look quickly at your finger. As the eyes converge to accomplish this the pupils become smaller. If the patient is blind, the test may still be carried out by getting him to hold up his own finger about a foot in front of his face, and then asking him to 'look at the finger'.

The *Argyll Robertson pupil* is the classical pupillary abnormality in neurosyphilis. The term is used to describe a pupil which is small and irregular, and which reacts briskly to accommodation but which does not react to light directly or consensually. The pupil dilates slowly or imperfectly to atropine. The abnormality is typically bilateral but it is frequently more obvious on one side.

Hippus is a term applied to alternate rhythmic dilatation and constriction of the pupil, either in response to light or spontaneously. It is rarely of clinical significance, although it may be unusually prominent in cases of retrobulbar neuritis, when it is usually accompanied by slow dilatation of the pupil, despite continuing illumination. This is known as an *afferent pupillary defect* (Gunn pupil).

Adie's pupil is an abnormality characterized by absent or delayed pupillary constriction with light or with accommodation/convergence. Once constricted the pupil dilates only very slowly, either in response to darkness or to far gaze. The abnormality is thus variable and this has led to its confusion with the Argyll Robertson syndrome. The pupil in Adie's syndrome varies in size from day to day but *never* reacts promptly to light. It is frequently unilateral and sometimes associated with absent tendon reflexes, often on the same side (Holmes–Adie syndrome). The distinction between the Argyll Robertson and Adie pupillary abnormalities is important since the latter, probably due to parasympathetic denervation, is usually of no clinical significance. The distinction may be made by instillation of sterile 2% methacholine into the conjunctival sac: the Adie pupil constricts but the Argyll Robertson pupil does not.

Paralysis of the cervical sympathetic (Horner's syndrome). The sympathetic nerve fibres supplying the pupil take origin in the lower cervical and upper thoracic regions of the spinal cord (ciliospinal centre), from which they emerge in the first thoracic nerve roots and pass to the sympathetic cord by the rami communicantes. From the cervical sympathetic chain the fibres pass along the internal carotid to the cavernous plexus, and thence via the ophthalmic division of the 5th to the eyeball. They convey the impulses which cause dilatation of the pupil and also supply the unstriped muscle in the insertion of the levator palpebrae into the upper lid.

Paralysis of the cervical sympathetic is recognized by the following signs: apparent enophthalmos; slight drooping of the upper lid, due to paralysis of the unstriped muscle fibres contained in it; contraction of the pupil with absence of dilatation on shading the eye or on instillation of cocaine; abolition of the ciliospinal reflex; and, less commonly, absence of sweating on the corresponding half of the face and neck, both in front and behind, extending as low as the 3rd rib and 3rd thoracic spine, and over the whole of the upper limb on the same side.

Dilatation of the normal pupil when the skin of the neck is pinched is due to reflex excitation of the pupil dilating fibres in the cervical sympathetic, and is abolished by lesions of that nerve and by some medullary cervical and upper thoracic cord lesions.

FIFTH OR TRIGEMINAL NERVE

Anatomy.   The *sensory root* takes origin from nerve cells in the Gasserian ganglion and enters the lateral surface of the pons at about its middle. The fibres which conduct impulses for light touch and postural sensibility terminate in a large nucleus in the pons situated lateral to the motor nucleus near the floor of the 4th ventricle, while the fibres for pain and thermal sensibility terminate in the 'descending' or bulbospinal root, which extends as low down as the 2nd cervical segment of the cord. Immediately distal to the trigeminal ganglion the nerve separates into its three divisions.

The *first or ophthalmic division* supplies the conjunctiva (except that of the lower lid), the lacrimal gland, the mesial part of the skin of the nose as far as its tip, the upper eyelids, the forehead, and the scalp as far as the vertex.

Lesions of this division result in loss of cutaneous and corneal sensibility and may cause trophic changes in the cornea, *neuropathic keratitis*. The corneal reflex is abolished.

The *second or maxillary division* supplies the cheek, the front of the temple, the lower eyelid and its conjunctiva, the side of the nose, the upper lip, the upper teeth, the mucous membrane of the nose, the upper part of the pharynx, the roof of the mouth, most of the soft palate, and the tonsils.

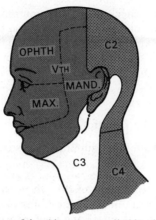

Fig. 8.11 Lateral view of the skin area supplied by the Vth cranial nerve and the 2nd, 3rd and 4th cervical segments.

Lesions of this division lead to loss of sensation in the above area and sometimes to loss of the palatal reflex.

The *third or mandibular division* is joined by the motor root. It supplies sensation to the lower part of the face, the lower lip, the ear, the tongue, and the lower teeth. It also supplies parasympathetic fibres to the salivary glands. The motor division supplies the muscles of mastication.

The *motor root* takes origin in a small nucleus lying medial to the chief sensory nucleus, and partly also from the mesencephalic root, which arises in the nerve cells scattered around the cerebral aqueduct. It emerges at the side of the pons, just anterior to the sensory division, passes underneath the trigeminal ganglion, and joins the mandibular division.

Paralysis of the whole 5th nerve leads to loss of sensation in the skin and mucous membrane of the face and nasopharynx as described above (Fig. 8.11). The salivary, buccal and lacrimal secretions may be much diminished and trophic lesions may be present. Taste is preserved, but lack of secretions may result in its subjective impairment.

Testing the motor functions

Ask the patient to clench his teeth: the temporal and masseter muscles should stand out with equal prominence on each side.

This is a sign better checked by palpation than by inspection. If there is paralysis on one side, the muscles on that side will fail to become prominent and, on opening the mouth, the jaw will deviate towards the paralysed side being pushed over by the healthy lateral pterygoid muscles.

Testing the sensory functions

The sensibility of the area supplied is tested in the usual way (p. 327).

Taste.   In suspected lesions of the 5th nerve the sense of taste should always be examined. These fibres pass from the lingual nerve into the chorda tympani and thence through the geniculate ganglion of the facial nerve and the nervus intermedius into the medulla oblongata. Rarely, these taste fibres may enter the brain stem with fibres in the maxillary division of the trigeminal nerve, rather than through the chorda tympani and the facial nerve. The taste fibres from the posterior third of the tongue enter by the glossopharyngeal nerve.

All the taste fibres enter the tractus solitarius and relay in the nucleus of the tract, whence further fibres pass upward in the gustatory fillets to the thalamus and thence to the foot of the post central gyrus. *Ageusia* or loss of taste occurs with lesions of the peripheral pathways concerned or with centrally placed pontine lesions which may involve the gustatory lemniscus.

To test the sense of taste, use strong solutions of sugar and common salt, and weak solutions of citric acid and quinine. These are applied by a glass rod to the surface of the protruded tongue and if the taste is recognized the patient writes down 'sweet', 'salt', 'sour' or 'bitter', as the case may be, *without* withdrawing the tongue. After each test the mouth must be rinsed. The quinine test should be applied last, as its effect is more lasting than that of the others. Both the anterior and posterior parts of the tongue should be tested. Taste may also be assessed using a weak galvanic current, Loss of taste may arise from lesions of the taste fibres in any part of their course. In addition to loss of taste, one should always ask the patient whether he has any abnormal taste sensations. These may form the aura of an epileptic fit, as in temporal lobe epilepsy.

Testing the corneal reflex

Twist a light wisp of cotton wool or cotton thread into a fine hair and lightly touch the lateral edge of the cornea at its conjunctival margin with the wisp, having asked the patient to gaze into the distance or at the ceiling. If the reflex is present the patient blinks. It is helpful to steady the hand by gently resting the little finger on the patient's cheek. The two sides should be compared. This can sometimes be done more easily by lightly blowing a puff of air into each cornea in turn. The cornea should not be wiped with the cotton and the central part of the cornea should never be touched, since to do so in the presence of corneal anaesthesia carries the risk of corneal ulceration and subsequent scarring.

SEVENTH OR FACIAL NERVE

Anatomy. The course of the fibres from the cortex to the nucleus of this nerve has already been described (p. 257). The nucleus is situated in the pons lateral to that of the 6th nerve. On leaving the nucleus the fibres wind round the nucleus of the 6th, and emerge medial to the 8th nerve, between the olive and restiform bodies.

The nerve then lies in close contact with the 8th and enters the internal auditory meatus with it so that a lesion of the one at this part often also affects the other. During its course through the temporal lobe, in close proximity to the aditus of the tympanic antrum, it gives off a branch to the stapedius muscle. It is joined by the chorda tympani which contains taste fibres from the anterior two-thirds of the tongue at the geniculate ganglion. In this part of its course the nerve is vulnerable to trauma and to oedema, since it is enclosed in a bony tube. It emerges at a point opposite the junction of the anterior border of the mastoid with the ear, and spreads out on the side of the face to supply the facial muscles.

Functions. The 7th is almost entirely a motor nerve. It supplies all the muscles of the face and scalp, except the levator palpebrae superioris. It also supplies the platysma. The chorda tympani travels with the facial nerve during part of its course and taste may therefore be lost on the anterior two-thirds of the tongue with lesions of the proximal part of the nerve. There is sometimes a small area of altered cutaneous sensation at the auricle in such cases.

Effects of paralysis.   These are usually at once seen on looking at the patient. The affected side of the face has lost its expression. The nasolabial fold is less pronounced, the furrows of the brow are smoothed out, the eye is *more* widely open than the other, and the mouth is somewhat drawn to the healthy side. The patient is unable to whistle; food is apt to collect between his teeth and his gums, and saliva and any fluid he drinks may escape from the affected angle of the mouth.

Testing the seventh nerve

1. Ask the patient to shut his eyes as tightly as he can. Note that the affected eye is either not closed at all—in which case the eyeball rolls upwards to make up for the failure of the lid to descend (*Bell's phenomenon*)—or, if the eye is closed, the eyelashes are not so much buried in the face as on the healthy side. Try also to open the eyes while the patient attempts to keep them closed. If the orbicularis is acting normally, it should be almost impossible to open them against the patient's wish.

The effect of screwing the eyes tightly shut causes the corners of the mouth to be drawn upwards. In paralysis of the lower part of the face, the corner on the affected side is either not drawn up at all, or not so much as on the healthy side.

2. Ask the patient to whistle. He is unable to do so.

3. Ask him to smile or show his upper teeth. The mouth is then drawn to the healthy side.

4. Ask him to inflate his mouth with air and blow out his cheeks. Tap with the finger in turn on each inflated cheek. Air can be made to escape from the mouth more easily on the weak or paralysed side.

5. Test the sense of taste on the anterior part of the tongue.

Remember that *bilateral* facial weakness is difficult to recognize.

Signs of paralysis of the facial nerve in different parts of its course

Paralysis of the face presents different symptoms depending on whether the lesion is situated above the nucleus, at the nucleus or below it. The former constitutes upper motor neurone or *supranuclear facial paralysis*, the latter lower motor neurone or *infranuclear paralysis*.

The chief difference between the two forms is that in *supranuclear paralysis* the lower part of the face is chiefly affected; in *infranuclear paralysis* both the upper and lower parts are equally involved. This is because there is bilateral innervation of the muscles of the upper part of the face; a unilateral lesion, therefore, will only cause partial paralysis of one side. Sometimes a supranuclear lesion only affects the fibres concerned in emotional movement and this function should be assessed separately from voluntary movement. Taste is not affected in supranuclear lesions.

Infranuclear facial paralysis may be produced by a lesion of the nucleus or of the facial nerve itself.

A lesion inside the facial canal—unless it is towards the outer end—involves the fibres of the chorda tympani and therefore produces loss of taste sensation in the anterior two-thirds of the tongue.

Lesions of the nucleus or the nerve below it will result in atrophy of the facial muscles. Supranuclear lesions do not produce this effect.

Abnormal facial movements

The muscles supplied by the facial nerve are frequently affected by spasm or spasmodic movements. These may involve all the facial muscles, or groups of them only. The spasm may be either clonic or tonic. If present, the nature of the movements, their extent, the muscles affected by them, and any factors which modify them should be carefully noted.

THE EIGHTH OR VESTIBULOCOCHLEAR NERVE

Anatomy. This nerve consists of two sets of fibres. One supplies the cochlea and subserves the function of hearing; the other supplies the vestibule and semicircular canals and is the nerve of equilibration. The *auditory* fibres, which arise from the cochlear ganglion, enter the brain stem at the lower border of the pons and are distributed to the dorsal and ventral cochlear nuclei. The *vestibular* fibres take origin from the vestibular ganglion, and terminate in a group of nuclei in the pons and medulla.

The secondary auditory tracts, after partial decussation, terminate in the inferior colliculi and the medial geniculate bodies, and another system, that takes origin from these, passes through the internal capsule to the cortical centre for hearing, in the 1st and 2nd temporosphenoidal convolutions. Sounds received in one ear reach the opposite hemisphere of the brain, but owing to the partial decussation of the secondary auditory tracts neither unilateral cerebral nor brain stem lesions produce deafness in one ear.

The vestibular nerve is closely connected with the cerebellum. It also has cerebral connections.

Tests of hearing

Before testing a patient's hearing, exclude the presence of wax in the ear. This done, hearing can be tested with a slight sound such as that produced by rubbing the fingers lightly together, or by the ticking of a watch. Ask the patient to shut his eyes. Begin outside the probable range of hearing and bring the sound gradually nearer the ear, asking the patient to speak when he hears it. It is necessary to know at what distance the sound should be audible to a healthy ear. Test each ear separately, keeping one closed with your finger tip whilst the other is being examined.

If impairment of hearing is detected, it must be determined whether it is really due to disease of the vestibulocochlear nerve or merely to some affection of the middle ear. In order to settle this point, the *tuning-fork* test may be employed. When the fork is sounding strongly, hold it opposite the ear; if it can be heard, then place its base on the mastoid process in order to determine if its vibrations can be heard when conducted through bone. If the patient hears this, ask him to compare the relative loudness of the fork when heard through air and through bone, or to determine which can be heard the longer as the vibrations die out. This is *Rinne's test*. Normally, aerially conducted sounds are louder to the patient than those conducted through bone. In middle ear disease, air conduction is diminished or lost, while bone conduction remains normal. When the auditory nerve is affected, both air and bone conduction are diminished or lost.

Weber's test, though less reliable than Rinne's, should also be used. Strike a tuning-fork and place the end of it against the centre of the patient's forehead. If the deafness discovered by the watch or sound of the fingers rubbing together is due to an affection of the middle ear, the patient will hear the tuning-fork better on that side than on the healthy one. On the other hand, if the deafness is due to disease of the auditory nerve, the tuning-fork will only be heard on the healthy side. The test may also be carried out by means of the watch. In affections of the nerve, sounds will not be heard even close to the ear; in disease of the middle ear, they may be heard even more loudly than when similarly applied to the healthy side.

These tests are frequently unreliable.

Other points in favour of the deafness being due to a lesion of the nerve and not to disease of the middle ear are: (*a*) if the hearing is better in a quiet place; (*b*) if conversation is heard better than other sounds; and (*c*) if inflation of the middle ear renders the hearing worse.

Abnormal auditory sensations

The patient may complain of 'ringing in the ears' (*tinnitus*). The precise character of the sound varies in different cases. It may be of a humming, buzzing, hammering or whistling character. The presence or absence of this symptom should always be inquired for, and if present, whether it is constant, or in what circumstances it occurs. It is only rarely of diagnostic significance in neurological disease.

Hyperacusis, a disorder in which even slight sounds are heard with painful intensity, sometimes occurs when there is paralysis of the stapedius muscle due to a facial nerve palsy.

Hallucinations of sound may also be present, the patient fancying that he hears voices, bells etc. These occur chiefly in the psychoses, but they sometimes arise as epileptic aura when the causal lesion is situated in or near the auditory cortex.

Tests for vertigo

The patient will usually describe this as *giddiness* or *dizziness*. In order to constitute true vertigo, external objects should seem to move round him. Ask if this is the case and, if so, in what direction the objects seem to move. Ask also whether the vertigo causes him to fall to the ground. The distinction between giddiness and true vertigo is rarely of great importance. Both may occur in disease of the vestibular system and one should look, therefore, for signs of disease of the ear, 8th nerve or brain stem.

THE NINTH (GLOSSOPHARYNGEAL), TENTH (VAGUS) AND ELEVENTH (ACCESSORY) NERVES

Anatomy. The ninth, tenth and eleventh nerves arise, in order from above downwards, in an elongated nucleus in the floor of the 4th ventricle. They emerge by several roots along the lateral aspect of the medulla, beginning above in the groove between the olive and restiform bodies. The spinal part of the 11th emerges from the lateral column of the cord, beginning as low as the 6th cervical nerve; it passes up through the foramen magnum to join the medullary (accessory) part, and emerges with it through the jugular foramen. After emerging, its two divisions separate, the medullary or accessory portion joining the vagus and supplying motor fibres to the larynx and pharynx.

The glossopharyngeal nerve

The ninth (glossopharyngeal) is sensory for the posterior third of the tongue and for the mucous membrane of the pharynx. It is motor for the middle constrictor of the pharynx and for the stylopharyngeus. It contains the taste fibres for the posterior of the tongue (p. 304).

The 9th nerve is rarely paralysed alone. Paralysis can best be diagnosed by examining its sensory and reflex functions. Examine taste in the posterior part of the tongue (p. 304). Loss of it may occur with a lesion of the trunk of the glossopharyngeal nerve.

Tickle the back of the pharynx, and note if reflex contraction occurs. This is also a test of the vagus (below).

The vagus nerve

The *tenth* (vagus) is motor for the soft palate (with the exception of the tensor palati), pharynx and larynx. It is sensory and motor for the respiratory passages, the heart and (through the parasympathetic ganglia) for most of the abdominal viscera. The fibres for the soft palate, pharynx and larynx take origin in the nucleus ambiguus, emerge in the upper roots of the 11th, reach the pharyngeal plexus, and thence pass to the muscles of the palate, the constrictors of the pharynx, and to the larynx. The visceromotor and the cardio-inhibitory fibres are derived from the dorsal vagus nucleus in the floor of the 4th ventricle.

Paralysis of the vagus is obvious clinically only through its palatine and laryngeal branches.

The palate. Ask the patient whether he notices regurgitation of fluids through his nose when he tries to swallow. This is a common symptom in total paralysis of the soft palate, owing to defective elevation during swallowing. For a similar reason the patient is unable to pronounce words which require complete closure of the naso-pharynx. Thus 'egg' is sounded as 'eng', 'rub' becomes 'rum', and so on. In unilateral paralysis these symptoms are not observed.

For direct examination of the soft palate, place the patient facing the light with his mouth open and introduce a tongue depressor. The position of the uvula is unreliable, as deviation is not uncommon even in health. One must watch the movements of the palate during phonation. Ask the patient to say 'Ah!' and observe whether both sides of the palate arch upwards. If one side is paralysed, it will remain flat and immobile and the median raphe will be pulled towards the other side. In bilateral paralysis the whole palate remains motionless.

Remember that minor degrees of asymmetry of the palate and of the tongue occur as part of a hemiparesis due to an upper motor neurone lesion. This is not what is meant by palatal palsy since in the latter the lesion is invariably of lower motor neurone type.

The larynx. The superior laryngeal branch of the vagus is sensory for the larynx above the level of the true vocal cords and is motor for the cricothyroid muscle. Unilateral paralysis of the nerve does not produce any symptoms. Bilateral paralysis causes the vocal cords to be relaxed. The voice is therefore hoarse and deep and the utterance of high notes is impossible.

The recurrent laryngeal branch supplies sensation to the larynx below the level of the vocal cords and motor fibres to all the laryngeal muscles except the cricothyroid. Paralysis leads to appearances which can be recognized with the laryngoscope and which are described on p. 402. *The speech is characteristically blurred and ineffectual* and the patient cannot cough clearly. Bilateral paralysis may cause serious stridor or even respiratory obstruction.

The accessory nerve

The *eleventh* (accessory) nerve is purely motor in function, contributing to the innervation of the larynx and pharynx as well as the sternomastoid and trapezius. The spinal part of the nerve dips below the sternomastoid muscle about 2 cm below the tip of the mastoid process and re-emerges from underneath that muscle at about the middle of its posterior border. It supplies the sternomastoid and trapezius, which are also supplied by twigs from the cervical plexus.

Paralysis of the upper part of the trapezius is demonstrated by asking the patient to shrug his shoulders while the examiner presses downward on them. Paralysis of the sternomastoid causes weakness of rotation of the chin towards the opposite side.

THE TWELFTH (HYPOGLOSSAL) NERVE

Anatomy.   The twelfth nerve arises from a nucleus in the lower part of the floor of the fourth ventricle, close to the midline. It emerges between the anterior pyramid and the olive. It is a purely motor nerve, supplying the tongue and the depressors of the hyoid bone.

Test.   Ask the patient to put out his tongue as far as possible. If the hypoglossal is paralysed the tongue, instead of being protruded straight, is pushed over to the paralysed side. Be careful not to mistake an apparent deviation of the tongue, really due to the mouth being twisted to one side, for a real deviation. Such an apparent deviation occurs in facial paralysis. Ask the patient to move his tongue from side to side, and to lick each cheek with it; observe whether he can do so freely. Strength may also be assessed by pressing against the tongue with a finger as the patient protrudes it into each cheek in turn. Note whether there is any wasting of the tongue, and whether there is any tremor or fasciculation of it. The presence of wasting indicates that the lesion is either nuclear or infranuclear (lower motor neurone). Fasciculation must be assessed with the tongue relaxed in the mouth, not when protruded.

MOTOR FUNCTIONS

The motor system should be examined with the following aspects of motor function in mind:
  1. Bulk of muscles

2. Tone of muscles
3. Strength of muscles
4. Reflexes
5. Coordination of movement
6. Gait
7. Involuntary movements

BULK OF MUSCLES

The bulk of the muscles is most easily estimated by inspection and palpation. Wasted or atrophic muscles are not only smaller, but also softer and more flabby than normal when they are contracted. When muscular wasting is accompanied by fibrosis, as in muscular dystrophy or polymyositis, the muscles feel hard and inelastic; they become shortened and it is not possible to stretch them passively to a normal degree. *Contracture* is then said to be present. Contractures may also occur as a result of prolonged hypertonia in a group of muscles.

Muscular atrophy is not only caused by neurological disorders. Generalized muscular wasting is seen in cachexia of any cause. Localized muscle atrophy may be due to injury or disease of a joint; this occurs, for example, in the thenar muscles in association with arthritis of the 1st metacarpophalangeal joint or in the quadriceps in patients with diseases of the knee. In such instances strength is well preserved in relation to the degree of muscular wasting. Some patients with *muscular dystrophy* develop large muscles (pseudohypertrophy) due to pathological changes in the muscles themselves. The calves, buttocks and infraspinati are particularly affected. These enlarged muscles are weak in spite of their size.

TONE OF MUSCLES

Muscular tone is a state of tension or contraction found in healthy muscles. An increase in tone is called *hypertonia* and a diminution *hypotonia*. The degree of tone is estimated by handling the limbs and moving them passively at their various joints. The maintenance of tone is dependent on a spinal reflex arc: afferent fibres from the primary and secondary endings of the muscle spindles entering the spinal cord and synapsing with the anterior horn cells, from which efferent fibres arise and pass to the muscles. Tone is diminished or lost if this reflex arc is damaged. *Hypotonia* therefore occurs in affections of the lower motor neurone, of the afferent sensory pathways, as in tabes, and in cerebellar disease in which suprasegmental mechanisms are abnormal. Tone may be reduced in sleep and by certain drugs.

Muscle tone is also regulated by corticospinal and extrapyramidal pathways.

Hypertonia following lesions of the corticospinal system (upper motor neurone lesions) is termed *spasticity* and it has a characteristic distribution; the upper limbs are held in flexion and the lower limbs in extension with the feet in plantar flexion (physiological extension). Spasticity is a term which should only be used to describe a state of increased tone which is of 'clasp-knife' type when the limb is fairly rapidly flexed or extended. These are the lengthening and shortenings reactions described by Sherrington. Spasticity is therefore a form of rigidity which is *stretch sensitive*. Moreover it can usually be shown that the degree of increased tone developed during any given passive stretch is velocity-dependent, i.e. it is proportional to the speed of the applied stretch.

Hypertonia resulting from disease of the basal ganglia is termed *extrapyramidal rigidity*. The hypertonia is more uniform, but often it is so distributed as to produce a general attitude of flexion of the limbs and trunk as in Parkinson's disease. The resistance to passive movement is regularly or irregularly variable and is aptly described as like a lever rubbing on the teeth of a cogwheel (cogwheel rigidity). It can usually be enhanced by asking the patient to clench his fist on the opposite side. Sometimes a plastic type of rigidity is found in which the resistance developed to passive movement is uniform during all phases of the applied movement. This is often referred to as *paratonic rigidity* or '*Gegenhalten*'. It is found in catatonic states, in patients with clouded or confused intellects from any cause and, commonly, in dementia. It should not be regarded simply as evidence of 'lack of cooperation'. Its physiological basis is unknown. In *hysterical rigidity* the resistance to passive movement increases in proportion to the effort applied by the examiner. The increased resistance is usually developed in a characteristically jerky fashion.

When the muscles are *hypotonic*, there is little or no resistance to passive movement of the limb and when handled or shaken the unsupported part flops about inertly. Hypotonic muscles are abnormally soft to palpation. The outstretched hypotonic upper limb may assume an abnormal posture, as in cerebellar disease or chorea. It is hyperextended at the elbow, the forearm is over-pronated, the wrist flexed, and the fingers hyperextended at the metacarpophalangeal joints.

STRENGTH OF MUSCLES

Much the quickest and most reliable method of making a quick or preliminary assessment is to watch the patient walking, jumping, hopping, standing up from lying and sitting positions and dressing or undressing. These movements require proximal and distal strength and coordination of a considerable degree and much can be learnt by observing them carefully. The strength of individual muscles can then be assessed as required. Each movement made during this assessment is tested by comparison with the examiner's own strength or by comparison with what he judges to be normal in a person of comparable build to the patient. It therefore requires practice and experience. It will be found that very simple requests produce better results than long explanations: a demonstration or gesture is often more effective than any verbal explanation. Remember that most patients have no knowledge of anatomy.

Testing the muscles of the upper limb

Abductor pollicis brevis.   This is an important muscle as it is supplied by the median nerve which is commonly damaged by compression in the carpal tunnel at the wrist. The patient is asked to abduct his thumb in a plane at right angles to the palmar aspect of the index finger. The muscle can be seen and felt to contract.

Opponens pollicis.   Ask the patient to touch the tip of his little finger with the point of this thumb.

First dorsal interosseous.   Ask the patient to abduct his index finger against resistance.

Interossei and lumbricals.   Test the patient's ability to flex his metacarpophalangeal joints and to extend the distal inter-phalangeal joints. The interossei also adduct and abduct the fingers. When these muscles are paralysed and power is retained in the long flexors and extensors of the fingers, a claw-hand or deformity is produced. The first phalanges are overextended and the distal two are flexed. The fingers are slightly separated.

Flexors of the fingers. Ask the patient to squeeze your fingers. Allow him to squeeze only your index and middle fingers—this is sufficient to assess strength of grip without his painfully crushing your fingers.

Flexors of the wrist. Ask him to bring the tips of his fingers towards the front of the forearm.

Extensors of the wrist. Ask the patient to make a fist, a movement which results in firm contraction of both the flexors and extensors of the wrists, and try to forcibly flex the wrist against his effort to maintain his posture. It should be almost impossible to overcome the wrist extensors of a healthy man or woman. The wrist flexors can be similarly tested.

Slight weakness of the extensors of the wrist may be elicited by asking the patient to grasp something firmly in his hand. If the extensors are weak the wrist becomes flexed as he does so, because the flexor muscles are then stronger than the extensors.

Weakness or paralysis of the extensors of the wrist as in radial nerve palsy leads to *wrist-drop*.

Brachioradialis. Place the arm midway between the prone and supine positions; then ask the patient to bend up the forearm, whilst you oppose the movement by grasping the hand. The muscle, if healthy, will be seen and felt to stand out prominently at its upper part.

Biceps. Ask the patient to bend up the forearm against resistance, with the forearm in full supination. The muscle will stand out clearly.

Triceps. Ask the patient to straighten out his forearm against your resistance.

Supraspinatus. Ask the patient to lift his arm straight out at right angles to his side. The first 30° of this movement is carried out by the supraspinatus. The remaining 60° is produced by the deltoid.

Deltoid. The anterior and posterior fibres help to draw the abducted arm forwards and backwards respectively.

Infraspinatus. The patient is asked to tuck his elbow into his side with the forearm flexed to a right angle. He is then asked to rotate the limb outwards against the examiner's resistance, the elbow being held against the side throughout. The muscle can be seen and felt to contract.

Pectorals. Ask the patient to stretch his arms out in front of him, and then to clap his hands while the observer endeavours to hold them apart.

Serratus anterior. When this muscle is paralysed the scapula is 'winged', the vertebral border projecting. The patient is unable to elevate his arm above a right angle, the deformity becoming more apparent as he tries to do so. Pushing forwards with the hands against resistance, such as a wall also brings out the deformity.

Latissimus dorsi. The patient is asked to clasp his hands behind his back while the observer, standing behind the patient, offers passive resistance to the downward and backward movement; alternatively the two posterior axillary folds can be felt as the patient coughs.

Testing the muscles of the trunk

Weakness of the muscles of the abdomen is shown by the patient's inability to sit up in bed from the supine position without the aid of his arms. *Babinski's 'rising up sign'* consists in making the patient lie on his back with the legs extended and rise up without using his hands. In organic spastic paralysis of a leg the affected limb will rise first, but in hysterical paralysis this does not occur.

Paralysis of a portion of the anterior abdominal wall can be detected by the displacement of the umbilicus that occurs when the patient attempts to lift up his head from the pillow against resistance. With paralysis of the lower segment the umbilicus moves upwards, but when the upper segment is affected the umbilicus is pulled downwards. This is sometimes known as *Beevor's* sign: it is a useful sign since it may indicate the level of a lesion in spinal cord disease.

To test the *erector spinae* and muscles of the back, make the patient lie on his face and try to raise his head from the bed by extending the neck and back. If the back muscles are healthy, they will be seen to stand out prominently during this effort.

The method of detecting paralysis of the *diaphragm* has already been described (p. 187).

The *trapezius* is tested in its upper part by asking the patient to shrug his shoulders while the observer tries to press them down from behind. In its lower part it can be tested by asking him to approximate the shoulder blades.

The cranial musculature has already been described (p. 275).

Testing the muscles of the lower limb

The intrinsic muscles of the foot cannot be easily examined. When the interossei are weakened or paralysed a 'claw-foot', analogous to the 'claw-hand', may develop. Rarely this deformity occurs in patients with spastic hemiparesis of very long duration; this is due to a form of dystonia and not to muscular weakness.

Dorsiflexion and *plantar flexion* of the feet and toes are tested by asking the patient to elevate or depress the part against resistance.

Extensors of knee. Bend up the patient's knee, and then, pressing with your hand on his shin, ask him to try to straighten it out again.

Flexors of knee. Raise the leg up from the bed, supporting the thigh with your left hand, holding the ankle with your right. Then ask the patient to bend his knee.

Extensors of the thigh. The knee being extended, lift the patient's foot off the bed, and ask him to push it down against resistance. If the extensors of the hip are paralysed he will be unable to do so.

Flexors of the thigh. With the leg extended ask the patient to raise his leg off the bed against resistance.

Adductors of the thigh. Abduct the limb and then ask the patient to bring it back to the middle line against resistance.

Abductors of the thigh. Place the patient's legs together and ask him to separate them against resistance.

Rotators of the thigh. With the lower limb extended on the bed, ask the patient to roll it outwards or inwards against resistance.

Grading of weakness. The Medical Research Council Scale is usually used to grade muscle weakness:

Grade 0	Complete paralysis
Grade 1	A flicker of contraction only
Grade 2	Power detectable only when gravity is excluded by appropriate postural adjustment
Grade 3	The limb can be held against the force of gravity, but not against the examiner's resistance
Grade 4	There is some degree of weakness, usually described as poor, fair or moderate strength
Grade 5	Normal power is present

The term *hemiplegia* is applied to a condition in which there is paralysis of one side of the body, especially of the arm and leg, and usually also of the face. If the paralysis of the arm and leg is on one side, and that of some of the muscles supplied by the motor cranial nerves on the other, the condition is one of *crossed paralysis*. This is a sign of disease in the brain stem. The term *paraplegia* is applied to a paralysis of both legs; the term *monoplegia* to a paralysis of one limb, which may be the arm (*brachial monoplegia*) or the leg (*crural monoplegia*). In *quadriplegia* all four limbs are weak.

The detection of hemiplegia in a patient who is comatose may be difficult. However, if the paralysis is of recent onset, one can usually detect hypotonia in the paralysed limbs. If his arm, for example, is raised from his side and allowed to drop, it falls, if it is paralysed, as if it did not belong to him; the sound arm also falls, but not in such an utterly limp fashion. The face is asymmetrical, the angle of the mouth more open on the paralysed side, and the affected cheek moves loosely outwards and inwards with respiration. The abdominal and tendon reflexes may be absent on both sides, but an extensor plantar response can usually be obtained on the hemiplegic side (see Reflexes, p. 312).

Myasthenic weakness

In *myasthenia gravis* weakness, which commonly affects the external ocular and bulbar muscles more than the rest of the skeletal musculature, is characteristically exacerbated or provoked by pro-longed contraction or exercise of the affected muscles. The degree of detectable weakness therefore varies during the course of the day. This is referred to as *myasthenic weakness*. A similar form of weakness in which there is an initial increase of strength with contraction, occurs as a rare phenomenon in carcinomatous neuromyopathies.

Myotonia

In certain myopathies and muscular dystrophies, of which *dys-trophia myotonica* is the best known, relaxation after contraction of muscle is impaired. The phenomenon is worse when the affected muscles are cold and it is therefore often best demonstrated in the hand. Ask the patient to grip your hand firmly and then let go *suddenly*. His grasp is maintained for a moment and then is slowly and gradually released. Myotonia can be demonstrated in the tongue and in other muscles, e.g. the thenar eminence, by lightly striking the muscle with a small patellar hammer. A dimple of contraction appears and relaxes only slowly.

REFLEXES

Tendon reflexes

If the tendon of a lightly stretched muscle is struck a single, sharp blow with a soft rubber hammer (thus suddenly stretching the muscle and exciting a synchronous volley of afferent impulses from the primary sensory endings of the muscle spindles in the stretched muscle), the muscle contracts briefly. This is the monosynaptic stretch reflex. It is a test of the integrity of the afferent and efferent pathways, and of the excitability of the anterior horn cells in the spinal segment of the stretched muscle. Properly performed, examination of the tendon reflexes offers a reliable and reproduc-ible method of assessment of the integrity of this system of neurones and their higher connections, and it is therefore very important to become skilled in the techniques for eliciting these reflexes.

Always use the same type of hammer; always examine these reflexes in the same manner, standing on the same side of the bed:

always make sure the patient is warm and comfortable and re-assure him that the hammer is soft and not an offensive weapon. When examining the tendon reflexes in the legs care taken to allow the patient's genitalia to be properly covered is repaid by more easily elicitable reflexes. The patient should be asked to relax or to 'let the muscles go to sleep'.

Knee jerk. The knee jerk is the best known of the tendon reflexes. The patellar hammer derives its name from its invention as an instrument for eliciting this reflex, the first tendon reflex to become a regular part of the neurological examination. The knee jerk consists of a contraction of the quadriceps when the patellar tendon is tapped. The spinal segments concerned are the 2nd, 3rd and 4th lumbar. It is best tested with the patient supine. The examiner's hand is passed under the knee to be tested and placed upon the opposite knee; the knee to be tested rests on the dorsum of the observer's wrist. The patellar tendon is struck midway between its origin and insertion. Following the blow there will be a brief extension of the knee from contraction of the quadriceps. The reflex can sometimes be more easily elicited with the patient sitting up, his legs dangling freely over the edge of the bed.

The briskness of the knee jerk varies greatly in different indi-viduals. In health it is hardly ever entirely absent. Sometimes, as in the case of the other tendon reflexes, one is unable to elicit it without applying *reinforcement* (Jendrassik's manoeuvre). This is done by asking the patient to make some strong voluntary muscu-lar effort with the upper limbs; for example to hook the fingers of the two hands together and then to pull them against one another as hard as possible. While he is doing this, a further attempt is made to elicit the knee jerk. Reinforcement acts by increasing the excitability of the anterior horn cells, and by increasing the sen-sitivity of the muscle spindle primary sensory endings to stretch (by increased gamma fusimotor drive).

Ankle jerk. Place the lower limb on the bed so that it lies everted and slightly flexed. Then, with one hand, slightly dorsiflex the foot so as to stretch the Achilles tendon and, with the other hand, strike the tendon on its posterior surface. A sharp contraction of the calf muscles results. This reflex can also be conveniently elicited when the patient is kneeling on a chair. It depends upon the 1st and 2nd sacral segments.

Triceps jerk.   Flex the elbow and allow the forearm to rest across the patient's chest. Tap the triceps tendon just above the olecranon. The triceps contracts. The reflex depends upon the 6th and 7th cervical segments. Care must be taken to strike the triceps *tendon* and not the belly of the muscle itself. All muscles show a certain amount of irritability to direct mechanical stimuli; but this is a direct response, not a stretch reflex.

Biceps jerk.   The elbow is flexed to a right angle and the forearm placed in a semipronated position; the examiner then places his thumb or index finger on the biceps tendon and strikes it with the patellar hammer. The biceps contracts. The 5th and 6th cervical segments of the cord are concerned.

Supinator jerk.   A blow upon the styloid process of the radius stretches the supinator causing supination of the elbow. This reflex depends on the 5th and 6th cervical segments.

With lesions at this level the supinator reflex may be lost but, when it is tested, brisk flexion of the fingers is seen. This phenomenon is known as *inversion* of the reflex and it is evidence of hyperexcitability of the anterior horn cells below the C5/6 level. The responsible lesion is in the C5/6 spinal segments.

Jaw jerk.   Ask the patient to open his mouth, but not too widely. Place one finger firmly on his chin and then tap it suddenly with the other hand as in percussion. A contraction of the muscles that close the jaw results. This jerk is sometimes absent in health and is increased in upper motor neurone lesions above the 5th nerve nuclei.

Clonus.   The phenomenon of clonus is often elicitable when the tendon reflexes are exaggerated as a result of a pyramidal lesion.

Ankle clonus. Bend the patient's knee slightly and support it with one hand, grasp the forepart of the foot with the other hand and suddenly dorsiflex the foot. The sudden stretch causes a reflex contraction of the calf muscles which then relax, but continued stretch causes a regular oscillation of contraction and relaxation which is called *clonus*. *Sustained* clonus is abnormal, and is evidence of an upper motor neurone lesion. It is then always associated with increased tendon reflexes (hyperreflexia) and an extensor plantar response. *Unsustained clonus* may occur in healthy persons, particularly in those who are very tense or anxious.

Grading the reflexes. The tendon reflexes may be graded:

0	Absent
1	Present (as a normal ankle jerk)
2	Brisk (as a normal knee jerk)
3	Very brisk
4	Clonus

Abnormal tendon reflexes. The tendon reflexes are diminished or absent with lesions affecting the afferent pathways, the anterior horn cells themselves, or the efferent pathways (lesions of the lower motor neurone). For example, in tabes dorsalis the posterior roots are affected; in poliomyelitis the anterior horn cells are diseased; and in most peripheral neuropathies both the efferent (motor) and afferent (sensory) nerve fibres are abnormal. In all these conditions certain tendon reflexes may be absent.

Hyperreflexia occurs with upper motor neurone lesions (at all levels above the anterior horn cells). It may also occur with anxiety or nervousness, in thyrotoxicosis and as a manifestation of tetanus. Hyperreflexia is therefore only of pathological significance if it is asymmetrical or if it is associated with other signs of an upper motor neurone lesion (spasticity, weakness or an extensor plantar response).

In cerebellar disease the reflexes may have a characteristic *pendular* quality. This is clearly evident only when there is a severe cerebellar ataxia and it is not a sign of diagnostic importance. It may be considered a manifestation of hypotonia.

In myxoedema both the contraction and relaxation phases of the tendon reflex may be prolonged. The relaxation time can be estimated by simple observation with surprising accuracy in relation to the normal and is a sensitive and reliable clinical index of hypothyroidism. This is sometimes called a *myotonic reflex*. It is also found in hypothermic patients.

Superficial reflexes

The plantar reflex. Assessment of the plantar reflex is of great clinical importance, not least because it is an objective response which can be easily compared by various observers. To elicit it the muscles of the lower limb should be relaxed. The *outer edge of the sole of the foot* is stimulated by gently scratching a key or a pin along it from the heel towards the little toe and then medially across the metatarsus. In healthy adults even a slight stimulus produces a contraction of the tensor fascia lata, often accompanied by a slighter contraction of the adductors of the thigh and of the sartorius. With a slightly stronger stimulus, flexion of the four outer toes appears, which increases with the strength of the stimulus till all the toes are flexed on the metatarsus and drawn together, the ankle being dorsiflexed and inverted. This is called the *flexor plantar response*. With still stronger stimuli withdrawal of the limb occurs. It is doubtful that the plantar reflex is ever completely absent in healthy subjects.

Babinski's sign. In lesions of the corticospinal system an abnormality in the plantar response was first described by Babinski. Extension of the great toe precedes all other movement. It is followed by spreading out and extension of the other toes, dorsiflexion of the ankle and flexion of hip and knee. The small amount of movement at the ankle is less conspicuous than the brisker movement of the normal response.

This *extensor plantar response* (so called because the movement described is extension according to anatomical terminology, although the reflex is, in reality, part of the nociceptive flexion withdrawal response described in the decerebrate preparation by Sherington), is most easily elicited by stimulation of the *outer part of the sole*. With slight corticospinal lesions, it may be evoked from this region alone when a normal flexor response is obtained by stimulating the medial edge of the sole. If the lesion is progressive, the area in which the extensor plantar reflex can be excited (receptive field) increases and spreads first inwards and over the sole of the foot, and then upwards along the leg to the knee or even the groin. For this reason extension of the great toe, generally associated with some dorsiflexion of the foot, can sometimes also be obtained by squeezing the calf or pressing heavily along the inner border of the tibia (*Oppenheim's sign*), or by pinching the calcaneus tendon (*Gordon's reflex*).

In adults, the extensor plantar response occurs only in cases of disease involving corticospinal pathways, but in children below the age of one year the extensor response is the normal response. The flexor response appears in the subsequent 6–12 months as myelination of the corticospinal pathways is completed.

Table 8.4. CHIEF SUPERFICIAL REFLEXES OF SPINAL ORIGIN

Reflex	How excited	Result	Level of cord concerned
Anal	Stroking or scratching the skin near the anus	Contraction of anal sphincter	3rd and 4th sacral segments
Bulbocavernosus	Pinching dorsum of glans penis	Contraction of bulbocavernosus	3rd and 4th sacral segments
Plantar	Stroking sole of foot	Movements of toes, of toes and foot, or leg	Lower part of lumbar enlargement (5th lumbar and 1st sacral segments)
Cremasteric	Stroking skin at upper and inner part of thigh*	Drawing upwards of testicle	1st and 2nd lumbar segments
Abdominal	Stroking abdominal wall below costal margin, at level of umbilicus and in iliac fossa	Contraction of abdominal muscles	7th to 12th thoracic segments
Scapular	Stroking skin in interscapular region	Contraction of scapular muscles	5th cervical to 1st thoracic segment

* The cremasteric reflex can often be most easily elicited by pressing over the sartorius in the lower third of Hunter's canal.

Flexor spasms may occur during testing of the plantar reflex. These consist of an exaggerated extensor plantar response, the whole limb being suddenly drawn up into flexion and the large toe extended. This is the fully developed human counterpart of Sherrington's nociceptive flexation withdrawal response. It is common in spinal cord disease and in some patients with bilateral upper motor neurone lesions at a higher level. Flexor spasms are often particularly severe in the presence of posterior column disease (as in multiple sclerosis or subacute combined degeneration), or when there is a constant stimulation of small unmyelinated fibre input to the spinal cord, as in the presence of bedsores or urinary tract infection in a patient with a cord lesion. *Extensor spasms*, conversely, are more likely to occur when posterior column function is normal.

Superficial abdominal reflexes.   These are elicited by allowing the patient to lie, relaxed and in a supine position, with the abdomen uncovered. A light stimulus, such as a key or a thin wooden stick, is passed across the abdominal skin in the plane of the dermatome from the outer aspect towards the midline. A ripple of contraction of the underlying abdominal musculature follows the stimulus. These reflexes are absent in upper motor neurone lesions above their spinal level. In disease of the thoracic spine they may indicate the segmental level of the lesion by their absence below this level.

It is often impossible to obtain them in anxious patients, in the elderly or obese and in multiparous women.

Corneal reflex.   See p. 297.

Palatal reflex.   See p. 303.

Sphincteric reflexes

This term includes the reflexes necessary for swallowing, micturition and defaecation. They depend upon complex muscular movements excited by increased tension in the wall of the viscus concerned.

One should ascertain from the patient whether he has any difficulty in swallowing (*dysphagia*), noting especially whether there is any regurgitation of food through the nose. As a rule patients with neurological disorders causing dysphagia complain of difficulty in swallowing liquids, whereas those with mechanical oesophageal obstruction complain they cannot swallow solids.

Defaecation. The patient should be questioned as to any difficulty and as to the presence of rectal and anal sensation. Incontinence of faeces should be noted.

The reflex action of the anal sphincter may be tested by introducing the lubricated gloved finger into the anus and noting whether contraction of the sphincter occurs with normal force, whether it is weak or paralysed, or whether any spasm is excited. The activity of the reflex may also be tested by gently pricking the skin near the anus. A brisk contraction of the sphincter should immediately occur, i.e. the *anal reflex*. In addition, the anal spincter contracts briskly in response to a sudden cough.

Micturition. The patient should be questioned as to difficulty in controlling or initiating micturition and as to whether bladder and urethral sensation are normal. Retention and incontinence or urgency of micturition should be noted.

Incontinence in neurological disorders may be due to overflow from an atonic distended bladder in which sensation has been lost. In this case the bladder will be enlarged to palpation or percussion and suprapubic pressure may result in the expulsion of urine from the urethra. Incontinence may also be due to *reflex incontinence*, either occurring at regular intervals as the bladder partially fills, or precipitately and unexpectedly in response to a sudden noise, to movement or to exposure to cold.

COORDINATION OF MOVEMENT

By coordination is meant the smooth recruitment, interaction and cooperation of separate muscles or groups of muscles, in order to accomplish a definite motor act. If such coordination is imperfect, motor performance becomes difficult or impossible and *ataxia* is said to be present.

The coordination of groups of muscles is the product of various factors, among which are the afferent impulses coming from the muscle spindles and joint receptors, cerebellar function and the state of tone of the muscles. When ataxia is present it is not always easy to say which of these factors is at fault. The movements that constitute a motor act can be controlled and directed by vision, but sight itself is not concerned in the coordination of most normal movements. When, however, there is loss of the sense of position of a limb or joint, the sensory defect may be compensated for by vision, and the disturbance of movement may become apparent only when the eyes are closed or the patient is in the dark. Such ataxia occurs typically in tabes dorsalis, when position sense is diminished or lost in the legs. Before ataxia can be ascribed solely to cerebellar disease, therefore, it is important to ascertain whether joint position sense is impaired, or not. Proximal weakness may mimic cerebellar ataxia, but this can usually be distinguished easily when muscular strength is tested.

How to test coordination

In the upper limbs.   Ask the patient to touch the point of his nose first with one forefinger and then with the other; or ask him to touch first his nose, then the examiner's forefinger with his own index finger. If he performs these movements naturally and without making random errors no incoordination is present. He may then be asked to perform the same actions with his eyes closed; any additional irregularity of the movements can be due only to disturbance of the sense of position.

It is often useful to watch the patient dressing or undressing, handling a book or picking up pins.

In the lower limbs.   If the patient is able to walk, a good test in the lower limbs consists of asking him to walk along a straight line. If incoordination is present he will soon deviate to one side or the other.

If he cannot walk, ask him, as he lies in bed to lift one leg high in the air, to place the heel of this leg on the opposite knee and then to slide the heel down his shin towards the ankle. In cerebellar ataxia a characteristic, irregular, side to side series of errors in the speed and direction of movement occurs. The test should be performed *with the eyes open*.

Another method is to ask the patient to describe a circle in the air with his toe or forefinger. If he is able to describe circles accurately coordination is good.

A special and very useful sign of cerebellar ataxia is *dysdiadokokinesia*; it consists of inability to execute rapidly repeated movements. The patient is asked to flex his elbows to a right angle and then alternately to supinate and pronate his forearms as rapidly as possible 'as though screwing in a light bulb'. All normal persons can do this very rapidly but usually slightly less rapidly with the left than with the right arm. When, however, dys-diadokokinesia is present the movements are slow, awkward and incomplete, and often become impossible after a few attempts. The rhythm of the movement becomes characteristically irregular. The sign can also be elicited by asking the patient to tap the examiner's palm with the tips of his fingers as fast as possible. Minor degrees of ataxia can then be both felt and heard.

Romberg's sign is often regarded as a special test for the coordination of the lower limbs. It is, however, *a test for loss of position sense* (sensory ataxia) in the legs and not a test of cerebellar function. However, patients with severe aural vertigo or cerebellar ataxia may also show some instability in the test.

The patient is asked to stand with his feet close together and if he can do this, he is then asked to close his eyes. If Romberg's sign is present, as soon as his eyes are closed he begins to sway about or may even fall. *The essential feature of the sign is therefore that the patient is more unsteady standing with his eyes closed than when they are open.* In the presence of sensory ataxia, as in tabes dorsalis, the patient is unable to maintain his posture without the aid of vision on account of defective position sense in his legs.

GAIT

The character of a patient's gait is often important in diagnosis, but particularly in cases of neurological disease. The legs must be fully exposed, the patient wearing only underpants. The feet should be bare. The patient is asked to walk away from the observer, to turn round at a given point and then to come towards him again.

The points to be noted are:

1. Can the patient walk at all? If he can:

2. Does he walk in a straight line or does he tend to deviate to one side or the other? To bring out this point, ask him to walk along a straight line, e.g. a crack in the floor.

3. Does he tend to fall and, if so, in what direction?

The next point to be decided is whether the gait conforms to any of the well recognized abnormal types. Before deciding this, *be quite sure* that the peculiarity in the patient's gait is not due to some surgical cause or to local disease of a joint, e.g. osteoarthritis of the hip. Examination of the bones and joints will eliminate such sources of error.

Common disorders of gait due to neurological disease are:

Spastic gait. The patient walks on a narrow base, has difficulty in bending his knees and drags his feet along as if they were glued to the floor.

The foot is raised from the ground by tilting the pelvis, and the leg is then swung forwards so that the foot tends to describe an arc, the toe scraping along the floor.

This gait is seen most characteristically in patients with corticospinal lesions. The *hemiplegic gait* is essentially a spastic gait in which only one leg is affected.

The gait in *sensory ataxia* may be described as 'stamping'. The patient raises his feet very suddenly, often abnormally high, and then jerks them forward, bringing them to the ground again with a stamp, and often heel first. If he watches the ground, he may be fairly steady, as he can use his eyes in place of his position sense, but he becomes severely ataxic when his eyes are closed or if he walks in the dark. This gait is best seen in tabes dorsalis. Other signs of loss of postural sensibility will be present.

The gait of *cerebellar incoordination* may be described as a 'drunken' or 'reeling' gait and requires no further description. Patients with this gait walk on a broad and irregular base, the feet being planted widely apart. The ataxia is equally severe whether the eyes are open or closed.

This gait occurs in disease of the cerebellum or cerebellar tracts and other signs of ataxia will be present.

Festinant gait. This occurs in Parkinson's disease. The patient is bent forwards, and advances with rapid, short, shuffling steps, so that 'he looks as if he were trying to catch up with his centre of gravity', and his arms do not swing. In some cases, if he is suddenly pulled backwards, he begins to walk backwards, and is unable to stop himself (*retropulsion*).

The *waddling gait* is like the gait of a duck. The body is usually tilted backwards, with an increase of lumbar lordosis; the feet are planted rather widely apart and the body sways from side to side as each step is taken. The heels and toes tend to be brought down simultaneously. This gait disorder is due to difficulty in maintaining truncal and pelvic posture because of proximal muscular weakness. It occurs, therefore, in the myopathies and the muscular dystrophies. A similar gait may occur with bilateral disease of the hip joints (Trendelenberg's sign).

The *high-stepping gait* is a device adopted by the patient to avoid tripping from his toes catching the ground. It occurs when there is weakness of the extensor muscles of the feet for example in common peroneal nerve palsy.

INVOLUNTARY MOVEMENTS

Involuntary, unintended movements occur, either at rest or during voluntary movement, in a number of different diseases of the nervous system. The different clinical varieties of involuntary movement are not specific disease entities, but represent clinical patterns of involuntary movement observed in many patients. Most are due to diseases of the basal ganglia and extrapyramidal system.

Epilepsy

The possibility that an involuntary movement limited to one side of the body, or to one limb, might be due to focal epilepsy should always be considered. Very rarely such an attack may continue for hours or even days (*epilepsia partialis continua*). The movement is usually complex and repetitive. It may be exacerbated by arousal or by handling or touching the limb and it will usually be relieved by anticonvulsant drugs. The movement differs from the involuntary movement disorders principally by its stereotyped repetitiveness.

Myoclonus

Myoclonus is a rapid, irregular jerking movement of the limb or of the whole body, often occurring in response to extraneous stimuli, such as a sudden loud noise. A sudden start when surprised, or the bodily jerks which occur on falling asleep or waking, are common varieties of myoclonus experienced by most normal people. In exaggerated form these jerks of *flexion myoclonus* may occur as a manifestation of major epilepsy or in some patients with degenerative disorders of the cerebellum. Generalized flexion myoclonus also occurs in certain types of encephalitis, when it often exhibits an obvious periodicity. Less commonly, irregular myoclonic jerks may occur in a single limb or a ripple of jerky irregular contraction may pass through the muscles of a limb. Myoclonus can occur with lesions at many levels in the nervous system and it does not, therefore, have localizing value.

Tremor

Regular or irregular distal movements having an oscillatory character are classified as tremors. The tremor of *anxiety* is usually fine and rapid, but it may be coarse and irregular. The tremor found in *thyrotoxicosis* is characteristically rapid. Coarser distal tremor, often exaggerated in awkward postures, as when the out-stretched fingers are held pointing at each other in front of the patient's nose and usually relieved to some extent during move-ment, occurs as a familial disorder: *benign essential tremor*. This tremor is often coarse, but usually irregular, and it is present both at rest and during movement. It must therefore be distinguished from parkinsonian and cerebellar tremors. The latter is present only during movement (*intention tremor*) and the former is accom-panied by signs of extrapyramidal disease. *Senile tremor* is similar to benign essential tremor. *Hysterical tremor* tends to involve a limb or the whole body and it is, characteristically, worsened by the examiner's attempt to control it.

The tremor of *parkinsonianism* is usually easily recognizable. It consists of a rapid rhythmic alternating tremor, predominantly in flexion/extension but often with a prominent rotary component between finger and thumb (*pill-rolling tremor*). More proximal muscles may be involved, and the lips and tongue are frequently affected. The tremor is invariably more severe in the arm than in the leg. It is often strikingly unilateral and is invariably associated with other symptoms and signs of extra-pyramidal disease, such as hypokinesia, cogwheel rigidity, postural abnormalities and gait disorder.

Athetosis

Athetosis is a writhing movement, usually more pronounced in distal than in proximal muscles, in which the play of movement is very complex but often seems to consist of a relatively constant interaction between two postures, those of *grasping and avoiding* (see p. 268). The fingers are alternately widely extended, the arm following into an extended, abducted and externally rotated posture, and then the fingers clench, often trapping the thumb in the palm, and the limb flexes slightly and internally rotates. In very severe forms of this disorder, as for example in *dystonia musculorum deformans* (torsion dystonia) the trunk and axial musculature is also affected and the patient may scarcely be able to stand.

Athetosis may be unilateral or generalized. The latter form is usually associated with degenerative disease of the basal ganglia. Very rarely it may occur as a paroxysmal phenomenon.

Chorea

The word means 'a dance'. The involuntary movements are brief, fluid and often difficult, at first, to discern. Ordinary voluntary movements, such as walking or picking up a cup and saucer, may be embellished with smooth, rapid extra little flourishes of movement. Muscular tone is often decreased. The outstretched upper limbs may assume a hyperpronated posture and little flicks of movement of the digits or wrist may occur. At rest the patient appears 'fidgety' and 'unable to sit still'. The movements often appear less obvious during voluntary movement, and are increased by agitation or nervousness. Chorea occurs as part of an inherited presenile dementia (*Huntington's chorea*), associated with rheumatic fever (*Sydenham's chorea*) and rarely in pregnancy and after certain *drugs* (phenothiazines). It may also occur with other systemic diseases, e.g. thyrotoxicosis and systemic lupus erythematosus, and in old age (*senile chorea*). Unilateral chorea may occur with deeply placed lesions in one hemisphere.

Dyskinesia

In the past this word was reserved for *phenothiazine-induced* involuntary movements, which particularly affect the pharyngeal perioral musculature, and also for *levodopa-induced* axial torsional movements. Latterly the word has come to be used simply to describe any involuntary movement.

Dystonia

This word is used to describe an abnormally maintained posture, often associated with a plastic rigidity. The dystonias are closely related to choreoathetosis, but the term can also be used to describe the flexed posture of Parkinson's disease (flexion dystonia) or the hemiplegic posture (hemiplegic dystonia).

Hemiballismus

This is a peculiar and unique involuntary movement, almost invariably unilateral and affecting the arm more than the leg, in which the limb is flung rapidly, and often with great force, from full extension into abduction and external or internal rotation. The movements may be so violent as to result in serious injury to the limb and in loss of weight. The disorder is associated with lesions in the region of the subthalamic nucleus.

Tics

These are simple normal movements which become repeated unnecessarily to the point that they become an embarrassment or a source of or reaction to psychiatric problems. They can be readily imitated in contrast to the other involuntary movement disorders. Head nodding is a common example.

Myokymia

This is a persistent twitchy and often rhythmical movement of the periorbital muscles. It may occur as a benign phenomenon in fatigued or anxious people. It is sometimes due to lesions in the facial nerve or its nucleus.

Metabolic flap (asterixis)

An irregular, abrupt, brief loss of posture, especially evident in the outstretched hands or tongue occurs in decompensated hepatic failure (*hepatic flap*) and in other metabolic disorders, e.g. uraemia, poisoning with hypnotic drugs, and in respiratory failure.

Tetany

Tetany, commonly due to hypocalcaemia or alkalosis, can be recognized by the characteristic posture of the affected hand. The fingers and thumbs are held adducted and extended; the wrist is usually moderately flexed. The toes may be similarly affected (carpopedal spasm). Ischaemia of the affected limb, produced by a sphygmomanometer cuff inflated above the arterial pressure for 2 or 3 minutes will augment this sign or produce it if it is not already present (*Trousseau's sign*). Another useful test is to tap lightly with a patellar hammer in the region of exit of the facial nerve from the skull, about 3–5 cm below and in front of the ear. The facial muscles twitch briefly with each tap (*Chvostek's sign*).

SENSATION

The following different forms of sensation are usually tested:

1. *Tactile sensibility*. This includes light touch and pressure, and tactile localization and discrimination.
2. *Position sense*, and the appreciation of passive movement.
3. *Recognition of the size, shape, weight and form of objects*.
4. *Appreciation of vibration*.
5. *Pain*.
6. *Temperature*.

The presence or absence of any abnormal sensations should be noted.

These 'sensory modalities' do not necessarily represent different, discrete sensory functions but, rather, are commonly experienced sensations in normal life. Perception depends on a complex physiological interaction of afferent input at many levels in the nervous system and, in some instances as in the recognition and naming of objects, it depends also on the ability to manipulate the object felt. Perception of vibration, for example, does not depend on a special set of nerve fibres responsible only for transmitting vibration sense to the central nervous system, but rather is a form of sensation subjectively similar to light touch which, in clinical practice is found to be disturbed when there is a lesion of the large diameter, afferent fibres in the peripheral nerves, posterior columns or, more rarely, at a higher level than this.

Begin testing sensation with touch and position sense. Use a pin later, when you have gained the patient's confidence. Always apply the sensory stimulus first to an area of impaired sensation and mark out its borders *from the abnormal to the normal*. The patient should readily note the sudden change to normality.

Areas of diminished sensation should be carefully, *but quickly*, mapped out so that their distribution in relation to root lesions, peripheral nerve lesions or lesions in the central nervous system can be studied. It is important to do this quickly, accurately and, as far as possible, without repetition. The longer the time spent on this the more confusing will be the result: it requires great concentration and cooperation from the patient and from the examiner.

Inconsistency in the patient's replies may be due to fatigue, poor cooperation, dementia or undue suggestibility. This can be checked by asking the patient to say 'now' whenever he feels the stimulus, his eyes being shut; by examining a related form of sensation such as temperature sense in the case of pinprick, or position or vibration sense in the case of light touch; or by exhorting the patient to be very careful to make the correct response. Never make much of small differences. Remember that many patients will experience changes in the acuteness or sharpness of a pin between the nail bed and the dorsum of the finger, or at about the level of the clavicle when the stimulus ascends the anterior chest wall. The pulp of the fingers is rather insensitive to pain, but very sensitive to light touch and discriminative tests such as two point discrimination. Vibration sense is best perceived over a bony prominence. On the whole it is better to test sensation with the patient's eyes open. During most sensory testing it should not affect the result to have the patient actually watching the procedure. It can be a frightening experience to be suddenly pricked with a pin when one's eyes are closed and such surprises, which destroy a patient's confidence in the examiner, should always be avoided.

Tactile sensibility

Use a wisp of cotton wool or the tip of your index finger.

Ask the patient to indicate whether he feels the touch, and if it feels normal. If not, *how* is it abnormal? It may be abolished or reduced (*hypoaesthesia*), misperceived as a painful, irritating or tingling sensation (*hyperaesthesia*) or mislocalized. Very rarely there may be a delay between the stimulus and its recognition by the patient. Areas of diminished sensation should be carefully delineated and recorded.

Ability to discriminate between two points is tested by the use of blunt dividers. The patient is asked whether he is being touched with one or both points. Normally 2 mm of separation of the points can be recognized as two separate stimuli on the finger tips, and slightly more separation on the pulps of the toes. This is an excellent objective sensory test which is particularly useful in cases of posterior column or parietal cortical lesions; and in some peripheral nerve lesions (such as the carpal tunnel syndrome).

Position sense

Ask the patient to look away or shield his eyes. Explain that you will move his finger (or toe or elbow) up or down and ask him to tell you which way it has been moved. He should be able to recognize movements of only a few degrees at all joints, including knee, ankle, elbow and wrist, in addition to the more commonly tested fingers and toes. It is sometimes helpful to ask the patient to imitate with the opposite limb or digit the position of the limb or digit being tested. It is essential that the patient be relaxed and that he allows the limb to be moved *passively*.

When the position sense is disturbed in the upper limbs, the outstretched fingers may twist, rise and fall when held with the eyes closed. These involuntary movements (pseudo-athetosis) occur unknown to the patient and disappear almost completely when the patient watches the position of his fingers. Patients with defective position sense may be unable to manipulate small objects, fasten buttons and so on without visually observing their movements (sensory ataxia)

The *appreciation of movement* is closely related to the sense of position and can be tested at the same time. Gradually move a digit or limb into a new position, with the patient's eyes closed and ask him to say 'now' as soon as he recognizes the movement. Note the angle through which the limb was moved. If the appreciation of movement is diminished this angle is many times greater than that in a normal limb. Movements of less than 10° can be appreciated at all normal joints. Finally test that the patient can recognize the direction of the movement, that is, whether the joint is flexed or extended. Patients can sometimes recognize the occurrence of a movement but not its direction.

Recognition of size, shape and form

These faculties can be tested most accurately in the hands with the eyes closed. To test size, place in the patient's palm objects of the same shape, but of different sizes, for example small rods or matches of different length. Ask him to say which is the larger. The objects should be applied consecutively.

To test recognition of shape familiar objects such as coins, a pencil, a penknife, scissors, etc. are placed in the hand, and the patient is asked to identify them or to describe their form. Loss of this faculty is known as *astereognosis*. It may occur, with parietal lesions, when position sense and light touch are normal, although there is usually some defect in these modalities. When astereognosis occurs with posterior column lesions position sense, vibration sense and light touch are invariably profoundly disturbed.

Appreciation of vibration

If the foot of a vibrating tuning-fork is placed on the surface of the body the vibrations can be felt, provided they are sufficiently strong. This is a valuable test, as the ability to appreciate vibration may be lost in various diseases, as in tabes dorsalis, in peripheral neuritis and in posterior column disorders. A tuning fork of 128 Hz (middle C) should be used. Vibrations of higher frequency are more difficult to perceive. If the patient perceives the vibration ask him to say when he ceases to feel it. If the examiner can then still perceived it, the patient's perception of vibration is impaired. There is often some loss of vibration sense in the feet and legs in old age.

Pain

Pain may be evoked either by a cutaneous stimulus as the prick of a pin, or by pressure on deeper structures, such as muscles or bones. Sensibility to superficial and to pressure pain should be tested separately.

Superficial pain. The point of a pin should be used as the stimulus. Care must be taken that the patient distinguishes between the *sharpness* of the point (that is, its relative size) and the *pain* which the prick evokes; it often happens that, even when sensibility to pain is abolished, he can recognize that the stimulus is pointed, and thus confuse the observer by calling it 'sharp'.

Pressure pain is examined by squeezing the muscles or the Achilles tendon. Abolition of pressure pain is often the most prominent sensory disturbance in tabes dorsalis.

Absence of sensibility to pain is termed *analgesia*; partial loss of pain sensibility is called *hypoalgesia*; and an exaggerated sensibility, so that even a mild stimulus causes an unnatural degree of painful sensation, is known as *hyperalgesia*. This occurs in some patients with spinal cord disease, for example in tabes dorsalis, and in certain patients with deep-seated parietal or thalamic lesions (thalamic pain). The pain experienced has a peculiar, ill-localized and persistent character. It often has a burning quality and it may occur as an intractable spontaneous phenomenon or only in response to cutaneous stimuli.

Temperature sense

Temperature sense is conveniently examined by using test tubes containing warm and cold water. The part to be tested is touched with each in turn, and the patient says whether each tube feels hot or cold.

Other disturbances of sensation

The phenomenon of *sensory inattention* is sometimes found in patients with lesions of the parietal lobe; it is demonstrated as follows. The patient is asked to close his eyes. Homologous points on opposite sides of the body are stimulated simultaneously by touch or with pins. The patient is asked to indicate which side, or sides are touched and, in the presence of sensory inattention he fails to perceive the stimulus on the abnormal side. This is sometimes called *sensory extinction. Bilateral simultaneous sensory stimuli* can also be studied when testing vision and hearing and a similar defect may be found. In the presence of hemisensory loss, of course, the sign is invalid.

Some patients with parietal lesions will also show *spatial summation*, a sensory abnormality in which a stimulus is only perceived if an area of skin larger than a certain critical area is stimulated, or *temporal summation* in which an ill-localized and often perverted or painful sensation is felt after rapidly repeated stimuli. Single stimuli will be missed. These abnormalities are part of a perceptual defect related to sensory *agnosia*, a disorder in which the patient is unaware of the nature or the severity of his sensory disorder. In its most extreme form there may even be denial of illness (*anosognosia*). In patients with higher perceptual defects of this type a number of other bedside tests may be useful. These include *constructional tests* such as the patient's ability to draw a map of his surroundings, to copy a complex figure (for example, two interlocking, irregular pentagons), to draw a clock face or a human face, or to draw more complex figures, for example a house. Visual and tactile memory can be tested by variations of these tests. Constructional ability is particularly impaired with right parietal lesions (*constructional apraxia*).

SIGNS OF MENINGEAL IRRITATION

Neck stiffness

The patient is asked to flex his neck as fully as he can to ascertain the degree of movement possible, and then to relax. The examiner then passively flexes the neck. The chin should normally touch the chest without pain.

In meningeal irritation the test causes pain in the neck, sometimes radiating down the back, and the movement is resisted by spasm in the extensor muscles of the neck. Neck rigidity is also caused by diseases of the cervical spine. Head retraction is an extensive degree of neck rigidity.

Kernig's sign

Kernig's sign is tested by passively extending the patient's knee when his hip is fully flexed. This movement causes pain and spasm of the hamstrings in meningeal irritation affecting the lower part of the spinal subarachnoid space. It is a less sensitive test than neck rigidity.

These two tests depend upon the fact that stretching the spinal nerve roots in conditions of meningeal irritation causes a reflex muscular spasm. They are positive in meningitis and subarachnoid haemorrhage, but also in patients with 'meningism', a state of irritation of the meninges, seen most commonly in young children with acute fevers; and in some patients with raised intracranial pressure in whom herniation of the cerebellar tonsils into the foramen magnum has begun.

Straight leg raising

This test is used in patients with sciatica. The sciatic nerve and its roots are stretched by passively elevating the patient's extended leg with the hand, which is placed behind the heel. The movement is restricted by pain in conditions in which the spinal roots are involved as in protrusion of a low lumbosacral intervertebral disc.

SPECIAL INVESTIGATIONS

The following special methods of investigation are in common use.

LUMBAR PUNCTURE

This is a procedure used for obtaining samples of cerebrospinal fluid (CSF) which requires some experience. It should be carried out under supervision in the first instance. It is performed as follows:

Mark out the 3rd and 4th lumbar spines. The 4th lumbar spine usually lies in the plane of the iliac crests. The puncture may be made through either the 3rd or 4th interspace. The patient should be lying on his side on a firm couch, with the knees and chin as nearly approximated as possible. His back should be right at the edge of the couch and it is *important that its transverse axis*, i.e. a line passing through the posterior superior iliac spines, *should be vertical*. Local anaesthesia may be produced by injecting 2% sterile procaine, first raising a bleb under the skin, and, when this is insensitive, anaesthetizing the whole dermis. It is not necessary to inject procaine into the deep ligaments. This procedure usually causes more pain than it relieves. A special needle about 8 cm in length should be used. The stylet should fit accurately and should not protrude through the bevelled cutting edge of the needle.

Push the needle firmly through the skin in the middle line or just to one side of it and press it steadily *forwards and slightly towards the head*, the bevel pointing towards the side on which the patient is lying. When the needle is felt to enter the spinal cavity the stylet is withdrawn and the CSF which escapes is collected in 3 sterilized stoppered test tubes. If any blood is present, a marked difference in the amount in the first and subsequent tubes indicates that the blood is due to trauma from the puncture. The patient should lie flat for 8 to 24 hours afterwards.

It is sometimes useful to have a manometer connected with the needle, so that the pressure of the fluid can be measured at the time of puncture. If this is done, the patient's head must be on the same level as the sacrum and he must be breathing quietly and with his muscles relaxed. The neck and legs should be slightly extended. The normal pressure is from 60 to 150 mm of fluid.

Queckenstedt's test can be used to detect a block to the circulation of fluid in the spinal canal. With the needle and manometer in position and the patient breathing quietly as described above, an assistant compresses one or other, but not both, jugular veins. This causes a sudden increase in intracranial pressure, which is immediately seen in the manometer as a sudden rise of cerebrospinal fluid pressure, followed by an equally rapid fall when the pressure on the vein is released. A similar sudden rise and fall is seen if the patient is asked to cough and this is a useful check that the needle tip is in free communication with the sub-arachnoid space.

With slight degrees of block there may be a rise of pressure in the manometer followed by a very slow fall when the pressure on the vein is released; and with more severe block no rise of pressure will be seen when the jugular vein is compressed.

This test is now rarely used since it has largely been superseded by myelography. *It should never be carried out in the presence of raised CSF pressure* since it may then precipitate transtentorial or tonsillar herniation.

Much the commonest cause of a 'dry-tap', the failure to obtain CSF, is an incorrectly performed puncture, and this is usually due to the patient not being in the correct position. The needle will then not be introduced at right angles to the transverse axis of the back, and will miss the spinal canal. Occasionally, however, a 'dry-tap' is due to a complete block to the flow of CSF through the spinal canal. In this circumstance urgent myelography is required and for this procedure *cisternal puncture* may be required. This should only be performed by an experienced physician or surgeon. It is best undertaken under radiographic control

Lumbar puncture should *never* be performed in patients in whom raised intracranial pressure is suspected. The fundi should *always* be examined before a lumbar puncture is performed in order to exclude papilloedema.

Abnormalities of the fluid

Normal cerebrospinal fluid is clear and colourless like water. Any yellowness is pathological and is due either to old haemorrhage, jaundice or excess of protein. In *Froin's syndrome* a pronounced yellow colour (xanthochromia) is associated with great excess of protein and the formation of a coagulum. It is a very rare phenomenon. Even slight increases in CSF protein, however, cause a noticeable increase in viscosity of the fluid when it is gently shaken, and an excessive frothiness of its surface.

Turbidity of the fluid may be due to the presence of white blood cells, either as a result of infection or of subarachnoid haemorrhage. If it does not clear on standing it is due to micro-organisms.

The presence of *blood* may be due to injury to a vessel by the needle or to subarachnoid haemorrhage. In the latter case the blood is more uniformly mixed with the fluid, and the supernatant fluid, after centrifugation, is yellow.

Cytological examination of a turbid fluid is of great importance. A centrifugal deposit should be examined with Leishman's stain in order to obtain an idea of the character of the cells present; and by Gram's and Ziehl-Neelsen's methods for bacteria. Cell counts are performed with a counting chamber and must be done immediately the fluid has been collected. Counts done some hours later give inaccurate results because the leucocytes stick together and to the sides of the tube, and endothelial cells break up in a short time. If any clot has formed an accurate cell count cannot be obtained but the cells in the clot can be stained and examined. Normal fluid contains 2–5 lymphocytes/μl.

An excess of cells ('*pleocytosis*') is described as being of polymorphonuclear type, if these cells are above 75% of the total and of lymphocytic type if more than 90% are lymphocytes. Bacterial meningitis is associated with a polymorphonuclear pleocytosis, virus meningitis and syphilis with a lymphocytic one, and tuberculous meningitis with either a lymphocytic or a mixed type.

The CSF should also be examined bacteriologically and chemically.

Normal cerebrospinal fluid contains only a trace of albumin and hardly any globulin, the *total protein* being not more than 40 mg/100 ml. In some neurological diseases, particularly in multiple sclerosis and in many acute and subacute virus infections, the globulin fractions in the cerebrospinal fluid are altered. The *Lange test* takes advantage of this. Varying dilutions of cerebrospinal fluid are mixed in ten tubes with a colloidal gold suspension of constant strength. The degree of precipitation which results is expressed by arbitrary figures 0–5, 0 representing no change and 5 complete precipitation. The CSF IgG concentration can also be directly estimated by immunoelectrophoresis and in many laboratories this estimation has replaced the Lange test.

Glucose is present in normal cerebrospinal fluid in a concentration of 2·5–4·2 mmol/l, which is about a half to a third of the blood glucose concentration. In purulent, tuberculous or fungal meningitis and rarely in carcinomatous meningitis the CSF sugar is reduced to less than half of the blood glucose. It is also low if the patient is hypoglycaemic.

One or more of the tests for syphilis are often performed on the cerebrospinal fluid.

The typical changes in the CSF in various neurological diseases are summarized in Table 8.5.

THE ELECTROENCEPHALOGRAM (EEG)

Electrodes applied to the patient's scalp pick up small changes of electrical potential, which after amplification are recorded on paper. The EEG is of particular value in the investigation of epilepsy and in the localization of cerebral tumours and other expanding intracranial lesions.

THE ELECTROMYOGRAM (EMG)

Electrical activity occurring in muscle during voluntary contraction, or in denervated muscle during rest, can be recorded with

Table 8.5. TYPICAL CHANGES IN THE CEREBROSPINAL FLUID IN VARIOUS DISEASES

Disease condition	Physical characteristics	Cytology	Protein (g/l)	Glucose (mmol/l)	Tests for syphilis	Stained deposit	Culture	Lange curve
Normal	Clear and colourless	0–5 cells/μl	0·1–0·4	2·5–4·2	Negative	No organisms	Sterile	0000000000 0000110000
Meningitis								
Bacterial	Yellowish and turbid	Polymorphs 200–2000 Lymphocytes 5–50	0·5–2·0	<2·0	Negative	Bacteria	Positive	0001344310
Tuberculous	Colourless sometimes viscous	Polymorphs 0–100 Lymphocytes 100–300	>0·5	<2·0*	Negative	Tubercle bacilli in films in some cases	Positive by special methods	0001344310
Viral (includes poliomyelitis)	Usually clear	10–100 mixed cells at first, becoming lymphocytic in 36 hours	0·1–0·6 Poliomyelitis 0·3–0·2, remaining high 6–8 weeks	2·5–4·2	Negative	No organisms	Sterile	0001344310
Multiple sclerosis	Clear and colourless	Rarely 5–15 lymphocytes	0·1–0·6 rarely higher	2·5–4·2	Negative	No organisms	Sterile	Paretic type of curve in 50% of cases
Syphilis								
GPI	Clear and colourless	5–100 lymphocytes	0·4–1·0	2·5–4·2	Positive	No organisms	Sterile	5555432100
Tabes	Clear and colourless	5–100 lymphocytes	0·3–0·6	2·5–4·2	20% negative by reagin tests†	No organisms	Sterile	0123210000
Meningeal	Clear and slightly turbid	10–50 polymorphs 50–500 lymphocytes	0·5–2·0	May be slightly low	Positive	No organisms	Sterile	0123210000

* CSF glucose is usually about half the blood glucose. Simultaneous blood and CSF glucose estimations should always be performed.
† Nearly all are positive by FTA-ABS or TPHA.

needle electrodes inserted percutaneously into the belly of the muscle, or with surface electrodes (silver discs attached to the skin overlying the muscle with a salty paste), amplified and displayed as an auditory signal through a suitable loudspeaker and as a visual signal on a cathode ray oscilloscope. They may be recorded on magnetic tape or by photography. Analysis of such electrical activity is useful in the diagnosis of primary diseases of muscle (*myopathies* and *dystrophies*) and of lower motor neurone lesions (*denervation*).

The speed of conduction of afferent impulses (*sensory nerve conduction velocity*) and efferent impulses (*motor nerve conduction velocity*) in peripheral nerves can be estimated using an electrical nerve stimulation technique and suitable recording electrodes and amplifying or digital averaging equipment. These measurements are useful in the diagnosis of peripheral nerve disorders, particularly those due to local compressive lesions as, for example, carpal tunnel syndrome.

NEURORADIOLOGY

Apart from routine radiographs of the skull and spine a number of *contrast techniques* are useful.

Myelography

This is a method for demonstrating the subarachnoid space in the spinal canal. A lumbar or cisternal puncture is performed with the patient on the myelogram table in the X-ray department and 2–10 ml of a special radiopaque contrast medium or 10–25 ml of oxygen or air (radiolucent or negative contrast) are injected into the subarachnoid space. By tilting the table the contrast medium can be made to flow up and down the spinal canal under direct vision, preferably using TV amplification; and radiographs can be taken of regions of deformity or obstruction to the flow of contrast. This is a very useful method for accurate localization of tumours in the spinal canal.

Computerized axial tomography (CT scanning)

CT scanning provides tomographic sections of the brain of very high resolution, without the need for contrast procedures. A crystallographic X-ray detection device is used instead of conventional X-ray film and a photographic picture is produced by computerized averaging techniques. The method greatly reduces the need for air encephalography and angiography.

Angiography

This is a method for studying the intracranial and extracranial vessels. A suitable radiopaque contrast medium is injected percutaneously into a carotid artery in the neck, or into a vertebral artery either by direct puncture or by catheterization of a major vessel such as the femoral, axillary, brachial or subclavian arteries. Radiographs are taken in various planes in the following few seconds as the contrast medium traverses the cerebral circulation. The arterial, capillary and venous circulations can be studied and abnormalities of the distribution, size, position and lumen of these vessels can be seen.

The technique is particularly useful for diagnosis of aneurysms, arteriovenous malformations and cerebral tumours. It is also useful in cerebral vascular disease. General anaesthesia is usually preferred.

Air encephalography (AEG)

5–30 ml of air or oxygen, injected as in myelography by lumbar puncture, are allowed to flow from the spinal canal into the subarachnoid cisterns of the posterior fossa, thus outlining the cerebellar hemispheres and brain stem. By judicious positioning of the head, it is then made to enter the ventricular system. In this way the fourth ventricle, the aqueduct and the third and lateral ventricles can be studied. A series of anteroposterior, postero-anterior, lateral and oblique radiographs are taken, often using tomographic techniques and a very accurate demonstration of the anatomy of the brain itself can be obtained. It is sometimes necessary to supplement AEG by the additional instillation of 2–5 ml of radiopaque contrast medium (Myodil encephalography).

Air encephalography may be dangerous in the presence of raised intracranial pressure and in these patients, as in many of those with hydrocephalus, the injection of air or Myodil may be made through frontal or parietal burr holes, directly into the ventricles (*air* or *Myodil ventriculography*). With increasingly accurate angiographic technique and the more general availability of computerized axial tomography this investigation is less often necessary now than formerly.

Very careful positioning of the head is required for air encephalography and special mechanical chairs are used in many departments to facilitate this. It is usual therefore to perform the investigation under general anaesthesia.

Diagnostic ultrasound

A pulsed ultrasonic beam is directed through the head in a lateral direction from one temporal region to the other. Reflections are recorded by a second transducer on the same side of the head. The position of the ultrasonic midline can be compared with that of the third ventricular walls and, occasionally, of the walls of the lateral ventricles themselves. The technique requires practice but it is particularly useful in the management of patients unconscious after head injuries. Unlike the radiographic procedures described above it is 'non-invasive' and can be repeated as often as necessary.

ROUTINE EXAMINATION OF THE NERVOUS SYSTEM

A detailed examination of the whole nervous system is time-consuming and something of an ordeal for the patient. There follows a scheme for a quick routine examination, which will be found useful in the examination of patients not suspected of neurological disease, and will also indicate what functions require detailed examination in those with such disease.

Mental state

Much useful information can be obtained during history taking and physical examination; no specific questions need usually be asked.

Is the history given *accurately*, *concisely* and *with insight*? Or is the patient *concrete*, *circumlocutory* or *vague*?

Is his *memory* normal?

Is he *neatly dressed* and *well cared for*?

Is his *behaviour* normal?
Is he *aphasic* or *dysarthric*?
Is he *confused*?
Can he *find his way* in and out of the room?
Can he *dress* and *undress* himself?

Gait

Is it *spastic, hemiparetic, ataxic* or *parkinsonian*?
Is there a *foot drop*?

Cranial nerves

Test *ocular movements*, looking for nystagmus.
Test *facial movements*.
Test *tongue protrusion* and *palatal movement*.

Visual fields

These, like aphasia, may provide absolute evidence of disease above the tentorium cerebelli.
Is there a *hemianopia*?
If so, is it *homonymous, bitemporal, unilateral* or something else?
Is *central vision* normal? This is crudely assessed by testing the visual acuity. Can he read small print with or without glasses?

Fundi

Is *papilloedema* present?
Is *optic atrophy* present?
Are there *hypertensive, uraemic* or *diabetic* changes present?

Motor

Is there any *weakness* of the outstretched upper limbs?
Is there *distal or proximal weakness* or *wasting*?
Is *muscular tone* normal, spastic or extrapyramidal in type?
Look for *cerebellar ataxia* in the limbs.
Assess the *tendon reflexes* and *plantar responses*.

Sensory

Test *position sense* in the fingers and toes and vibration sense in the feet (posterior columns).

Test *pin-prick* in the four limbs and on the face (lateral spinothalamic tracts).

Light touch need only be tested if the patient complains of numbness.

General

Examine the *skull*, *spinal movements* and *posture*.
  Look for *cutaneous naevi*.
  Listen for *bruits in the neck*.

9

The unconscious patient

History
Examination
Diagnosis of brain death

Coma is a common medical problem. Diagnosis can usually be accomplished at the bedside, provided attention is given both to the history and examination. In this chapter clinical methods relevant to diagnosis of the comatose patient will be described.

Consciousness is a state of normal cerebral activity in which the patient is aware of himself and of his environment and is able to respond to changes both within himself, for example hunger, and in his environment. *Sleep*, although a state of altered consciousness, is obviously a normal variation in consciousness. The sleeping patient can be roused, both spontaneously and in response to external stimuli, to a full state of wakefulness. Altered consciousness resulting from brain disease may take the form of a *confusional state*, in which the patient is alert but agitated, frightened, and disorientated in time, space and person. Such patients usually show evidence of misperception of their environment, and hallucinations and delusions may occur. Confusional states must be carefully distinguished from aphasia, in which a specific disorder of language is the characteristic feature, and from continuous temporal lobe epilepsy, a form of focal status epilepticus in which the behavioural disorder is often accompanied by aphasia if the epileptic focus is left-sided. Usually this can be recognized by the occurrence of frequent but slight myoclonic jerks of facial and, especially, perioral muscles and by variability in the patient's confusion from moment to moment during the examination. *The examiner should always pause and observe an unconscious patient for a few moments before disturbing him.*

A state of abnormal drowsiness is often found in patients with space-occupying intracranial lesions or metabolic disorders before stupor or coma supervenes. The patient appears to be in normal sleep but cannot be easily wakened and, once awake, tends to fall asleep despite attempts to continue conversation or clinical examination. Further, while awake such patients can usually be shown to be disorientated; higher intellectual function, such as the ability to perform abstract tasks or to make judgements, is disturbed. By *stupor* is meant a state of disturbed consciousness from which only vigorous external stimuli can produce arousal. Arousal from stupor is invariably both brief and incomplete. In *coma* the patient is unrousable and unresponsive to all external stimuli. It is sometimes helpful to recognize states of light and deep coma to indicate the degree of abnormality in patients in whom coma is becoming progressively deeper, but this distinction is necessarily difficult to define.

The objective of examination of the unconscious patient is to achieve a diagnosis and so to plan management. Coma may be due either to metabolic or structural disease of the brain; it is only very rarely a psychogenic disorder. Coma results from lesions affecting the brain widely, diffusely or multifocally, and from lesions of deep centrally placed structures in the diencephalon or brain stem (Table 9.1). For example, supratentorial mass lesions, such as tumours, may damage deep diencephalic structures, while subtentorial neoplasms may directly damage the brain stem reticular formation. Metabolic disorders, for example hypoglycaemia, hypnotic drugs or hypoxia, widely depress brain function. It is important to distinguish supratentorial from subtentorial space-occupying lesions because coma due to the former has a better prognosis.

Table 9.1. OUTLINE OF CAUSES OF COMA

Metabolic	*Structural*
drug overdosage (including alcohol)	meningitis
hypoglycaemia	encephalitis
diabetes mellitus	other infections (e.g. cerebral malaria)
renal failure	subarachnoid haemorrhage
hepatic failure	epilepsy
hypothermia	head injury
hypothyroidism	pituitary apoplexy
cardio-respiratory failure	hypertensive encephalopathy
hypoxic encephalopathy	

Supratentorial lesions	*Subtentorial lesions*
cerebral haemorrhage	cerebellar haemorrhage
cerebral infarction with oedema	pontine haemorrhage
subdural haematoma	brain stem infarction
extradural haematoma	tumour
tumour	cerebellar abscess
cerebral abscess	secondary effects of trans-tentorial herniation of brain due to cerebral mass lesions

HISTORY

The history is of very great importance and attempts should always be made to find family or other witnesses of the onset of the coma. Coma occurs suddenly in vascular disorders such as sub-arachnoid haemorrhage or stroke, especially with cerebral or cere-bellar haemorrhage. A history of trauma with concussion or fol-lowed a few days later by fluctuating drowsiness and stupor, suggesting sub-dural haematoma, should never be regarded lightly. Concussion followed by a brief lucid interval before rapidly deepening coma suggests extra-dural haematoma. A history of headache before coma supervenes is frequent in patients with intracranial space-occupying lesions of any cause. Seizures of recent onset, whether focal or generalized, strongly suggest cere-bral disease, which may be due to tumour, encephalitis, abscess or trauma. Patients with drug-induced coma may be known by neighbours, family, medical attendants or the ambulance driver to have taken drugs by the presence of drug containers or alcohol in their homes. A history of depression might be known. A search of the patient's clothing may reveal hospital out-patient attendance cards, unfilled prescriptions, drugs or even syringes. Diabetic or epileptic patients sometimes carry some form of identification either in their clothing or as a wristband or necklace. *If there is any suspicion whatsoever that the patient might be hypoglycaemic, a blood sample should be taken for blood glucose estimation and then 20 g of 50% glucose given intravenously, before any diagnostic tests are undertaken.* Hypo-glycaemia is characterized by a stupor or coma from which the patient can be roused to a resentful and aggressive state of partial awareness, with pallor and sweatiness, bounding pulse, and often focal or generalized seizures. It is important to try to discover whether the coma was of gradual or sudden onset; the latter clearly suggests vascular disease. Before examination commences the doc-tor must make sure that the patient is breathing adequately, that the pulse and blood pressure are satisfactory and that the patient is not bleeding rapidly. If oxygenation is not satisfactory, whatever the breathing pattern, oxygen should be administered. If the patient is clearly in status epilepticus this must be treated appropriately immediately, and clinical examination continued afterwards.

GENERAL EXAMINATION

Certain general features of the patient's clinical state are of great importance. Does the patient appear clean, well nourished and generally cared for, or are there signs of social decline such as a dishevelled appearance, lack of personal cleanliness, malnutrition or infestation? Is there evidence of trauma or exposure? A rapid search must be made for fractures and, especially, for signs of cranial trauma. Bruises in the scalp are difficult to recognize but scalp oedema or haematoma can usually be palpated and bruising of the skin behind the pinna, called a battle sign, is a useful sign of basal or temporal skull fracture. Likewise, bleeding from the external auditory meati is a reliable sign of cranial trauma, with basal skull fracture. Pallor, circulatory failure and other evidence of shock must be recognized and a search made for external or internal haemorrhage, especially if trauma is suspected. In drug-induced coma there may be signs of repeated intravenous injections under conditions of imperfect sterility, causing venous thrombosis in forearm or antebrachial veins. The odours of alcohol, uraemia, diabetic acidosis and hepatic coma may be recognizable in rare instances. The sterterous, rapid respiration of acidotic coma (air hunger), usually due to diabetes, can be quickly recognized (see below). The presence of jaundice, liver palms, Dupuytren's contraction or spider naevi, even in the absence of hepatic enlargement raise the suspicion of hepatic coma. Meningitis can usually be recognized by the presence of drowsiness, lethargy or stupor with fever and signs of meningeal irritation (p. 332). The pulse may be unexpectedly slow in relation to the fever in pyogenic meningitis, although the respirations are usually rapid. Seizures and focal neurological signs may develop and there is usually a history of headache and neck stiffness, perhaps with vomiting. Further, there may be a skin rash, or a primary site of infection such as otitis media or sinusitis may be apparent. The ocular fundi must always be examined by ophthalmoscopy for signs of papilloedema, retinal haemorrhages or exudates, or intra-arterial emboli, which appear as luminescent, highly refractile yellow or white plaque-like material occluding vessels.

CONSCIOUSNESS

Examination of the unconscious patient should be directed towards defining the state of consciousness, as described above, particularly noting any variation or tendency to improve or deteriorate during the period of observation. *Change in level of consciousness is the single most important piece of information which will indicate the need for a change of management.* It is important to note exactly the *degree of responsiveness to external stimuli*, including conversation, calling the patient's first name, a sudden loud noise, a flash of light, contactual or painful stimulation, passive movement of the limbs and deep noxious stimuli such as squeezing the achilles tendon, sternal pressure applied with a hard blunt object or supra-orbital pressure from the examiner's thumb. Special attention must also be directed to *pupillary reaction and ocular movements*, both volitional and reflex, to the *pattern of breathing* and to *motor responses*, either spontaneous or reflexly evoked.

Pupils

Pupillary size and responsiveness to light should be noted. If the pupils are unequal a decision as to which is the abnormal must be made. Usually the large pupil indicates the presence of a third nerve palsy, whether from damage to the third nerve from pressure and displacement, or from a lesion in the mesencephalon itself, but occasionally the smaller pupil may be the abnormal pupil from a Horner's syndrome. If the larger pupil does not react to light it is likely that there is a partial third nerve palsy on that side. If the smaller pupil also fails to react to light this may be the mid-position pupil of complete sympathetic and parasympathetic lesions, indicating very extensive brain stem damage. Pupillary dilation in response to neck flexion or to pinching the skin of the neck is not a reliable phenomenon.

In drug-induced coma and in most patients with metabolic coma the pupillary responses to light are normal. Exceptions to this rule are glutethimide poisoning and very deep metabolic coma, in which the pupils may become dilated and, rarely, may become unreactive to light. In pontine and in thalamic haemorrhage the pupils may be very small, like a pin point, and unreactive to light.

Ocular movements

In comatose patients the eyes become slightly divergent at rest. If there is a pre-existent strabismus, deviation of the ocular axes may be pronounced, both at rest and during reflex ocular movements. If the patient is too drowsy or stuporose to test voluntary or following eye movements *'doll's head' movements* should be tested. If possible the patient should be placed on his back, although the test can be carried out in any position. The examiner grasps the patient's head with both hands, using the thumbs to gently hold the eyelids open, and firmly rocks the patient's head from side to side through about 70°, and then from passive neck flexion to passive neck extension. The patient's eyes tend to remain in the straight ahead position despite these passive movements of the head, a phenomenon like that found in some children's dolls. The patient's eyes tend to deviate in the opposite direction to the induced head movement. This movement depends on intact vestibular reflex mechanisms, and is thus a test of the peripheral sense organs involved, the labyrinths and otoliths, and their central connections in the brain stem, including the vestibular nuclei, the medial longitudinal fasciculi and the third, fourth and sixth cranial nerves and their nuclei. Sometimes lesions in these structures can be recognized during the doll's head test by the presence of disturbances in ocular movements consistent, for example, with a sixth or third nerve palsy. Absence of the reflex on one side indicates an ipsilateral pontine lesion, but complete absence of doll's head movements may be found with both extensive structural lesion in the brain stem and in deep metabolic coma. In most patients with drug-induced coma however, doll's-head ocular movements are intact.

Caloric reflexes may similarly be used as a test of brain stem function. Irrigation of the external auditory meatus on one side with at least 20 ml of ice-cold water induces slow conjugate deviation of the eyes towards the irrigated side after a few seconds' delay. In the awake or drowsy patient this slow, tonic, deviation is masked by a fast, coarse nystagmus towards the opposite side. Normal caloric nystagmus is characteristically also found in cases of psychogenic coma. After a few minutes' delay the opposite ear should also be tested. It is important to inspect the tympanic membrane on each side *before* irrigating the external auditory meatus since it is unwise to perform this test in the presence of a large perforation, or if there is an active otitis media.

Occasionally, in patients with infarction or other structural lesions in the posterior fossa *spontaneous ocular movements* may be observed. These may be accompanied by marked ocular divergence, sometimes with elevation of one eye and depression of the other. Rarely there may be a spontaneous 'see-saw' nystagmus in which one eye rotates up and the other down, the movements alternating at a very slow rate. Rapid ocular oscillations may occur especially after poisoning with tricyclic anti-depressant drugs, and a slow, once or twice a second, conjugate downward bobbing movement is sometimes a sign of cerebellar haemorrhage or tumour. In thalamic haemorrhage the pupils are pin point, and the eyes seem to be looking downward as if at the patient's own nose. Rapid conjugate lateral movement, at a rhythm and rate reminiscent of cerebellar nystagmus, occurring in an unconscious patient, should suggest focal motor seizures originating in the contralateral frontal lobe. Such seizures are often accompanied by deviation of the head and eyes in the direction of the 'nystagmoid movement', but not necessarily by a fully developed focal seizure involving face and limbs on the same side. Nystagmus itself cannot occur in the comatose patient because it requires ocular fixation to develop the fast, corrective phase.

Pattern of breathing

Depressed, but regular breathing at a normal rate occurs in most drug-induced comas, but Cheyne-Stokes respiration can occur in coma of any cause, especially if there is coincidental chronic pulmonary disease. In Cheyne-Stokes respiration, breathing varies in regular cycles. A phase of gradually deepening respiration is followed, after a period of very deep rapid breaths, by a phase of slowly decreasing respiratory excursion and rate. Respiration gradually becomes quieter and may cease for several seconds before the cycle is repeated (see Chapter 6). Deep sighing, rapid breathing at a regular rate should immediately suggest metabolic acidosis. Diabetic ketoacidosis or uraemia are the commonest causes of this acidotic (Kussmaul) breathing pattern, but a similar pattern may occur in some patients with respiratory failure, and in deep metabolic coma, especially hepatic coma. Deep, regular breathing may also occur with rostral brain stem damage, whether due to reticular pontial infarction or to central brain stem dysfunction secondary to trans-tentorial herniation associated with an intra- or extra-cerebral space-occupying lesion. This breathing pattern is called *central neurogenic (pontine) hyperventilation*. Interspersed deep sighs or yawns may precede the development of this respiratory pattern. Rapid shallow breathing occurs if central brain stem dysfunction extends more caudally to the lower pons. When medullary respiratory neurones are damaged, for example by progressive trans-tentorial herniation, irregular breathing (*ataxic respiration*) may develop. Irregular, slow, deep gasping respirations, sometimes associated with hiccups, suggest terminal medullary failure. In patients with raised intracranial pressure, these abnormal breathing patterns are often associated with other evidence of brain stem dysfunction, including a rising blood pressure, a slow pulse, flaccid limbs, absence of reflex ocular movements and dilation of the pupils.

It should be apparent from the foregoing description that changing patterns of respiration in an unconscious patient, particularly the development of central neurogenic hyperventilation, provides important and relatively objective evidence of deterioration. It must be recognized, however, that these changes in respiratory pattern may occur in structural lesions with raised intracranial pressure, in brain stem infarction and in some varieties of metabolic coma, especially hepatic coma. They are thus indicative of brain stem dysfunction, but not of its causation.

Motor responses

It is often difficult to elicit signs of focal cerebral disease in the unconscious patient. If progressive brain stem dysfunction from raised intra-cranial pressure with trans-tentorial herniation has occurred, focal signs indicative of the causative lesion may no longer be recognizable. However, papilloedema is usually present in such cases. In the drowsy or stuporose patient it may be possible to recognize a hemianopia by testing to menace or, sometimes, by testing for optokinetic nystagmus (p. 291). Visual threat, or menace, consists of testing the patient's response to rapid movement of the examiner's hand towards the patient's face, in first the left, and then the right field. Normally this threat induces rapid eye closure or a flinch. It is necessary to obtain the patient's attention transiently to assess any meaningful response and the test is, unfortunately, only rarely useful. Hemiplegia may be evident either from abnormal flaccidity of the arm and leg on the affected side or, in the stuporose or lightly comatose patient, by absence of spontaneous movements on that side. Noxious stimuli, for example pinching the skin of the forearms and thighs, deep rubbing pressure with a hard object applied to the sternum or, often most effective, lightly pricking the skin and mucous membranes near the nasal orifices on both sides will fail to induce movement of the paralysed limbs. Sometimes in a patient with a dense hemiplegia the cheek blows flaccidly in and out with each breath on the side of the hemiplegia. The tendon reflexes may be asymmetrical, but in most comatose patients both plantar responses are extensor (see p. 316). It should be noted that *asymmetry* of these motor responses is the important feature to assess.

In both structural lesions and metabolic disorders coma may be accompanied in its terminal stages by decorticate or decerebrate postures. These may occur asymmetrically and may be apparent, at first, only when induced by noxious external stimuli, such as deep sternal pressure or pinching the skin or achilles tendon. Decorticate and decerebrate postures are features of severe upper brain stem dysfunction and are thus usually found in association with pupillary abnormalities, absence of doll's-head and caloric reflexes and a disturbed breathing pattern. Decerebrate and decorticate postures are found much more commonly with structural coma than with metabolic coma, and thus do not usually occur in patients with drug-induced coma unless there has been additional hypoxic or ischaemic brain injury.

DIAGNOSIS OF BRAIN DEATH

With the advent of improved methods of intensive care, and especially of positive pressure ventilation in patients in whom spontaneous respirations have ceased, it has become important to define new criteria for the diagnosis of death. This has become important not only because of general recognition that brain death may have occurred in certain patients whose respiration has been maintained with a ventilator, although both the body temperature and the systemic circulation continue to be maintained spontaneously, but also because it has become possible to transplant organs, for example the kidney, from such patients to others. In both these situations the *diagnosis of brain death must be certain* before any decision is made to cease attempts to keep the patient alive. A conference of the Royal Colleges and Faculties of the United Kingdom considered this problem in 1976 in the light of previous attempts to define brain death, the changing needs of medical practice, and public concern about the issue and agreed the following guidelines.

A. Conditions under which the diagnosis of brain death should be considered.
   1. The patient is deeply comatose.
      a. There should be no suspicion that this state is due to depressant drugs.
      b. Primary hypothermia as a cause of coma should have been excluded.
      c. Metabolic & endocrine disturbances that can be responsible for or can contribute to coma should have been excluded.
   2. The patient is being maintained on a ventilator because spontaneous respiration had previously become inadequate or had ceased altogether.
      a. Relaxants . . . & other drugs should have been excluded as a cause of respiratory failure.
   3. There should be no doubt that the patient's condition is due to irremediable structural brain damage. The diagnosis of a disorder that can lead to brain death should have been fully established.

B. Diagnostic tests for confirmation of brain death
   ALL BRAINSTEM REFLEXES ARE ABSENT
   1. The pupils are fixed in diameter & do not respond to sharp changes in the intensity of incident light.
   2. There is no corneal reflex.
   3. The vestibulo-ocular reflexes are absent.
   4. No motor responses within the cranial-nerve distribution can be elicited by adequate stimulation of a somatic area.
   5. There is no gag reflex or reflex response to bronchial stimulation by a suction catheter passed down the trachea.
   6. No respiratory movements occur when the patient is disconnected from the mechanical ventilator for long enough to ensure that the arterial carbon dioxide tension rises above the threshold for stimulation of respiration.

C. Other considerations
  1. Repetition of testing
     The interval between tests must depend upon the primary
     pathology & the clinical course of the disease ... In some
     conditions the outcome is not so clearcut, and in these cases it
     is recommended that the tests should be repeated. The inter-
     val between tests depends upon the progress of the patient &
     might be as long as 24 hours ...
  2. Integrity of spinal reflexes
     It is well established that spinal-cord function can persist
     after insults that irretrievably destroy brainstem func-
     tions ...
  3. Confirmatory investigation
     It is now widely accepted that electro-encephalography is not
     necessary for the diagnosis of brain death ... Other investig-
     ations such as cerebral angiography or cerebral blood-flow
     measurements are not required for the diagnosis of brain
     death.
  4. Body temperature
     ... it is recommended that it should be not less than 35°C
     before the diagnostic tests are carried out.
  5. Specialist opinion & the status of the doctors concerned
     Only when the primary diagnosis is in doubt is it necessary to
     consult with a neurologist or neurosurgeon.
     Decision to withdraw artificial support should be made after
     all the criteria presented above have been fulfilled & can be
     made by any of the following combination of doctors:
     a. a consultant who is in charge of the case & one other
        doctor;
     b. in the absence of a consultant, his deputy, who should
        have been registered for 5 years or more & who should
        have had adequate experience in the care of such cases, &
        one other doctor.

(From The Lancet 1976, 2, 1069–1070)

These recommendations fall into three groups, parts A, B and C.
The patient must be deeply comatose and on a ventilator, and it
must be clearly established that the patient's coma is due to
irremediable structural brain damage (part A). Drug-induced coma,
hypothermia and metabolic causes of coma and relaxant drugs, as
a cause of ventilatory failure must have been clearly excluded. If
these conditions are fulfilled brain death may be diagnosed if no
brain stem reflexes can be demonstrated (part B). Repeated tests

are necessary but the interval between such tests depends on the pathology and the course of the disease. Purely spinal reflexes can persist after total brain stem destruction but it must always be remembered that decorticate and decerebrate postures are far from necessarily irreversible phenomena and therefore that their presence does not inevitably indicate that brain death has occurred. Indeed, many authorities would not allow a diagnosis of brain death if such reflexes persisted. All these tests should be carried out at a body temperature not less than 35°C.

Electroencephalographic and other studies, such as angiography, are not necessary for diagnosis of brain death but absence of brain electrical activity in an electroencephalogram, recorded for not less than 20 minutes at an amplification of 5 μV/cm provides very strong confirmatory evidence of cerebral death, provided that depressant drugs have not been given. In the past, it has been recommended that such an iso-electric electroencephalogram should be recorded twice not less than six hours apart before brain death is diagnosed, but this is no longer regarded as necessary in the United Kingdom. It is recommended that at least two doctors, one registered for not less than five years, should be concerned in the diagnosis of brain death before a decision to withdraw artificial support is made.

10

The locomotor system

The bones
The joints
The gait
Some investigations used in rheumatic diseases

The locomotor system includes the muscles, bones and joints. The examination of the muscles has been considered in the previous chapter.

THE BONES

In examining the *long bones* of the limbs, look for any alterations in shape or outline, for localized swellings in the bone, for signs of fracture and for evidence of undue tenderness. In osteitis deformans (Paget's disease) the bones are both deformed and enlarged. Alteration in the shape of the bones occurs in rickets. Localized swellings may be caused by infections, cysts or tumours. Spontaneous fractures may occasionally assist in the diagnosis of secondary carcinoma, generalized osteitis fibrosa (hyperparathyroidism), osteogenesis imperfecta or multiple myeloma. Undue tenderness of the bones is found with infection, in generalized osteitis fibrosa, myelomatosis, occasionally in carcinomatosis of bones, and very rarely in leukaemia.

The *vertebral column and skull* demand special attention. Note the presence of any local projections or angular deformity of the vertebral spines, which vertebrae are involved and at what level the projection is most prominent. Landmarks are C7 (vertebra prominens) and the last rib, articulating with the 12th thoracic vertebra. In many cases, however, the last rib cannot be distinctly felt and is therefore rather untrustworthy as a guide.

Note also any curvature of the spinal column as a whole, or of part of it, distinguishing such general curvature from the local projections referred to above.

The curvature may be in an anterior, posterior or lateral direction. Anterior curvature (extension deformity) is termed *lordosis* and is commonest in the lumbar region. General posterior curvature (flexion deformity) is spoken of as *kyphosis*. It occurs most typically in the thoracic region in old persons and must be distinguished from the localized angular deformity of Pott's disease (spinal tuberculosis). Lateral curvature is termed *scoliosis*, and may be towards either side. It is always accompanied by a rotation of the bodies of the vertebrae in such a way that the spines come to point towards the concavity of the curve, i.e. the curvature is greater than it appears from inspection of the posterior spinous processes. Kyphosis and scoliosis may often be combined.

Test the movements of the spine (p. 360). Note the exact site of any pain and observe whether it is accompanied by reflex muscle spasm. Painful restriction of movement of the cervical and lumbar spine is an important sign of *cervical and lumbar spondylosis* but may also be found in disc or other mechanical disorders of the back or neck. The spine may be fixed in *ankylosing spondylitis*, as may also the costovertebral joints (chest expansion reduced to less than 5 cm).

THE JOINTS

These should be examined by inspection and palpation, and by tests for their range of movement. It is best to proceed in a routine manner, e.g. the jaw, cervical spine, shoulder girdle and upper limb, thoracic and lumbar spine, pelvis and lower limb, so that inconspicuous but important joints like the temporomandibular, sternoclavicular and sacroiliac will not be overlooked. Always compare the corresponding joints on the two sides of the body.

On inspection and palpation look for enlargement or irregularity of the joint; for redness, tenderness and heat; and note whether the overlying skin is dry or moist. Tenderness may be recorded in four grades, depending upon the patient's reaction to firm pressure of the joint between finger and thumb. Grade 1 tenderness: the patient says the joint is tender. Grade 2: the patient winces. Grade 3: the patient winces and withdraws the affected part. Grade 4: the patient will not allow the joint to be touched. Grade 4 tenderness only occurs in gout, rheumatic fever or suppurative arthritis. In gout the skin overlying the affected joint is dry, whereas in suppurative arthritis or rheumatic fever it is moist.

Look for Heberden's nodes which are bony outgrowths from the base of the distal phalanges of the fingers found in some patients with osteoarthritis. Rheumatoid subcutaneous nodules may be detected by running the examining thumb from the point of the elbow down the proximal portion of the ulna. Look for gouty tophi on the helix of the ear as well as over joints. Muscle wasting may be a pointer to disease of a nearby joint.

If the joint is enlarged, determine whether the enlargement is due to effusion into the joint space, when it normally has a characteristic shape and fluctuation can often be elicited; to thickening of the tissues, such as occurs in rheumatoid arthritis; to irregular bony thickening by osteophytes such as occurs in osteoarthrosis; to enlargement of the ends of the bones, such as occurs in pulmonary osteoarthropathy; or to complete disorganization of the joint with absence of pain sense such as occurs in neuropathic (Charcot's) joints.

If tenderness is present localize it as accurately as possible and determine particularly whether it arises in the joint or in neighbouring structures, e.g. in the supraspinatus tendon rather than in the shoulder joint. Feel the joint with one hand, while it is moved passively with the other. A grating or creaking sensation known as *crepitus* may be felt. This often indicates osteoarthrosis, but not invariably so, for crepitus is commonly felt in the shoulder joints of older persons, whereas osteoarthrosis of these joints is rare.

In examining joints for the range of movement an estimate of the degree of limitation present based on previous experience or on comparison with the normal side may often be sufficient, but for accurate description the actual range of movement should be measured with a protractor or goniometer. Testing the range of *passive* movement is generally more informative than observing *active* movement, although it is sometimes useful to test the latter as well. Gentleness must be exercised, particularly in the case of painful joints. Limitation of movement in a joint may be due to pain, muscle spasm, contracture, inflammation or thickening of the capsules or periarticular structures, effusion into the joint space, bony overgrowths, bony ankylosis, or to painful conditions quite unconnected with the joint.

In describing the range of movement of joints the scheme shown in the following pages (modified by permission of the authors and publishers, from E. F. Cave & M. R. Sumner (1936) *J. Bone Jt Surg.*, XVIII, 455) will be found useful. All motion should be measured in degrees from a neutral or zero position which must be defined whenever possible.

Lumbar and dorsal spine (Fig. 10.1). Neutral position is a normal upright stance with head erect and chin drawn in. While the neck moves freely in all directions, the thoracic spine permits mainly rotation, while the lumbar spine can flex, extend and bend laterally. Remember to test costovertebral mobility by measuring chest expansion, and test for sacroiliac irritability by pressing

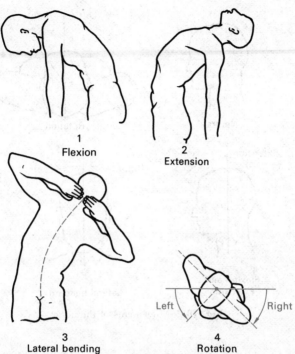

Fig. 10.1 Movements of the lumbar and dorsal spine.

firmly over the centre of the sacrum with the patient prone. Adequate exposure is essential. Test:

1. Flexion
2. Extension
3. Lateral bending
4. Rotation (patient seated)

Cervical spine (Fig. 10.2).

1. Rotation
2. Flexion
3. Extension
4. Lateral bending

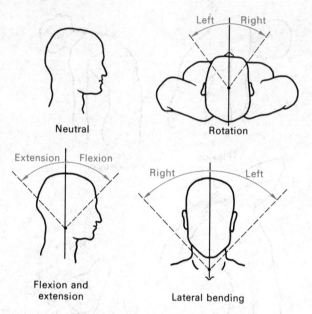

Neutral

Rotation

Flexion and extension

Lateral bending

Fig. 10.2 Movements of the neck.

Shoulder (Fig. 10.3).   Neutral position is arm to side, elbow flexed to 90° with forearm pointing forwards. Because the scapula is mobile, true shoulder (humeroscapular) movement can be assessed only by the examiner anchoring the scapula. Test:

1. Flexion
2. Extension
3. Abduction
4. Rotation in abduction
5. Rotation in neutral
6. Elevation (this is partly shoulder girdle motion as compared with 1–5 which are pure humeroscapular movements)

Elbow (Fig. 10.4).   Neutral position is with forearm in extension. Test:

1. Flexion
2. Hyperextension

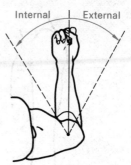

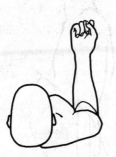

Neutral

Rotation in neutral

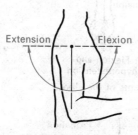

Flexion and extension

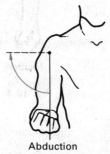

Abduction

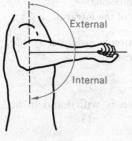

Rotation in abduction

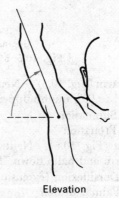

Elevation

Fig. 10.3 Movements of the shoulder.

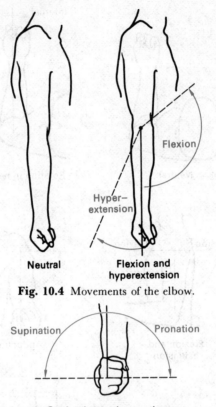

Neutral   **Flexion and
                      hyperextension**

Fig. 10.4 Movements of the elbow.

Supination and pronation

Fig. 10.5 Movements of the forearm.

Forearm (Fig. 10.5).   Neutral position is with arm by side, elbow flexed to 90°, thumb uppermost. Test:

1. Supination
2. Pronation

Wrist (Fig. 10.6).   Neutral position is with hand in line with forearm and palm down. Test:

1. Dorsiflexion (extension)
2. Palmar flexion
3. Ulnar deviation
4. Radial deviation

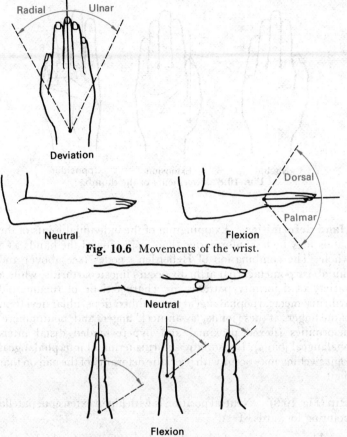

Fig. 10.6 Movements of the wrist.

Fig. 10.7 Movements of the fingers.

Fingers (Fig. 10.7). Neutral position is with fingers in extension. Test the flexion at metacarpophalangeal joints.

Thumb (carpometacarpal joint) (Fig. 10.8). Neutral position is with thumb alongside forefinger and extended. Test:

    1. Extension
    2. Flexion—measured as for the fingers
    3. Opposition
    4. Abduction (not illustrated) is movement at right angles to plane of palm

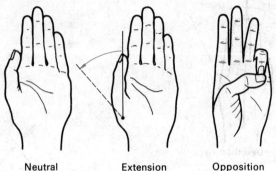

Neutral   **Extension**   **Opposition**
Fig. 10.8 Movements of the thumb.

Hand deformities.   Examination of the individual joints of the hands may be less informative than inspection of the hands as a whole. The combination of Heberden's nodes (see above) and thumb carpometacarpal arthritis occurs in osteoarthritis, while a variety of deformity patterns are characteristic of rheumatoid arthritis: metacarpophalangeal joint subluxations, ulnar deviation of the fingers at these joints, 'swan-neck' fingers and 'boutonnière' deformities (flexed proximal and hyperextended distal interphalangeal joints). In psoriatic arthritis terminal interphalangeal joint swelling may occur with psoriatic deformity of the nail on that digit.

Hip (Fig. 10.9).   Neutral position is with hip in extension, patella pointing forwards. Test:

1. Flexion measured with knee bent. Opposite thigh must remain in neutral position
2. Abduction, measured from a line which forms an angle of 90° with a line joining the anterior superior spines
3. Adduction, measured in the same manner
4. Rotation in flexion
5. Rotation in extension

Additional examinations of the hip joint:

1. Testing for extension. Attempt to extend the hip with the patient lying in the lateral position on the opposite side. Extension

should normally be at least 30° from the neutral position. This movement is lost early in hip joint disease and the loss is associated with a flexion deformity and a 'waddling' gait.

2. Measurement of 'true' and 'apparent' shortening. If the length of the legs is measured from the anterior superior iliac spine to the medial malleolus on the same side, any difference is referred to as 'true' shortening, and almost invariably indicates disease of the hip joint or the neck of the femur on the shorter side. If the

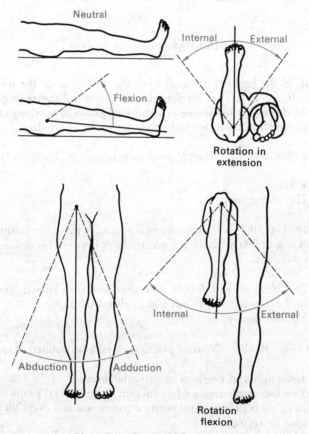

Fig. 10.9 Movements of the hip.

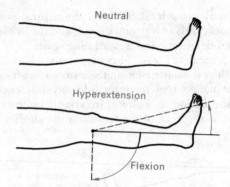

Fig. 10.10   Movements of the knee.

length of the legs is measured from the umbilicus to the medial malleoli, any difference is referred to as 'apparent' shortening and may be due either to disease as mentioned above or to tilting of the pelvis, usually due to an adduction deformity of the hip.

Knee (Fig. 10.10).   Neutral position is complete extension. Test:

1. Flexion
2. Hyperextension

Ankle (Fig. 10.11).   Neutral position is with the outer border of foot at angle of 90° with the leg, and midway between inversion and eversion. Test:

1. Dorsiflexion, with foot in inversion; test with knee in flexion and extension to exclude tight calf muscles.
2. Plantar flexion

Foot (Fig. 10.12).   Neutral position cannot be defined. Test:

1. Inversion and eversion at sub-talar joints
2. Forefoot adduction and abduction at mid-tarsal joints, with os calcis held in neutral position (inversion and eversion may also be tested)
3. Flexion at metatarsophalangeal and interphalangeal joints

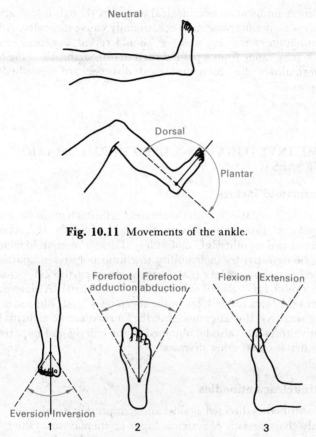

Fig. 10.11 Movements of the ankle.

Neutral

Dorsal

Plantar

Forefoot adduction | Forefoot abduction

Flexion | Extension

Eversion | Inversion

1

2

3

Fig. 10.12 Movements of the foot.

THE GAIT

When one studies the gait, it is well to have the legs fully exposed. The patient should therefore be unclothed or else wear a small triangle or bathing slip. The feet should be bare. Ask the patient to walk away from you, to turn around at a given point and then to walk towards you again.

Abnormalities of the gait are usually due either to local lesions in the lower limbs or to neurological disorder, though intoxication, hysteria or malingering may occasionally cause difficulty. A full examination of the legs and feet should reveal any local cause, which may range from a painful corn to osteoarthrosis of the hip. Abnormalities due to neurological disorder are described in Chapter 8.

SOME INVESTIGATIONS USED IN RHEUMATIC DISEASES

Rheumatoid factors

About 80% of patients with rheumatoid arthritis have in their sera *antiglobulins* (autoantibodies in the IgM, IgG or IgA classes directed against other IgG molecules). These 'rheumatoid factors' may be detected by their ability to clump polystyrene particles coated with human IgG (*Latex test*) or sheep erythrocytes coated with rabbit IgG (*Rose-Waaler, DAT or SCAT tests*). A significant titre in the latex test is 1/80, in the sheep tests 1/32. The former is more sensitive, the latter more specific for rheumatoid arthritis but positive tests may also be obtained in the elderly and in patients with hepatic and other diseases.

Antinuclear antibodies

Autoantibodies directed against antigens present in cell nuclei are highly characteristic of systemic lupus erythematosus. Other systemic connective tissue diseases may give results which are positive, usually less strongly so. Three laboratory tests are most commonly used:

Antinuclear factor test (ANF).   An immunofluorescent technique which is highly sensitive, easy to perform and therefore useful as a screening test. The significance increases with the titre. It is always positive in active SLE.

DNA binding test.   A radioisotope immunochemical technique detecting antibodies to native (double-stranded) DNA. Expressed as 'percentage binding', results over 30% are positive and the significance increases with higher figures up to 100%. This is the most specific laboratory test for active SLE.

LE cell test. The original test is time-consuming to perform. Peripheral blood 'buffy layer' cells which have been incubated are smeared and stained. Ingestion of nuclear material by leucocytes produces the characteristic 'LE cell'.

Uric acid determinations

A consistently normal plasma uric acid level (below 375 μmol/litre in women and 425 μmol/litre in men) effectively excludes the diagnosis of (untreated) gout. Raised levels occur in a wide variety of circumstances and, in themselves, do not establish the diagnosis of gout. On a low purine diet the 24 hour urinary urate excretion should not exceed 600 mg. Higher levels indicate 'overproducers' of urate who may be at risk of stone formation.

Synovial fluid examination

Synovial fluid may be obtained for examination from any joint in which it is clinically detectable. The knee is the most convenient source: after infiltration with 1% local anaesthetic, a 21 gauge needle is inserted on the medial aspect between the patella and the femoral condyle. The aspirated fluid should be placed in a plain sterile container; if a cell count is required, some should also be mixed with EDTA anticoagulant.

Synovial fluid examination is diagnostic in two conditions: bacterial infections and crystal synovitis, and every effort should be made to obtain a fluid when either of these is suspected. Polarized light microscopy can differentiate between the crystals of urate in gout and those of calcium pyrophosphate dihydrate in pseudogout. Outside these conditions synovial fluid examination is unlikely to be diagnostic: frank blood may point to trauma, haemophilia or villonodular synovitis, while inflammatory (as opposed to degenerative) arthritis is suggested by an opaque fluid of low viscosity, with a total white cell count over 1000/ml, neutrophils over 50%, protein content over 35 g/litre, and the presence of a firm clot.

Antistreptolysin-O (ASO) test

The presence in the serum of this antibody in a titre greater than
1/200 (reported as the reciprocal, i.e. '200') or, more significantly,
a rising titre, indicates a recent haemolytic streptococcal infection.
A positive test does not establish a diagnosis of rheumatic fever,
but a negative test makes this diagnosis unlikely.

11

Examination of the eye, ear, nose and throat

THE EYE

Before examining the various parts of the eye, one should test the visual acuity, and, when relevant, the colour sense and the extent of the visual fields.

Test for distant vision

Visual acuity is measured with Snellen's test-types, a series of letters of varying sizes so constructed that the top letter is visible to the normal eye at 60 metres, and the subsequent lines at 36, 24, 18, 12, 9, 6 and 5 metres respectively. Visual acuity (V) is recorded according to the formula $V = d/D$, where d is the distance at which the letters are read, and D that at which they should be read. The patient is normally placed at a distance of 6 metres from the test types ($d = 6$) and each eye is tested separately. The patient reads down the chart as far as he can. If only the top letter of the chart is visible, the visual acuity is 6/60. A normal person should be able to read at least the seventh line, i.e. a visual acuity of 6/6. A person with an uncorrected refractive error may have a subnormal visual acuity, and a rough estimate of his corrected visual acuity may be obtained by asking him to view the chart through a pin-hole aperture. If the visual acuity is less than 6/60, the patient is moved towards the test-types until he can read the top letter. If the top letter is visible at 2 metres, the visual acuity is 2/60. Visual acuities of less than 1/60 are recorded as '*counting fingers*' (CF), '*hand move-ments*' (HM), '*perception of light*' (PL) or '*no perception of light*' (no PL).

If the patient wears glasses, the type of lens he is wearing may be determined as follows. Hold the lens in front of the eye and look at an object through it. Then move the lens in front of the eye and look at an object through it. Then move the lens from side to side and watch the object. If the latter seems to move in the opposite direction to the lens, the lens is convex; if in the same direction, it is concave. Patients with myopia use concave (diverging) lenses and those with hypermetropia convex (converging) ones.

In order to tell whether a lens is spherical or cylindrical, look at a straight object through it and then slowly twist the lens round. If the lens is cylindrical, the object will appear to take up an oblique position. Patients who are astigmatic need cylindrical lenses.

Test for near vision

Visual acuity at the ordinary reading distance is assessed with reading test types of varying sizes, the notation being based on the printers' 'point' system. The smallest print used is N5. The near vision is recorded as the smallest type which the patient can read comfortably.

COLOUR SENSE

Colour sense is most easily tested by the use of pseudo-isochromatic plates, the best known being those of Ishihara. People with defective colour vision confuse certain colours. Pseudo-isochromatic plates are so constructed that a person with normal colour vision will read a different number on the same plate.

The most common anomalies of colour vision are various types of red–green deficiency, inherited as sex-linked recessive conditions, which occur in about 8% of males and 0·5% of females in this country. People with blue–yellow deficiencies and with total colour-blindness are rare.

VISUAL FIELDS

The testing of the visual fields is described on p. 278.

EXAMINATION OF THE EYE

After the visual functions have been tested, the eyes should be examined systematically. The shape and position of the eyelids should be noted. Mongolian races have a long narrow palpebral aperture with an upward and outward obliquity and a characteristic fold of skin along the upper lid. The highest point of the aperture is at the junction of its middle and inner thirds, whereas in mongolism (Down's syndrome) the oblique palpebral aperture is short and wide with its highest point at the centre of the lid.

Ptosis, or drooping of the upper lid, may be congenital or acquired. A congenital ptosis may be unilateral or bilateral, whereas an acquired ptosis is usually unilateral if due to paralysis of the third cranial nerve or of the cervical sympathetic, and usually bilateral if due to myopathy.

Lid retraction is present if a band of white sclera is visible above the iris when the eyes are looking straight ahead. Lid retraction, which is usually due to thyrotoxicosis, is often associated with infrequent blinking and with lid-lag, i.e. the upper lid seems to lag behind the eyeball when the patient looks downwards. Patients with thyrotoxicosis frequently also have a slight degree of forward displacement of the eyeball (exophthalmos). Some patients with thyrotoxicosis or some whose thyrotoxicosis has been successfully treated medically or surgically, develop a more severe and progressive form of exophthalmos, which may be associated with ocular palsies. Exophthalmos also results from space-occupying lesions in the orbit, and an apparent exophthalmos may be present when the eye is longer than normal, as in myopia.

The presence of an inflammation of the margins of the lids (marginal blepharitis) should be noted, together with any abnormality in the position of the lid margins, i.e. eversion (ectropion) or inversion (entropion) of the lashes.

The lacrimal gland.   The lacrimal gland is examined by pulling up the outer part of the upper lid while asking the patient to look downwards and inwards. Acute inflammations (dacryoadenitis) result in a tender swollen gland with oedema of the upper lid and localized conjunctival injection. Chronic dacryoadenitis, a painless enlargement of the lacrimal gland which is frequently bilateral, occurs in the reticuloses, sarcoidosis and tuberculosis. Tumours of the lacrimal gland produce a hard swelling of the gland associated with proptosis.

The conjunctiva.   The conjunctiva lining the eyeball (bulbar conjunctiva) and that lining the inner surface of the eyelids (palpebral conjunctiva) should be examined. In order to examine the palpebral conjunctiva of the lower lid, the lower lid should be pulled down while asking the patient to look upwards. To expose the palpebral conjunctiva of the lower lid, ask the patient to look downwards, then place the right thumb at the upper part of the upper lid and pull it upwards so as to evert the eyelashes. Grasp the lashes between the forefinger and thumb of the left hand and evert the lid by rotating it round the right thumb. The conjunctiva may be pale in anaemia, jaundiced, or injected in conjunctivitis. Marked injection of the bulbar conjunctiva with a mucopurulent discharge suggests a severe bacterial inflammation; marked injection with a little serous discharge is indicative of a viral infection; slight oedema of the conjunctiva with a milky hue suggests an allergic condition. Follicles on the upper palpebral conjunctiva occur in trachoma, whereas their presence on the lower palpebral conjunctiva suggests an allergic condition or a conjunctivitis of viral origin.

Conjunctivitis. In conjunctivitis the injection is maximal in the fornices (the junction of bulbar and palpebral conjunctiva), and this appearance must be distinguished from the circumcorneal injection that occurs in keratitis, anterior uveitis and acute glaucoma. In circumcorneal injection there is a narrow band of dilated blood vessel around the limbus, and the injection is minimal in the fornices.

Inflammations of the cornea. Inflammations of the cornea (keratitis) may be superficial or deep, and are accompanied by circumcorneal injection. Superficial keratitis and corneal ulcers result in breaches in the corneal epithelium, and these breaches will stain with fluorescein. A drop of fluorescein is instilled into the conjunctival sac and the excess dye is then washed out with normal saline. Breaches in the corneal epithelium are stained green. Deep keratitis results in a hazy cornea, often with an intact epithelium; it is usually caused by a viral or syphilitic infection. Both keratitis and trauma to the cornea may result in corneal opacities; small opacities are described as nebulae, larger ones as leucomata.

Arcus senilis. Arcus senilis is a crescentic opacity near the periphery of the cornea. It usually starts at the lower part of the cornea, extending to form a complete circle. It is common in old people, but may occur in the young (arcus juvenilis). It does not appear to have any significance.

Anterior uveitis. In anterior uveitis (iridocyclitis) circumcorneal injection also occurs. In addition, white specks may be visible on the posterior surface of the cornea (keratitic precipitates); there may be an exudate in the anterior chamber, and the pupil may be

constricted and irregular due to the formation of adhesions between the edge of the pupil and the anterior surface of the lens
(posterior synechiae). Other abnormalities of the pupils are
described on p. 291.

Ocular tension.   The ocular tension may be roughly assessed by
palpating the eyeball, although even with practice only gross
variations from normal can be appreciated. The sclera is palpated
with the two forefingers through the upper lid with the patient
looking downwards, the other fingers resting on the patient's
forehead. The degree of fluctuation gives an indication of the
ocular tension. More accurate measurements of ocular tension can
be made with Schiøtz or applanation tonometers. A diminished
tension occurs in diabetic coma and in severe dehydration from
any cause. A myopic eye frequently feels softer than a normal one.
An increased ocular tension occurs in glaucoma.

The fundus

Examination of the fundus of the eye with an ophthalmoscope is an
essential part of every complete medical examination. Valuable
information may be obtained as to the state of the optic nerve head
and of the arteries and veins of the retina, in addition to the
detection of local ophthalmic conditions.

In routine medical examinations it is usually possible, with
practice, to examine the optic disc and surrounding retina without
dilating the pupil, but for a complete examination of the fundus the
pupils should be dilated by instilling a few drops of 1% cyclopento-
late (Mydrilate) or 2% homatropine into the conjunctival sacs. In
patients with a predisposition to closed-angle glaucoma an acute
attack may be precipitated when the pupils are dilated. Before a
mydriatic is instilled, the patient should be asked whether he has
ever seen haloes (coloured rings) around lights, and, if he has, this,
or the presence of a shallow anterior chamber, is a contra-
indication to the use of a mydriatic. After the examination of the
fundus has been completed, the effects of the mydriatic should be
counteracted by the instillation of a few drops of 2% pilocarpine.

The patient should be examined either sitting or lying down in a
darkened room. He is asked to look straight ahead and to keep his
eyes as still as possible. The ophthalmoscope is held a few centimetres from the patient's eyes, and a suitable plus lens is used in

the ophthalmoscope so that the iris is in focus. Opacities in the media of the eye (cornea, anterior chamber, lens, vitreous) will appear as black specks or lines against the red reflex of the fundus.

The ophthalmoscope should then be brought as close as possible to the patient's eye and the light directed slightly nasally. In this way the optic disc can be found, and in addition the light will not shine directly on the macula. If the patient's pupils are not dilated, shining a light on to the macula will make the pupils contract and may make the examination of the fundus difficult or impossible. If the optic disc is not in focus, the strength of the lenses of the ophthalmoscope should be gradually reduced until the disc becomes sharply focused. If the observer's eye is emmetropic and his accommodation is relaxed, the strength of the lens necessary to bring the fundus into focus gives an indication of the refractive error of the patient's eye. Plus lenses indicate hypermetropia, and minus ones myopia. The optic disc, the retinal blood vessels, the macular region and the periphery of the fundus should be examined in turn.

The optic disc

Shape.   The normal disc is round or slightly oval. If astigmatism is present, the disc may appear more oval than normal.

Colour.   The normal disc has a pale pink colour, distinctly paler than the surrounding fundus. The temporal side of the disc is usually paler than the nasal side.

In atrophy of the optic nerve, the disc becomes very pale and may even become white or greyish-white in colour. In oedema of the optic nerve-head, resulting from raised intercranial pressure (papilloedema) or from inflammation (papillitis), the disc is pinker than normal and may approach the colour of the surrounding retina. In pseudopapilloedema, a congenital anomally usually associated with hypermetropia, the disc may appear swollen and pinker than normal, but the retinal blood vessels are normal in appearance, corrected vision is normal and the condition is stationary.

Physiological cup.   In its central part there is usually a depression in the disc, the physiological cup. The cup is paler than the surrounding disc, and from it the retinal vessels enter and leave the eye. In glaucoma the cup may be greatly increased in size, and the retinal vessels will kink as they cross the edge of the disc. When the cup is deep (in advanced glaucoma), retinal vessels disappear as they climb from the floor to the rim, and reappear again as they bend sharply over the cup (Plate V).

Edge of the disc.   This is normally well defined. In normal eyes there is sometimes a white scleral ring, a dark pigmented ring, or a stippled choroidal ring surrounding the optic disc.

The retinal blood vessels.   These radiate from the disc, dividing dichotomously into many branches as they pass towards the periphery of the retina. The retinal arteries are narrower than the veins, are a brighter red in colour, and have a brighter longitudinal streak where light is reflected from their convex walls. Spontaneous retinal artery pulsation is an abnormal finding, and occurs in some cases of glaucoma and aortic regurgitation. Spontaneous venous pulsation is frequently seen in normal eyes; it never occurs in papilloedema. It is important to study the points where arteries and veins cross. Most frequently it is the artery that crosses the vein, and in normal eyes neither vessel shows any change in colour, diameter or direction.

The macular region.   This is situated about 1·5 disc diameters from the temporal border of the optic disc. It is recognized by being darker in colour than the surrounding fundus, and is frequently surrounded by a halo of annular light reflex. It is devoid of blood vessels. At the centre of the macular region is a small depression, the fovea, which is lighter in colour and often glistens. Pathological changes in the macular region are important, as they produce a greater reduction of vision than similar changes in any other part of the fundus.

The periphery of the fundus.   This area can be examined only if the pupil is dilated with a mydriatic. Certain disease processes start in this region, for example retinal tears and retinitis pigmentosa.

The following is a brief description of the chief changes met with in the fundus which are important medically.

Papilloedema (Plate V).   This is a passive oedema of the optic nerve head, most commonly due to raised intracranial pressure. There is an absence of inflammatory changes, and frequently there is little or no disturbance of visual function. In the initial stages of the condition there is an increased redness of the disc with blurring of its margins, the blurring appearing first at the upper and lower margins, particularly in the upper nasal quadrant. The physiological cup becomes filled in and disappears and the retinal veins are slightly distended. Spontaneous pulsation of the retinal veins is absent.

As the condition progresses the disc becomes definitely swollen. In order to measure the degree of swelling of the disc, it is necessary to start with a high plus lens in the ophthalmoscope and reduce the power of the lens until the centre of the disc is just in focus. The retina, a short distance from the disc, is then brought into focus by further reduction of the power of the lens. This further reduction indicates the degree of swelling of the disc (3 dioptres is equivalent to 1 mm of swelling).

If papilloedema develops rapidly, there will be marked engorgement of the retinal veins with haemorrhages and exudates on and around the disc, but with papilloedema of slow onset there may be little or no vascular change, even though the disc may become very swollen. The retinal vessels will, however, bend sharply as they dip down from the swollen disc to the surrounding retina. The oedema may extend to the adjacent retina, producing greyish-white striations near the disc, and a white macular fan between the fovea and disc may develop in some cases.

Papilloedema occurs frequently in cases of brain tumour, but is particularly liable to occur in children with tumours of the cerebellum and fourth ventricle. It is uncommon in patients with pituitary tumours. An acute form of papilloedema with haemorrhage extending into the vitreous is characteristic of subarachnoid haemorrhage. A subdural haematoma may produce a similar clinical picture to that of a cerebral tumour. Papilloedema is uncommon in acute meningitis, but is more common in subacute and chronic meningitis. It may be the only physical sign in benign intracranial hypertension. Papilloedema occurring in malignant hypertension is accompanied by arterial changes characteristic of this condition and the haemorrhages and exudates extend far beyond the region of the disc.

Optic neuritis. Inflammatory, demyelinating, or vascular disease may attack any part of the optic nerve, producing an optic neuritis, the characteristic symptom of which is loss of vision, presenting as either a central scotoma or complete blindness. There is often pain on moving the eye, and the pupil on the affected side shows an ill-sustained contraction to a bright light. It is customary to divide optic neuritis into papillitis and retrobulbar neuritis.

Papillitis.   This is present when the disease affects the optic nerve head, producing hyperaemia and some swelling of the optic disc. It must not be confused with papilloedema, in spite of their similar ophthalmoscopic appearances. The two conditions can usually be distinguished by the gross visual loss that occurs with papillitis, as compared with the often minimal loss in papilloedema. In papillitis the swelling of the optic disc is usually slight, the distension of the retinal veins is less marked than in papilloedema, and there may be signs of inflammation (hazy vitreous, retinal exudates).

Retrobulbar neuritis.   This is present when the disease process affects that part of the optic nerve behind the eye. The same severe visual loss occurs as in papillitis, but the optic disc appears normal in the acute stage of the disease. Both papillitis and retrobulbar neuritis may be followed by optic atrophy.

Optic atrophy.   In this condition the optic disc is paler than normal and may even be white (Plate V). Because of the wide variation in colour of the normal disc, a useful sign of optic atrophy is the reduction in capillaries on the disc. In optic atrophy the number of capillaries that cross the disc margin is reduced from the normal of 10 to 7 or less. From the appearance of the disc it is customary, although not always very useful, to divide optic atrophy into primary and secondary types. In the *primary* type the disc is flat and white with clear-cut edges. *Secondary* optic atrophy follows swelling of the optic disc, due either to papilloedema or to papillitis. The disc is greyish-white in colour; it may be slightly swollen and its edges are indistinct.

Optic atrophy may occur in a number of disorders, of which the following are a few.

1. Interference with the blood supply to the optic nerve, as in occlusion of the central artery of the retina

2. Pressure on the nerve, whether in its intra-ocular, intra-orbital, intracanalicular or intracranial portions
3. Following optic neuritis
4. Following trauma where the optic nerve or its blood supply is involved
5. In toxic conditions due to substances such as tobacco, alcohol, lead, etc
6. In certain congenital disorders, when it is frequently associated with other neurological signs
7. Following widespread chorioretinal inflammation or degeneration

Opaque or medullated nerve fibres. These usually present as one or more bright white patches radiating for a short distance from the optic disc (Plate V). The patch has a characteristic feathered edge and retinal vessels may disappear for a short distance within it. This condition is a harmless and stationary congenital anomaly.

A myopic crescent. This is a ring of exposed white sclera, usually on the temporal side of the optic disc (Plate V), but in some cases extending all round it. When marked it may be associated with other degenerative changes in the fundus, which, if they involve the macula, will result in reduction of central vision.

Retinal haemorrhages. These occur in a number of different conditions and are due to one or more of the following factors.

1. Increased blood pressure within the retinal vessels, as in hypertension and chronic nephritis
2. Abnormalities in the walls of the retinal vessels, as in arteriosclerosis, diabetes mellitus and occlusion of the central vein of the retina
3. Abnormalities in the circulating blood, as in severe anaemia, leukaemias, and bleeding diatheses
4. Sudden reduction in intra-ocular pressure, following a penetrating wound (surgical or traumatic) of the eye

When superficial, within the nerve fibre layer of the retina, the haemorrhages are elongated and 'flame-shaped', whereas when deep they are round blotches or spots. Subhyaloid haemorrhages, situated in front of the retina, are occasionally seen as very large round haemorrhages with a straight horizontal upper border; they sometimes occur in diabetic retinopathy and after a subarachnoid haemorrhage.

Retinal arteriosclerosis.   This occurs either as an exaggeration of the general ageing process of the body or in association with hypertension. It is characterized by (*a*) broadening of the arterial light reflex, producing a 'copper wire' or 'silver wire' appearance; (*b*) tortuosity of the vessels; (*c*) nipping, indentation or deflection of the veins where they are crossed by the arteries; (*d*) white plaques on the arteries; and (*e*) 'flame-shaped' haemorrhages and 'cotton-wool' exudates in the region of the macula.

Hypertensive retinopathy (Plate VI).   This is characterized by a generalized narrowing of the retinal arteries, particularly in the young patient. In older patients these changes are masked by the accompanying arteriosclerosis. If the hypertension is severe, fullness of the retinal veins and 'flame-shaped' haemorrhages occur around the optic disc, and there is retinal oedema extending towards the macula, sometimes accompanied by a star-shaped collection of white exudates around the macula. In malignant hypertension papilloedema is also present. The retinopathy seen in some cases of acute and chronic nephritis is due to the associated hypertension.

Diabetic retinopathy (Plate VI).   The fundamental change in this condition is the formation of capillary micro-aneurysms, seen as tiny red spots around the macula. Micro-aneurysms are not seen in such abundance in any other condition. Retinal haemorrhages and exudates may occur; the haemorrhages are punctate or round, and the exudates have a waxy yellow-white appearance. The haemorrhages may extend into the vitreous and result in a glial proliferation called retinitis proliferans, which may result in blindness by covering the macula or by causing a retinal detachment. Patients with diabetic retinopathy often have associated arteriosclerotic or hypertensive changes in their fundi.

Retinopathies in disorders of the haemopoietic system.   In severe anaemias the fundus may be paler than normal and a few small 'flame-shaped' haemorrhages and small woolly exudates may be present.

In polycythaemia the retinal vessels are dark, tortuous and

dilated. There may be oedema of the optic disc, and a few retinal haemorrhages may be observed.

In the leukaemias the retinal veins may be tortuous and dilated. In later stages of these diseases the arteries and veins may be yellowish in colour, and the fundus may have a generalized pallor. Retinal haemorrhages of various types may occur, the characteristic ones in leukaemia being round with a pale centre.

Occlusion of the central artery of the retina. The optic disc and surrounding retina are pale, and there is a cherry-red spot at the macula which contrasts with the milky pallor of the adjacent retina. The retinal arteries are narrow or even thread-like.

Occlusion of the central vein of the retina. There is intense swelling of the optic disc, with gross venous dilatation, and numerous retinal haemorrhages extend from the disc in all directions.

Choroiditis. In acute choroiditis there are one or more round or oval whitish patches in the fundus, lying deep to the retinal vessels. These patches have ill defined edges and the vitreous may be hazy. When the acute phase subsides, flat white scars with pigment around their edges are left. The numerous causes of choroiditis include tuberculosis, syphilis (which may cause a disseminated choroiditis), and toxoplasmosis (which characteristically produces lesions at the maculae).

THE EAR

EXAMINATION

A good history is the first essential for examination. Many diseases of the ear have an hereditary basis. In the case of suspected deafness in early childhood, the obstetric history is important. Not infrequently the symptoms of inner ear disease—deafness, tinnitus and vertigo—are due to disorder of the cardiovascular, central nervous or skeletal systems. An increasing number of drugs and medications can cause otological abnormality. Earache or mastoid pain is frequently referred from teeth, the temporomandibular joints, laryngopharynx or cervical spine. Psychiatric problems, especially anxiety and depressive states can present with ear symptoms. Occupational and social hazards include noise exposure, barometric pressure change and underwater swimming. The ear should never be considered in isolation.

Examination starts with inspection of the pinna (cartilaginous auricle), mastoid area, external auditory canal and tympanic membrane.

Congenital abnormalities such as microtia (small grossly deformed pinna) and complete atresia of the external canal are obvious. Lesser deformities such as bat-ears, accessory auricles between the tragus and the angle of the mouth, or pre-auricular sinus are familial disorders sometimes associated with developmental abnormality of the middle and inner ear.

Discharge from the ear, otorrhoea, should be noted. At one time this was so common that the ear was considered as an organ of excretion. It results from otitis externa or otitis media. In external otitis there is local irritation, pain and tenderness on moving the pinna. The infection is usually bacterial, sometimes fungal. It may be related to skin diseases such as seborrhoeic or contact dermatitis or to eczema or psoriasis. Furunculosis is very painful and may lead to local cellulitis or pre and post auricular lymphadenitis. The red tender swelling can mimic mastoiditis. Perichondritis is also a very painful complication of local infection or trauma. The pinna is red, hot and swollen. Gram-negative bacteria are usually responsible.

In acute suppurative otitis media, due to the common respiratory pathogens, the otorrhoea is mucoid or purulent in character. The complication of acute mastoiditis in childhood is rarely seen today in the UK. Apart from the redness and pitting oedema over the mastoid, there is marked tenderness on palpation. In chronic otitis media the discharge is frequently fetid, a mixture of Gram-negative organisms being found. In uncomplicated chronic mastoiditis there is no mastoid swelling or tenderness.

In all cases with otorrhoea, it is highly desirable that swabs of the discharge be submitted for culture and bacterial or fungal antibiotic sensitivity analysis.

Examination of the external auditory canal and tympanic membrane can be accomplished by the use of a head mirror with reflected light and an aural speculum. However, the student is advised to become familiar with the electric auriscope for this part of the examination. Practice is the only secret to success in identifying the normal and the abnormal. The auriscope should have a good light source, beamed out of the speculum end. It magnifies about 1·5 times. The pinna must be pulled upwards and backwards, to straighten the cartilaginous part of the external canal and align it with the medial bony part. To avoid causing discomfort the tip of the speculum must be inserted gently under direct vision. There are considerable anatomical variations. In the young child the tympanic part of the temporal bone has not fully developed and the drum, though lying more horizontally than the adult 55°–60°, is easier to inspect. In adults the curvature of the bony canal varies so that it may be difficult to visualize the antero-inferior part of the drum. The size of the speculum must vary with the dimensions of the canal. When a better view is required, or in order to carry out minor local procedures, the binocular operating microscope is employed. The magnification can be varied from 6 to 40 times.

The tympanic membrane

The normal drum has a translucent greyish appearance, rather like tightly stretched tissue paper (Fig. 11.1). It is almost circular,

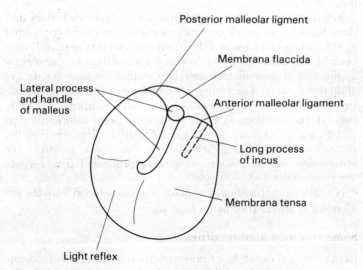

Fig. 11.1 Normal left tympanic membrane.

Posterior malleolar ligment

Membrana flaccida

Anterior malleolar ligament

Lateral process and handle of malleus

Long process of incus

Membrana tensa

Light reflex

about 1 cm in diameter, obliquely set and slightly concave. The much larger lower tense part has an outer cuticular layer continuous with the canal skin, a medial fibrous layer with both circular and radial fibres and an inner layer of mucosa continuous with the lining of the middle ear and Eustachian tube. The small flaccid part is devoid of a fibrous layer. In the fibrous layer is the prominent long process or handle of the malleus. The short process of the malleus and malleolar folds should also be recognized. The commonly described light reflex is seen better with the head mirror than with the auriscope. Sometimes the shadow of the long process of the incus may be seen through the posterior part of the membrana tensa.

Toilet and syringing

Vision of the external canal and drum is sometimes obstructed by wax, epithelial debris or pus. Toilet can be performed using the head mirror and twists of cotton wool on special applicators. Wax curettes are available. Suction clearance can be effected under the operating microscope. The ear can be syringed. These procedures, minor though they are, are best left to experienced nursing or medical staff.

Before syringing it is important to ascertain from the history that there has been no previous ear disease which might have resulted in a chronic perforation or a thin tympanic membrane scar. If time permits it is desirable to soften wax for a few days by the nightly application of olive oil. Commercially available wax 'solvents' are of doubtful value. The syringes should be reliable and the nozzle tightly attached. Water should be at body temperature. Only slight deviations from 37°C are required to cause caloric-induced vertigo and nystagmus. The stream of water is directed along the meatal wall and, being deflected by the drum, it forces the obstruction out. Excessive pressure or prolonged perseverence are contraindicated.

No early attempts should be made to remove blood from the ear after either direct trauma or head injury.

Some common abnormalities

In the external canal, bony exostoses are seen especially in swimmers (Fig. 11.2). In children under the age of 3 and in the

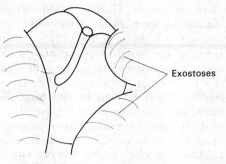

Fig. 11.2 Exostoses of the bony canal.

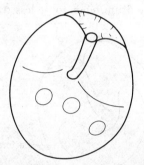

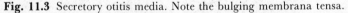

Fig. 11.3 Secretory otitis media. Note the bulging membrana tensa.

subnormal at any age, foreign bodies are sometimes seen. In the presence of suppuration the skin of the canal is hyperaemic and the surface of the drum is dull. In chronic suppurative otitis media a fleshy polyp may fill the external canal and even protrude at the meatus.

In acute suppurative otitis media, before rupture, the drum is red and bulging. An extremely common finding in all age groups, but especially in children, is secretory otitis media. A variety of appearances is encountered. The drum is dull and retracted from the negative middle ear pressure, and the handle of the malleus looks short. A fluid level, or air bubbles within the fluid, may be seen (Fig. 11.3).

Acute perforations, either traumatic or inflammatory, are centrally placed in the drum and usually small. Chrome perforations come in all sizes and shapes. They are commonly kidney shaped (Fig. 11.4). In chronic suppurative otitis media or chronic mastoiditis, perforations are normally marginal, involving the flaccid part of the drum or the postero-superior margin (Fig. 11.5). In chronic disease, cholesteatoma may be seen through the perforation; this has a white pearly appearance, the tissue consisting of onion-like layers of desquamated keratin from the epithelium which is growing in the middle ear and mastoid.

Scarring of the tympanic membrane is very common and takes on one of two appearances sometimes seen in the same ear. There may be an atrophic scar which is thin and excessively translucent due to loss of the fibrous layer; or there may be tympanosclerosis, a type of hyaline thickening of the drum which has a white chalky look. In old age the drum tends to be less translucent.

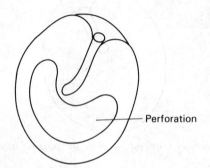

Fig. 11.4 Chronic centre perforation of the tympanic membrane.

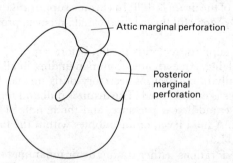

Fig. 11.5 Chronic suppurative otitis media.

THE INVESTIGATION OF HEARING AND HEARING LOSS

Hearing loss of one sort or another is remarkably common. The frequency of deafness at birth is of the order of 1 per 1000 while over the age of 65 years hearing problems occur in 30%. There have been remarkable advances in the audiological methods of investigation. The subject has graduated from an art to a science. Yet there is still a place for simple clinical evaluation.

The simplest method of testing is to use the human voice. This can give a fair measure of handicap. A normal conversation voice will be normally heard at about 20 feet and a soft whispered voice at 3 to 4 feet from the ear. With experience, the tester can soon learn to relate the hearing distances to the likely hearing level in decibels. The ear not being tested requires to be blocked or masked by noise.

The tuning fork tests are not yet obsolete. A 256 or 512 fork is best for clinical use. The Rinne test consists of comparing the hearing by air and by bone conduction (the base of the fork on the mastoid process). Normally air conduction is better than bone conduction (Rinne positive). This also applies in sensorial deafness. Bone conduction is better than air (Rinne negative) in middle ear or conductive deafness. One has to be careful about a false Rinne negative when, in the presence of severe to total deafness in one ear, the tuning fork vibrating on that mastoid process is really perceived by the opposite cochlea. The absolute bone conduction test compares the patient's hearing by bone conduction with the examiner's (assuming that it is normal). If the patient continues to hear after the examiner, there is an element of conductive loss; if the examiner continues to hear after the subject, there is some sensorineural loss. The third test commonly used is the Weber test. The base of the vibrating fork is placed anywhere on the mid-line of the skull or mandible. In conductive deafness it is heard in the deaf or deafer ear while in sensorineural deafness it is referred to the better ear.

A combination of soft whispered voice and tuning fork testing gives a good idea of the site and degree of hearing disorder and determines which specialized investigations are necessary.

Conductive deafness

The pure tone audiogram measures the threshold of hearing in decibels for the frequency scale 0·25 to 8 kHz. If there is an element of conductive loss, the air–bone gap is estimated from the pure tone threshold for bone conduction (Fig. 11.6). In the investigation of conductive disorders, the use of an acoustic impedance bridge gives valuable differential diagnostic information. The recordings are objective and can be carried out in a few seconds even in infancy or in the absence of patient cooperation. The principle involves measuring the acoustic energy not absorbed by the middle ear system and monitoring this change in energy absorption consequent upon applying graduated negative to positive pressure changes on the drum. The resultant tympanogram, which can be plotted on an 'X–Y' recorder, can differentiate ossicular fixation from loss and, in the former, can provide clues as to which ossicle is immobilized. It gives typical results in secretory otitis media. In otosclerosis, a dominant hereditary progressive stapedial fixation, it can indicate the likely operative findings.

Sensorineural deafness

In the great majority of patients with sensorineural deafness the lesion is in the cochlea and involves the hair cells and supporting structures or the stria vascularis. Deafness in this site is called

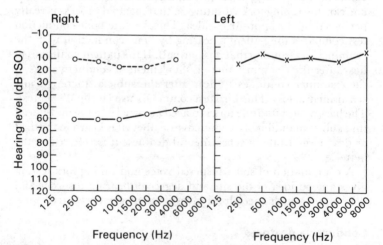

Fig. 11.6 Pure tone threshold for bone conduction showing conductive deafness.

sensory, end organ or cochlear. With many sensory disorders of long standing (e.g. noise-induced, ototoxic damage, late syphilis, presbyacusis, Menière's disease, etc.) the primary auditory neurones undergo secondary degeneration, especially in the basal coil (high tones). This produces a truly sensorineural hearing loss. Pure neural deafness is much less common. It can be further subdivided, according to the level of the lesion, into neural (e.g. tumours of the cerebello-pontine angle), brain stem (e.g. multiple sclerosis) or cortical. There are now a battery of both subjective and objective tests to help localize these disorders.

Sensory deafness is characterized by the presence of recruitment. This phenomenon, the presence of deafness at but not above the threshold, can be demonstrated by a number of tests, the oldest of which is the alternate binaural loudness balance test (Fig. 11.7). In the example shown both ears have a threshold hearing loss of 60 dB at 2 kHz. In the right ear this deafness remains above threshold (a neural loss) while in the left, at 90 dB, sounds are equally loud in the two ears (sensory loss).

When there is bilateral deafness the acoustic or stapedial reflex threshold (Fig. 11.8) can be used to localize the lesion. This employs

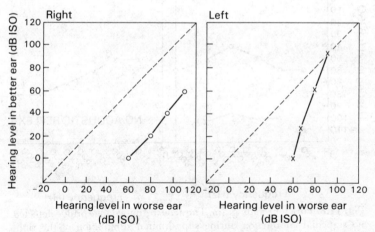

Fig. 11.7 The alternative binaural loudness balance showing sensory deafness. Frequency 2000 Hz.

the same principles: loud noises, stimulating a greater number of neurones over a wider area of the cochlear partition including those arising from the inner hair cells, cause the stapedial muscle to contract on both sides. The supraliminal stimulation is applied to one ear while the acoustic impedance bridge detects the stapedial contraction in the other ear (Fig. 11.8). In the example shown there is a sensory loss on the right and a neural loss on the left. The subjective levels of loudness discomfort give similar results.

Speech audiograms, apart from helping to localize the lesion, can give additional information (Fig. 11.9). Various types of recorded speech material can be used at graduated intensities and the percentage of correct 'words' or 'phonemes' repeated by the patient enable the graph to be drawn. There is overlap between c and d (Fig. 11.9) in the presence of sensorineural deafness. Some treatments of inner ear diseases are reflected in better speech discrimination without pure-tone threshold shift. The speech tests can therefore be used as a therapeutic as well as a diagnostic index.

There are several tests based on the presence or absence of abnormal adaptation to steady or interrupted (tone decay) tones.

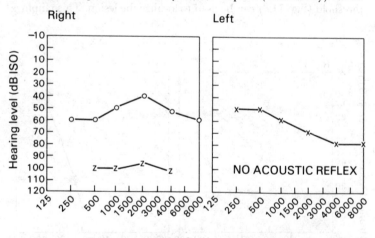

Fig. 11.8 Pure tone audiogram. The acoustic impedance bridge detected no stapedial contraction during supraliminal stimulation of the right side. (See text.) O — O, X — X: auditory threshold Z — Z: stapedius reflex.

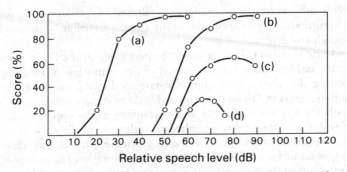

Fig. 11.9 Speech audiogram: (*a*) normal result. (*b*) conductive deafness. (*c*) sensory loss. (*d*) neural lesion.

Measurements of the different limits of intensity or frequency can be employed. Many of these tests are quite complex for the patient and they are not as reliable as objective methods of investigation.

The assessment of hearing in infants and young children is a specialized topic. Basically the clinical evaluation involves watching the infant's responses to carefully selected and monitored environmental sounds which are picked according to the age and development of the child. Intelligence assessment is also important. Deaf infants are mute or have delayed or faulty speech production.

The need for better evaluation of hearing in children has led to the development of electrical response audiometry. In response to acoustic stimulation of the auditory system, the various electrical potentials in the inner ear, the acoustic nerve, the cochlear nucleus, the superior olive, the inferior colliculus and the auditory cortex can be recorded. Far-field myogenic responses can also be detected.

Vestibular investigation

Many diseases of the middle and inner ear cause disturbance of the peripheral sensory vestibular organs whether in the semicircular canals or the static labyrinth. More centrally placed lesions in the vestibular nerve or nuclei also cause vertigo or vestibular ataxia. Nystagmus (p. 291) or abnormalities of induced nystagmus are frequently seen. The reader is referred to Chapter 8 for descriptions of nystagmus of brain stem, cerebellar, optic and optokinetic origin.

Acute vestibular lesions from the periphery to the brain stem cause sudden onset vertigo—a subjective sensation of rotation. During the acute phase objects rotate to the opposite side, the patient tends to fall to the same side, there is past pointing with both arms to the same side and nystagmus to the opposite side. Vestibular nystagmus is described according to the direction of the fast (central correction) component. In severity it has three degrees: third degree when present in any direction of gaze, second degree when the patient looks ahead and to the opposite side, and first degree when induced only by gaze to the opposite side from the lesion. The degrees give an indication of severity in relation to time.

A latent nystagmus of peripheral origin (including the vestibular nerves) can be elicited following recent or less severe vestibular lesions by the abolition of optic fixation. This is simply done by the use of Frenzel glasses. These have a 20 plus dioptre lens and an internal source of illumination. The patient wearing them can see little, yet the observer has an excellent magnified view of the eyes. A similar latent peripheral nystagmus can be demonstrated by electronystagmographic recording with the eyes closed or in darkness. Eye movements can also be observed with a special viewer in infra-red light.

The principle of abolition of fixation is an important one for differentiating peripheral from central nystagmus. Peripheral nystagmus is enhanced by the abolition of fixation, central nystagmus is diminished or even abolished.

Tests of positional nystagmus are simple to conduct. The patient is assisted by lying supine with the head hanging over the end of the examination couch, first with one ear and subsequently with the other ear dependent. In some peripheral disorders this causes intense vertigo and nystagmus of peripheral origin usually shows fatigue, i.e. it cannot be reproduced immediately by replacing the patient in the same position. With central lesions the nystagmus is more likely to be repeatable.

In the Hallpike caloric test the patient lies supine on a couch, with the head raised 30°, to bring the lateral semicircular canal into the vertical plane. The eyes are open and fixed on a mark on the ceiling. Each ear is tested separately first with water at 44°C and then at 30°C with an interval of a few minutes between each of the four tests. About 250 ml of water from thermostatically controlled tanks, is used each time, the fluid being run for 40 seconds. The caloric effect induces convection currents in the fluid of the semicircular canal causing vertigo and nystagmus which can be measured in different ways. The simplest measure is the duration of the nystagmus, normally about two minutes (Fig. 11.10). In disease states there may be diminished sensitivity or absence of responses on one or both sides, there may be a preponderance of nystagmus to one or the other side, or there may be any combination of these findings.

The data can be recorded on electronystagmographic tracings and analysed by the number of beats or alternatively by the velocity of the slow component of the nystagmus.

As in the case of spontaneous nystagmus, caloric-induced nystagmus can be significantly modified by the abolition of optic fixation (using Frenzel glasses or making recordings with the eyes closed or in darkness). In normal subjects and in ears affected by peripheral disease, the nystagmus is enhanced, while in central

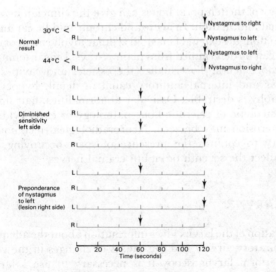

Fig. 11.10 Caloric tests.

lesions it is diminished or unchanged compared with recordings employing optic fixation.

Preponderance of caloric-induced nystagmus to the opposite side can result from lesions of the peripheral connections of the vestibular nuclei, but it is more likely to occur with central lesions, especially brain stem disorders. Preponderance of this nystagmus to the same side is sometimes seen in lesions of the temporal lobe of the brain.

Optokinetic or railway nystagmus is reproduced by sitting the patient about 3 feet from a rotating striped drum. The resultant eye movements are identical to vestibular nystagmus with slow and quick components. Altering the direction of rotation changes the direction of the nystagmus. Normally, with the same speed of rotation, recordings produce the same number of beats in both directions. Preponderance of optokinetic nystagmus to the same side is sometimes seen in lesions of the parietal lobe or their connections with the superior colliculus and medial longitudinal bundle. (See Chapter 8.)

Radiological examination

Radiology of the temporal bones can give the clinician invaluable additional information. In acute and chronic middle ear and mastoid infection, the extent of mastoid cellular involvement or of bone erosion can be determined from plain X-rays. Linear tomography shows more detail. To visualize the ossicles and cavities of the inner ear and internal auditory canal in detail, hypocycloidal tomography is desirable. Ossicular abnormalities, hair line fractures, osteolytic or sclerotic bone pathology or early evidence of tumour erosion may be seen. Neuroradiological techniques are necessary to confirm the presence of space-occupying lesions which affect the seventh or eighth cranial nerves.

THE LARYNX

Examination of the larynx gives information about the adequacy of the respiratory airway and the causes of changes in the voice.

To perform laryngoscopy it is necessary to use a laryngeal mirror. This is a rounded mirror set at an angle at one end of a long

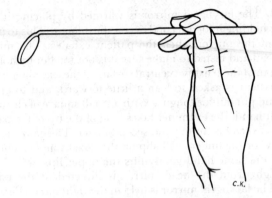

Fig. 11.11 Holding the laryngeal mirror.

thin metal handle (Fig. 11.11). The idea is to hold the back of the mirror lightly but firmly against the soft palate so that an image of the vocal cords will appear in the mirror.

The examiner seats himself facing the patient. He will have to sit very close to his patient, with his legs to the side nearest to the source of light. A standard lamp with a good bright beam is placed at the side of the patient, on a level with the patient's mouth and its beam is directed at the examiner. For a right-handed examiner the light is placed at the patient's left. The examiner may wear a face mask to protect himself should the patient cough directly at him during the examination; most patients with serious lesions of the larynx are very helpful and cooperative, but anxious patients with slight diffuse inflammation of the larynx may be very sensitive and cough easily. Next, the examiner places a head mirror on his forehead, over his right eye. A head mirror is concave and has a hole in the centre through which the examiner's right eye will inspect the image in the laryngeal mirror. The mirror is fastened to the head by a band, and can be adjusted easily because it is fitted with a ball-and-socket joint. The beam of light from the standard lamp is reflected on to this concave head mirror, then on to the laryngeal mirror, and so down to the larynx. The examiner's eye looks directly down the centre of this reflected light beam, and so the lighted image in the laryngeal mirror becomes clearly visible.

First the patient's mouth is inspected and any dentures are

removed. The laryngeal mirror is warmed by placing it in hot water, or holding it for a second over a spirit flame. This to prevent misting of the mirror when the patient exhales. The mirror is wiped clean and tested to make sure it is not too hot by holding it firmly against the sensitive ventral surface of the examiner's wrist.

The patient is asked to lean a little forward, and to open his mouth and put out his tongue. With a small square of clean gauze in the left hand, the examiner takes hold of the tip of the patient's tongue between his thumb and second finger. The gauze square is necessary, or the fingers will slip on the moist tongue. The index finger of the same hand gently lifts the upper lip.

The light from the head mirror is directed at the patient's mouth. The laryngeal mirror is held in the right hand (Fig. 11.11) and, very carefully in order to avoid touching the tongue, the small round mirror is placed deliberately and steadily against the soft palate near the base of the uvula. The shaft of light from the examiner's head mirror should now shine directly on to the laryngeal mirror, and the laryngeal mirror is gently adjusted until the vocal cords come into view.

Laryngoscopy requires no local analgesic in the great majority of examinations, but it does require the confidence of the patient in the examiner and the examiner's confidence in himself. The examiner must train himself to make rapid and accurate observations.

To facilitate matters, the patient is asked to continue breathing throughout the examination. If the patient is concentrating on breathing he will not think of retching or coughing. If movement of the cords is required, he is asked to say 'ee'.

The *larynx* should be inspected with great care (Fig. 11.12). The *epiglottis* lies in front, at the base of the tongue. Normally its upper curved edge is clearly seen, its colour is a pale yellow. Any abnormal position should be noted. The base of the *tongue* and the *valleculae* are next examined. Both *piriform fossae* are inspected, and the presence of excessive froth or mucus round the *oesophageal opening* behind the larynx, or in either piriform fossa, should suggest upper oesophageal obstruction or paralysis. In upper oesophageal obstruction, the saliva and mucus from the mouth and upper respiratory tract cannot get away easily, and may overflow into the larynx, explaining the patient's irritating cough.

The *vocal cords* are normally clear-cut, and of a pale-yellow

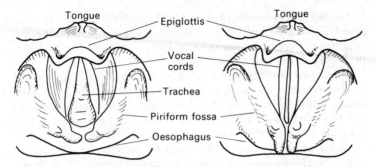

Fig. 11.12 The larynx as seen in the laryngeal mirror.

glistening appearance. The rest of the laryngeal mucosa is normally a moist pinkish-red colour. Between the vocal cords is seen the lumen of the *trachea*, and the outlines of the tracheal rings. The presence of any pus or mucus in the trachea and any narrowing of the tracheal inlet should be noted.

Displacement of the larynx suggests inflammation or new growth in the tissues closely adjacent to the larynx.

The *epithelium* should be inspected for any irregularity, ulceration, change of colour or presence of oedema. Raised irregular epithelium suggests malignant changes. Ulceration with oedema makes one think of tuberculosis if there is evidence of pulmonary infection. Oedema alone indicates inflammation or trauma, or both. Diffuse redness of sudden onset suggests acute laryngitis.

The *movement* of the larynx should be noted. The movement of both sides of the larynx should be symmetrical. When normal movement is absent, the examiner must ask himself whether some local condition, such as fixation due to malignant changes or myopathy, is preventing normal movement, or whether some lesion along the course of the recurrent laryngeal nerves is responsible. If loss of movement is caused by some local change, there will usually be signs of swelling, or obstruction, or ulceration; or there may be a past history of poliomyelitis or diphtheria.

If the larynx looks quite normal, except for the paralysis, common sites along the courses of the recurrent laryngeal nerves worthy of clinical examination are: (*a*) the thyroid gland; (*b*) the apices of the lungs and structures related to the under surface of the aorta; and (*c*) the cervical oesophagus.

Absence of movement of one or both cords should be carefully noted. If one arytenoid lies a little in front of the other, this is often suggestive of unilateral paralysis and this finding may be helpful if the larynx is difficult to examine.

In *unilateral paralysis* the examiner is struck by the overaction and compensation of the normal cord, which comes right across the middle line to meet the paralysed cord, if the patient endeavours to say the vowel 'ee'. It is this remarkable compensation which explains the apparently normal voice in unilateral paralysis and accounts for the tiredness of the voice towards the end of the day. There is usually no stridor and no apparent obstruction to the airway. Compensation is rapid. Some very temporary difficulty with swallowing is experienced due to unilateral paralysis of the upper sphincter of the oesophagus (cricopharyngeus) which is also supplied by the recurrent laryngeal nerve.

The extraordinary compensatory powers of the larynx are well seen in *bilateral paralysis* where, although the voice is undoubtedly weak, it is remarkably clear, those muscles not supplied by the recurrent nerves taking on added functions. Even when the complete larynx has had to be removed, because of malignant changes, and a permanent tracheotomy is the only respiratory passage, many patients develop an amazingly good voice. Folds in the pharyngeal walls are used for phonation and the relaxed oesophagus makes an efficient air reservoir.

In unilateral paralysis, the patient does not complain of shortness of breath on exertion; whereas in bilateral paralysis there is great narrowing of the laryngeal airway, because the main abductors of the cords are paralysed, and the patient does complain of real shortness of breath on exertion. There is usually acute distress if both cords are paralysed suddenly, but with reassurance, and when adaptation is established, most patients complain of little difficulty in breathing when at rest, or during light movement. The *stridor* during sleep is very inconvenient for others. There is no stridor in unilateral paralysis. It must be remembered that recovery does take place more often than is usually realized, in both unilateral and bilateral paralysis of the recurrent laryngeal nerves.

It is very important to examine the larynx in any case of *hoarseness* that has persisted for two or three weeks. Intermittent attacks of hoarseness, or loss of voice, with a complete return to normal between attacks, should suggest simple laryngitis or hysteria. If any growth is present on either vocal cord, the voice will never clear until the growth has been removed. Whenever the epithelium of the larynx is ulcerated or irregular, an X-ray of the lung fields, and tests for syphilis should be done before any question of biopsy is considered. If there is purulent sputum, this also should be examined.

Squamous carcinoma arising on the surface of a vocal cord is one of the commoner malignant tumours in men and is not rare in women. In chronic laryngitis there may be polypoid thickening at the anterior end of one or both cords. Nodules due to vocal strain and abuse are usually unilateral. Papillomas are seen in both children and adults. In all such cases direct laryngoscopy under general anaesthesia is indicated, with biopsy or excision of the lesion. Microlaryngoscopy is often employed today.

No laryngoscopy is complete without an examination of the *neck*. The position of the thyroid cartilage and trachea should be examined and any displacement noted. Movement of the larynx on swallowing should be free and any unusual lump or enlarged nodes must be felt for.

THE NASAL PART OF THE PHARYNX

Examination of the nasal part of the pharynx is carried out in much the same way as that described above for laryngoscopy, and with the same precautions; only here the mirror is smaller, and its handle is bent to avoid touching the tongue. The tongue may be depressed with a spatula, and the small mirror is placed just behind the soft palate facing upwards. The examination requires considerable skill and confidence, and, as with laryngoscopy, some patients are easy to examine, and some very difficult indeed.

The *posterior nares*, lying to either side of the sharply defined vomer, come into view in the mirror, and the posterior ends of the inferior and middle conchae can be seen. To either side lie the opening of the *Eustachian tubes*. The presence of any tumour or pus, or change in the normally pink moist epithelium should be noted, and in children the size of the adenoids should be assessed.

THE NOSE

The outside of the nose must be inspected first. Old scars may indicate past trauma. Recent cuts or bruising should be noted.

Redness or swelling may be caused by inflammation. Displacement of the *nasal bones*, to right or left, or depression of the bridge suggests trauma. If the bones are firm and painless, the injury will not have been of recent origin. Collapse of the bony or cartilaginous *bridge* may have followed necrosis. With a finger and thumb on the outside of each nostril, the anterior part of the cartilaginous *septum* can be palpated and any gross displacement or thickening of the septum detected.

The skin round the *nostrils* must be inspected for fissuring or redness. The presence of discharge, whether blood-stained, mucopurulent or watery, must be noted, and whether the discharge is confined to one nostril only or comes from both.

To inspect the *vestibule* of the nose and the nasal passages, a head mirror is needed. There are several advantages in using a concave head mirror for examinations of the nose, nasopharynx and larynx. The examiner can look right down the centre of the beam of light which his head mirror reflects into these narrow and darkened passages. Both hands of the examiner are free, and his eyes are shaded. Other forms of light such as torches or head lamps or lighted speculae can be tried, but they are not as satisfactory as the perforated head mirror with reflected light.

The vestibule of a small child's nose and the openings of its nasal passages can be inspected by tilting the nose upwards with a finger.

To examine an adult's nose properly a *nasal speculum* is needed. The speculum is held in the left hand (Fig. 11.13) and the light beam reflected from the head mirror is directed on to the patient's nostril. The speculum is closed, and gently introduced into the nostril. The spring is allowed to open a little, but never to its fullest extent. Gentleness is all important.

The skin of the vestibule extends inwards for about 1 cm, and it is well supplied with protective hairs, particularly in males. The skin of the nasal vestibule is heir to all the common skin diseases. There is a clear line where the pale skin meets the pink moist mucous membrane of the nasal passages. Medially lies the *nasal septum* which is commonly displaced by trauma. A haematoma of the nasal septum causes a swelling which is soft to the touch, unlike the normal septum, which is firm. Note the presence of any ulceration or perforation of the septum, or the presence of any bleeding point. Laterally, is seen the *inferior nasal concha*. This should be

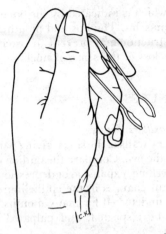

Fig. 11.13 Holding the nasal speculum.

moist and pink and, as its epithelium can become pale and greatly thickened in hay fever and asthma, comparison should be made with the normal. Above the inferior concha can be seen the anterior part of the *middle concha*. The presence of pus coming from under the middle concha strongly suggests purulent sinusitis, for most of the accessory nasal sinuses open under this concha. Nasal polyps appear as moist greyish swellings occluding the air passages. They are easily movable and painless, unlike the conchae, which are fixed and tender. Hyperaemia of the mucosa and the presence of mucopus in the nasal passages, probably indicates infection. A persisting one-sided blood-stained nasal discharge may indicate the presence of a foreign body or malignancy if present in an older person. The presence of any raised irregular or bleeding epithelium should be noted.

The *nasal passages* form part of the upper respiratory tract and should never be examined without reference to the lower respiratory tract. All air reaching the lungs has to pass through the nasal passages to be filtered, warmed and moistened, and any infection or obstruction in these passages may ultimately have some effect on the health and function of the lungs and bronchi. The presence of nasal obstruction must be noted. In children, mouth breathing due to nasal obstruction gives rise to a change in the pattern of facial expression, which is indicated by the open mouth and sagging of the facial muscles. The lips and mouth are dry.

Severe nasal obstruction may prevent air reaching the olfactory area, and so cause loss of the sense of smell.

THE NASAL SINUSES

To examine the *maxillary sinuses:*

1. Palpate the bony walls of the sinus, giving particular attention to the bone under the eye. Compare the outline on the two sides. Any tenderness, swelling, expansion or depression of bone must be observed. Malignant changes in the epithelium of the maxillary sinus may remain undetected for many months. The palate and alveoli must also be inspected, and palpated from inside the mouth.

2. Examine the nasal passages, to detect any evidence of pus or polyps appearing from any of the normal openings of the sinuses.

3. Transilluminate the sinuses. This is done by placing a strong light in the centre of the hard palate. Any upper denture should be removed. The patient closes the lips round the handle of the transilluminating lamp. The examination should be performed in a dark room. Light from inside the mouth shines through the hollow sinuses, producing a light in the bone under each eye, and a reddish reflection from the retinae.

Comparison between the two sides is made. Pus in the maxillary sinus throws a dark shadow. Patients will differ greatly in the thickness of their maxillary bones. Some transilluminate clearly, others with difficulty. Transillumination is a useful clinical aid, because if the sinuses are perfectly clear on transillumination, an X-ray may be unnecessary.

If any abnormal shadow is found, an X-ray of the sinuses will give additional information, and will help to confirm the clinical examination.

To transilluminate the *frontal sinuses*, the light is placed under the frontal ridge of the orbit. The *ethmoid* and *sphenoid* sinuses are best examined by X-ray, combined with clinical inspection of the nasal passages.

12

Examination of children

General examination
Special examinations
Developmental screening examinations
Examination of the newborn

The clinical examination of young children is a skill which must be learnt by experience. However, since children who object very strongly to being examined usually do so because they are afraid, the beginner can often achieve an adequate examination by patience and a gentle approach. The child and his mother should be greeted in a friendly manner and the child offered a selection of toys suitable to his age. The *history* is then taken from the mother incorporating the special questions set out on p. 21. While talking to the mother, the examiner should observe the patient and take note of certain points. Does the child look well or ill? Is he apathetic or alert, anxious or relaxed? Is there anything unusual about the facies? Are there any obvious physical deformities? Is the child well nourished or wasted? Is there any difficulty in breathing?

GENERAL EXAMINATION

The child should now be at ease and getting used to the strange surroundings. This is the time to record the respiration and pulse rates. The average respiratory rate in a normal newborn child is 40/minute; by the second year it has fallen to 25 or so, and by the fifth year to about 20. A raised respiratory rate in a child at rest usually indicates some disorder of the respiratory or cardiovascular systems. The normal pulse–respiration ratio is 3 or 4 to 1.

The pulse rate is counted in young infants by palpation or auscultation of the chest, in older children by palpation at the wrist. The average pulse rate at birth is about 130/minute, at 1 year 110, at 3 years 100, at 8 years 90, and at 12 years 80. During sleep the pulse rate falls about 10–20 beats/minute. The normal range for pulse rates is wide. Tachycardia is common and may be due to crying, excitement, exercise and fever as well as to various diseases. Bradycardia is rare and usually indicates some cardiac abnormality. Sinus arrythmia (see p. 232) is present in almost all children, but other irregularities of rhythm are uncommon even in the presence of cardiac disease. Always feel for the femoral pulses which are either absent or weak in coarctation of the aorta.

Examination should now proceed by the usual methods of inspection, palpation, percussion and auscultation; but no set routine can be followed and the examination is by regions rather than by systems. Each patient will, by his reaction to the various procedures, dictate the order of examination and even the position in which he will be examined. Young infants are usually examined on the mother's lap; older children who may not be prepared to lie down on a couch can be examined standing at the mother's side. Most children are prepared to have some of their clothes removed, although they are often modest and should be allowed to keep their pants on.

It is important to be gentle and to have warm hands. Begin by looking at and feeling the child all over. Observe the general state of development and nutrition. Is the skin dry or moist, and is there the normal degree of elasticity? Is there a rash present? Are there any bruises? Multiple bruises of different ages in children under the age of 3 suggest the possibility of non-accidental injury. The shape of the chest and abdomen should be noted. The abdomen is normally rather protuberant in young children.

Feel the head and the *anterior fontanelle*: this closes normally between 15 months and two years and delayed closure may be due to rickets or hydrocephalus. The posterior fontanelle is always small and closes by the second month. The degree of tension of the anterior fontanelle is important. In health it pulsates and is in the same plane as the rest of the surrounding skull. A depressed fontanelle is a sign of dehydration, and a tense bulging fontanelle indicates raised intracranial pressure. The fontanelle is normally tense when the child is crying. The *shape of the head* should be noted. It may be abnormally shaped, owing to premature fusion of the sutures. It is globular in hydrocephalus, and is often asymmetrical in normal infants who tend to lie persistently on one side (plagiocephaly).

Inspect the *eyes* for cataracts and conjunctivitis. In infants a squint may be detected by shining a light in front of the face. The light reflex should be at the same position on each cornea.

Examine the *limbs*. Look for wasting, swelling and tenderness, and for limitation of movement of joints. A painful limb may be immobile in infants (pseudo-paralysis) or cause a limp in older children. Feel the wrists for widening of the epiphyses of the radius and ulna which is a sign of rickets. Note the presence of deformities such as knock-knee, bow-legs and flat feet.

The *lymphatic glands* should be palpated. Small glands can normally be felt in the anterior and posterior triangles of the neck, the axillae and the inguinal regions. Lymph glands enlarge readily in children as a result of local conditions such as tonsillitis or generalized diseases such as rubella.

The *abdomen* cannot be palpated satisfactorily in a child who is crying or resisting. Small infants can be given a feed to stop them crying, but with an older child one must wait until he settles down before attempting to palpate the abdomen. Children from about 1 to 3 years old will often refuse to be examined lying down, but in this age group the abdomen can be palpated from behind when the child is standing on the mother's lap and looking over her shoulder. Palpation should be gentle and light. The liver edge can be felt quite easily and in young children normally extends down to 2 cm below the costal margin. The spleen when enlarged can be felt below the left costal margin. Slight enlargement of the spleen is common in children with infections of all types. Faecal masses can be felt in constipated children and a full or distended bladder presents as a firm mass arising out of the pelvis. Abdominal tenderness is best detected by watching the child's facial expression during palpation. Feel for testes in the scrotum but remember that an active cremasteric reflex may retract them into the abdomen.

The *thorax* should be inspected for deformity of the chest wall and for intercostal or subcostal recession, which indicates respiratory obstruction, chronic lung disease or a cardiac abnormality. Look also for the grunting respirations of the child with pneumonia. This is due to a reversal of the normal respiratory rhythm. The grunting expiration is followed by inspiration and then a pause. The thickening of the costochrondral junctions ('rickety rosary') which occurs in rickets can be seen and felt. Palpate the anterior chest wall for the cardiac impulse and for thrills. In children under the age of 6 or 7 years the cardiac impulse is normally in the fourth intercostal space, just to the left of the midclavicular line. In older children it is usually in the fifth space in the midclavicular line. Vocal fremitus is not a sign of great value in children.

Percussion of the chest should be light and in small children can be direct, that is to say the chest wall is tapped directly with the percussing finger without the use of a pleximeter finger. The chest is much more resonant in children than in adults.

A stethoscope with a small bell chest-piece is suitable for general auscultation of a child's chest. Listen for the breath sounds and for adventitious sounds. Because of the thin chest wall, breath sounds are louder in children than in adults, and their character is more like the bronchial breathing of adults (puerile breathing). Upper respiratory infections frequently give rise to loud coarse rhonchi, which may be conducted down the trachea and main bronchi.

The normal splitting of first and second heart sounds is easier to hear in children than in adults. Venous hums and functional systolic flow murmurs are often heard in normal children.

In older children examination of the *nervous system* can be carried out in the usual manner. In young children the extent of the neurological examination depends on their age and willingness to cooperate. If the child can walk, look for abnormalities of gait and the presence of a limp or ataxia. Note any abnormal movements. Tics or habit spasms are repetitive but purposeful movements, such as turning of the head or shrugging of the shoulders. Choreiform movements are coarse, involuntary, purposeless jerks which follow no particular pattern. These are best demonstrated by asking the child to hold out his arms in front of him. In this position the child with chorea adopts a characteristic posture, with the wrists in flexion and the fingers in hyperextension. Coordination is tested by some modification of the finger–nose test, for example reaching out to touch a toy held in the examiner's hand.

Muscle tone and muscle power should be assessed. The child with marked hypotonia will slip through one's hands when picked up under the armpits. Meningeal irritation or spasm of the spinal muscles is detected more readily by resistance to passive flexion of the head and neck (neck stiffness) than by testing for Kernig's sign.

Tendon reflexes are often difficult to elicit in normal children, and some time may be needed to find the correct position of the limb for this purpose. Only gentle percussion of tendons is required and this is often better done with the examiner's finger than with an adult-sized patellar hammer. The plantar responses are extensor in normal infants up to the age of about 18 months, but the persistence of an extensor response after the age of two years indicates an upper motor neurone lesion.

With a little ingenuity, most of the cranial nerves can be tested. For example, by getting a baby to follow a bright object moving in various directions the eye movements can be studied and the presence of nystagmus noted. Examination of the fundi is particularly difficult in infants, as they cannot fix their gaze. Infinite patience is needed for this manoeuvre, as it entails waiting with the ophthalmoscope in position for fleeting glimpses of the optic disc. Forcible attempts to keep the eyes open only make the procedure more difficult. Older children will often fix their eyes on a toy held up behind the examiner by an assistant.

The testing of vision, hearing and certain motor functions in young children is included in the developmental screening examination described on p. 423.

For the child the most unpleasant examinations are those of the *ears, nose, mouth* and *throat* and these should be left until last. With skill, gentleness and patience, even these procedures can usually be carried out without making the child cry. Start with the nose, which need only be examined superficially. By placing a shiny surface, such as a mirror, under the nostrils, patency of the nasal airways can be judged by the size of the area of clouding. With a good light, the appearance of the mucous membrane of the anterior nares can be inspected. Look for the pale swollen inferior turbinates which are characteristic of allergic rhinitis. Proceed next to examine the external auditory meati and tympanic membranes. Allow the child to see and handle the auriscope and

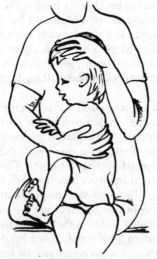

Fig. 12.1 Position for examination of the ear in infants.

speculum, using the instruments as a toy in a simple game for a few moments. If, in spite of these preparations, the child still resists, he will have to be held by his mother. Sit the child on her lap facing to one or other side, and get her to hold the child firmly with one arm around his head and the other around his upper arms and shoulders (Fig. 12.1). Held in this way, the child can be kept still long enough for the ear drums to be inspected.

The mouth and throat are examined in similar fashion. A cooperative child can be encouraged to 'show his teeth' and thus open his mouth without the use of a spatula, which so many children dread. The uncooperative or very young child must be held by the mother, as for the examination of the ears, but in this case the child sits facing the examiner. The use of a spatula may be unavoidable. Force it gently between the teeth and on to the tongue, which is then depressed. Note the state of the teeth, the tongue, and the mucous membrane of the mouth. Look for Koplik's spots, the pharyngeal lesions of chicken pox, and the white patches of thrush. Inspect the tonsils and the pharynx. Look for streaks of mucopus on the posterior pharyngeal wall (postnasal drip).

SPECIAL EXAMINATIONS

The following examinations need special mention.

Measurements

Measurements of weight and height are important in the examination of children. Height can be measured only in children over the age of about two years. Below this age supine length can be measured roughly with a tape measure or more accurately with a special measuring board. All measurements should be made under standard conditions, and children should be weighed unclothed. One of the particular features of childhood is that it is a period of growth, the pattern of which may be adversely affected by many disturbances of health. Heights and weights should be compared with those of healthy children of similar sex, age and build, and for this purpose the percentile charts (Figs 12.2–12.7) are invaluable.

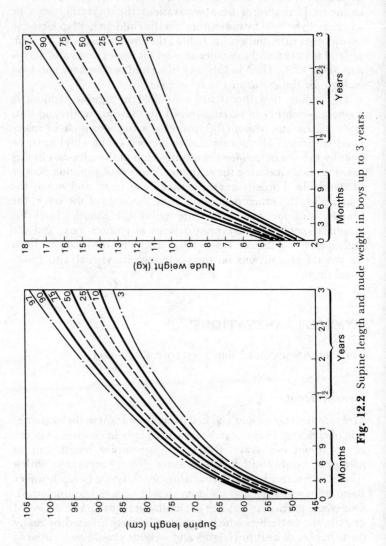

Fig. 12.2 Supine length and nude weight in boys up to 3 years.

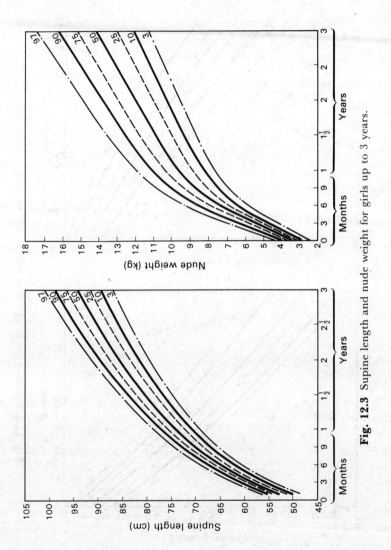

Fig. 12.3 Supine length and nude weight for girls up to 3 years.

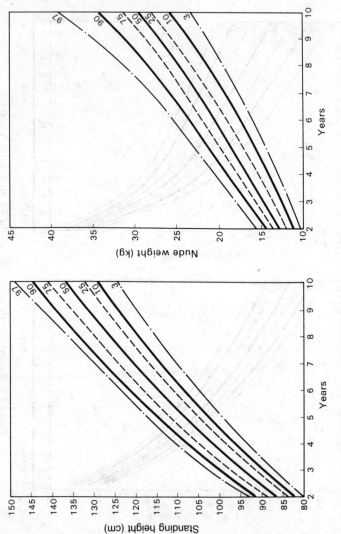

Fig. 12.4 Standing height and nude weight in boys aged 2 to 10 years.

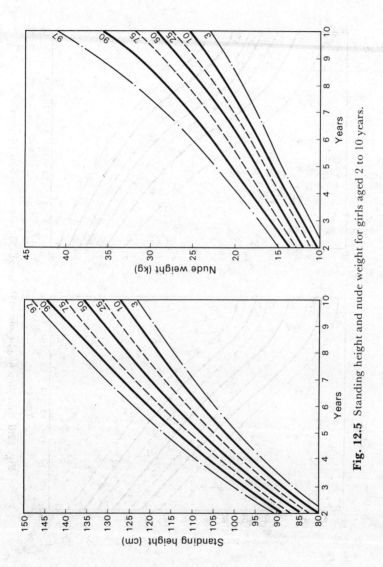

Fig. 12.5 Standing height and nude weight for girls aged 2 to 10 years.

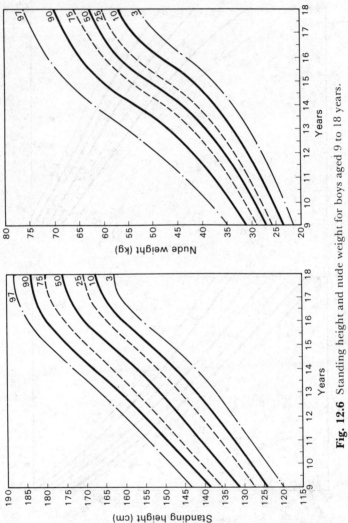

Fig. 12.6 Standing height and nude weight for boys aged 9 to 18 years.

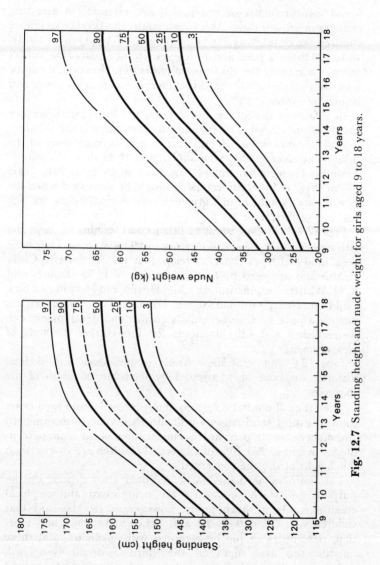

Fig. 12.7 Standing height and nude weight for girls aged 9 to 18 years.

Serial measurements over a period are essential in assessing changes in growth rates. As a rough guide, the average weight of children can be taken as 3 kg (7 lb) at birth, 6·5 kg (14 lb) at 1 year, 13 kg (28 lb) at 2 years and 22·5 kg (49 lb) at 7 years (the 'rule of seven' when using the old Imperial measure). However, it can be seen from the percentile charts that there is a wide range above and below the average.

In infants under the age of 2 years the head circumference should be measured. The standard measurement is the occipito-frontal circumference, which is the largest circumference of the head. The average head circumference at birth is 35 cm, at 3 months 41 cm, at 6 months 43 cm, at 1 year 46 cm and at 2 years 49 cm (Fig. 12.8). Hydrocephalus should be suspected when the rate of growth of the head is greater than is normal for the sex, age and size of the infant.

Figs 12.2–12.7 show standard heights and weights for boys and girls aged up to 3 years, 2 to 10 years and 9 to 18 years. They have been modified from charts developed at the Institute of Child Health and are used by kind permission of J. M. Tanner and R. H. Whitehouse, Institute of Child Health and Hospital for Sick Children, Great Ormond Street, London. The original charts include a page on which a child's growth and development can be recorded and full directions for the correct methods of measurement.

Figs 12.8 and 12.9 show head circumference and skeletal maturity (or bone age), assessed by the state of fusion of the epiphyses.

The range of normal is expressed in percentiles and each chart shows the third, tenth, twenty-fifth, fiftieth, seventy-fifth, ninetieth and ninety-seventh percentiles. The meaning of the tenth percentile for height is that 10% of all normal children are shorter than this height at the age concerned.

The limits of normality to be accepted must depend on the purpose for which the charts are being used and on local conditions. As a rough guide, however, it can be said that children who fall outside the area between the tenth and nine-tieth percentiles should be regarded with suspicion, and those outside the area between the third and ninety-seventh percentiles should be regarded as unhealthy unless proved otherwise.

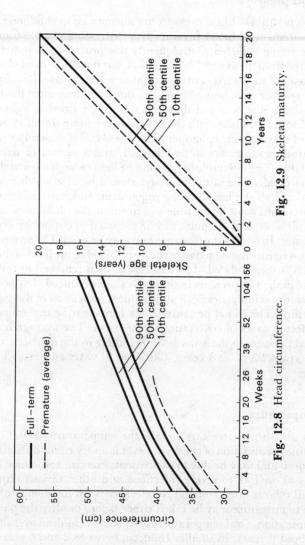

Fig. 12.9 Skeletal maturity.

Fig. 12.8 Head circumference.

Blood pressure

Abnormalities of blood pressure are uncommon in childhood, and measurement of blood pressure is a distressing examination for some young children. Consequently this procedure is sometimes omitted from the general examination, but it must be carried out in all cases of suspected cardiovascular or renal disease. Blood pressure readings are best obtained in most children after the main examination is over and the child is partially dressed. Allow the child to see and play with the cuff and give some simple explanation of what is going to happen. The size of cuff is most important if accurate readings are to be obtained, and a variety of sizes are available. The inflatable bag should be long enough to encircle the full circumference of the arm and should be of a width roughly equal to half the length of the upper arm. In small children and infants it may not be possible to determine the blood pressure by auscultation, and the pulse can be palpated to obtain the systolic pressure. In babies the flush method may be used. The arm is held up and tightly bandaged to exclude the blood to the level of the cuff which is then inflated. The bandage is then removed to reveal a white limb. The pressure in the cuff is slowly reduced. The point at which the skin flushes is an approximate indication of the systolic pressure. The blood pressure in the legs must be determined in suspected cases of coarctation of the aorta. The average level of blood pressure in the arms is 80/50 mmHg in the newborn, 85/60 at 4 years, 95/65 at 8 years, 100/70 at 10 years and 110/75 at 13 years.

Temperature

It is not always necessary to take the temperature as part of the routine examination of children. Fever is a very common finding in children and may be due to excitement, exercise and minor infections as well as to severe infections and other serious illnesses. Small infants often respond to infections with low temperatures. The temperature may be taken either before or after the physical examination. Oral temperatures are taken in children over the age of about 6 years. In smaller children, between 2 and 6 years, the thermometer can be placed in the axilla or groin. Rectal temperatures are taken in infants. The temperature in the axilla or groin is about 0·5°C lower and in the rectum about 0·5°C higher than the oral temperature. The temperature of normal children varies between 36·5°C and 37·5°C and is about 1°C higher in infants than in older children. Rapid rises of temperature to 39·5 or 40°C are sometimes associated with febrile convulsions in young children.

Rectal examination

Most children find rectal examination extremely unpleasant and small infants experience some pain from the procedure even when the little finger is used. One must use one's judgement, therefore, in deciding whether this examination should be inflicted on a child. Anal fissure is a common condition in childhood and can be detected by close inspection of the anal canal, the buttocks and anal orifice being gently held open with one hand on either side.

Stools

The stools of normal breast-fed infants may be loose and green or pasty and yellow. Infants feed on cow's milk preparations pass stools of a paler yellow colour and of a much firmer consistency. The character of the stool in older children is more variable than in adults.

Urine

Special techniques are required for the collection of urine specimens in infants who have not yet acquired sphincter control. It may be possible to 'catch' a specimen by holding the infant over a sterile container. Alternatively specially made sterile plastic containers with an adhesive opening can be applied to the washed genitalia. In the last resort bladder urine may be obtained by careful subrapubic aspiration.

DEVELOPMENTAL SCREENING EXAMINATION

Development is the normal process of maturation of function which takes place in the early years of life. It may be delayed by disease or adverse environment and the delay can be detected by developmental examination. A simple developmental screening examination should be carried out at regular intervals on all normal infants and as part of the clinical examination of infants presenting with symptoms.

It is usual to consider development under four main headings:

1. Movement and posture.
2. Vision and manipulation
3. Hearing and speech
4. Social behaviour

Screening for developmental delay involves testing the child's performance of a few skills in each of the four fields of development and comparing his achievements with those of average normal children of the same age. Children who appear to have delayed development on screening should be referred to an appropriate specialist for more detailed assessment.

Movement and posture

Head control.   By four months a baby will bring his head up in line with the trunk when pulled from supine to sitting, and when held in the sitting position will keep his head upright (Fig. 12.10). Before this age the head lags behind the trunk.

Sitting.   At seven months a baby begins to sit unsupported.

Standing and walking.   At nine months a baby can stand with support; at 10 months he takes a few steps with support and can crawl on hands and knees; at 13 months he begins to walk unsupported.

Vision and manipulation

Vision.   At eight weeks a baby lying supine will fix his gaze on a bright object dangling on a string 20 cm from his face and will move his head to follow it briefly. At six months he will follow a rolling ball at a distance of 3 m.

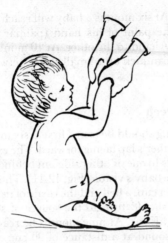

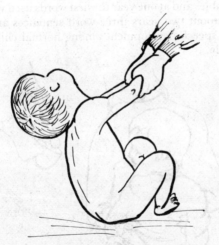

Fig. 12.10 Head control. *Above*. At 4 months the head is in line with the trunk when the baby is pulled to sitting. *Below*. Before the age of 4 months, the head lags.

Manipulation.   At six months a baby will reach out for an object and grasp it in the palm of his hand (palmar grasp) and will transfer it from one hand to the other. At 10 months he develops a pincer grasp and can pick up a small sweet between index finger and thumb.

Hearing and speech

Hearing.   Hearing should be tested first at six months. The baby is seated on his mother's lap facing forward. The examiner makes a series of soft sounds to one or other side but behind the mother and baby and out of the baby's vision (Fig. 12.11). The sounds used are a rattle, a spoon in a cup, a bell and the rustle of tissue paper. At six months the baby should turn to the source of sound when it is about 45 cm from his ear. At nine months he reacts more quickly and localizes the sound at a distance of 90 cm.

Speech.   By the age of nine months the infant is babbling with a series of syllables and at one year the first words used with meaning appear. By about two years three-word sentences are used. The variation in speech development among normal children is particularly wide.

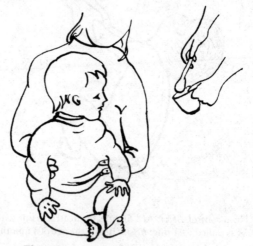

Fig. 12.11 Testing hearing at 6 months.

Social behaviour

One of the first social skills to be developed is smiling in response to a pleasurable stimulus which can be observed from about six weeks. At nine months a baby can hold and chew a biscuit. At 18 months he can drink from a cup, no longer puts objects into his mouth, and can build a tower of three cubes. At three years he can feed himself with a spoon and fork and makes a good attempt at dressing himself.

The range of normal developmental progress is wide and the milestones described above are achieved at the ages given by an average normal baby. Delay in all fields of development is more significant than delay in only one and severe delay is much more significant than slight delay. Allowance must always be made for those babies who were born prematurely, at least up to the age of one year by which time they should have caught up. The following is a list of some of the important milestones of development:

Milestones of development

3 weeks	Smiles
3 months	Holds head steady
4 months	Turns head to sound
5 months	Reaches out and grasps object
7 months	Sits unsupported
7 months	Transfers objects from one hand to the other
9 months	Stands with support
11 months	Crawls
12 months	Says 2–3 single words with meaning
13 months	Walks unsupported
15 months	Holds cup and drinks
18 months	Builds a tower of 3 cubes
2 years	Says 2–3 word sentences
3 years	Dresses himself

EXAMINATION OF THE NEWBORN

The routine examination of the newborn baby is designed to assess his general state of health and to detect congenital abnormalities.

It is usual to carry out one examination immediately after birth and another before discharge from hospital or on about the seventh day.

The routine measurements—weight, length and head circumference (occipito-frontal)—will usually have been taken by the midwife. Note the time of the first urine and meconium, which is the dark green sticky stool of the newborn baby in the first few days of life.

General inspection of the baby will indicate whether or not he is in good general condition, i.e. active and with a strong cry. Look for *abnormal facial features* such as those of Down's syndrome and for *external abnormalities* such as cleft lip, neural tube defects along the length of the spine, and abnormalities of the genitalia such as hypospadias and hydrocoele. The testes can usually be felt in the scrotum at birth. Remember to examine the *palate* for clefts, and the *anus* which may be imperforate.

Examine the *eyes* with an assistant who will gently hold the lids apart, and look for conjunctivitis, clouding of the cornea which suggests glaucoma and for lens opacities (cataract).

Observe the colour of the *skin*. Peripheral cyanosis is a common finding in normal newborns but central cyanosis indicates cardiac or respiratory disease. So-called physiological jaundice is present after 48 hours in most pre-term and some full-term babies but severe jaundice on the first or second day is usually due to some haemolytic disorder. Look for birth marks which are either pigmented lesions or haemangiomata. Most babies have a collection of dilated capillaries on the upper eyelids or at the nape of the neck which fade after a few weeks. Some babies develop crops of small papules on the trunk during the first week (erythema toxicum) but these fade quickly and are of no significance. 'Mongolian Blue Spot' is the name given to dark blue areas of racial pigmentation seen over the sacral area or on the back or legs in babies of African, Asian or Oriental origin.

Breast enlargement with exudation of a milky fluid from the nipples is sometimes seen in newborn babies of both sexes. This is due to the effect of transferred maternal hormones and disappears in a few days without causing problems.

The *head* should be inspected and palpated. There is considerable normal variation in the size of the fontanelles and in the width of the sutures. A cephalhaematoma is a subperiosteal haematoma which appears a few days after birth as a large cystic swelling limited to the area of one of the bones of the skull vault. The caput succedaneum is an area of oedema of the scalp over the presenting part of the head. It pits on pressure and is not fluctuant.

It is essential to examine the *hips* of all newborn infants in order to detect actual or potential dislocation. The infant is laid on his back with hips and knees flexed. The examiner grasps the thighs with the middle fingers over the greater trochanters and the thumbs over the lesser trochanters (Fig. 12.12). Pressure with the fingers will replace a dislocated femoral head and pressure with the thumbs will dislocate an unstable joint. Both abnormal movements will be associated with a pronounced and palpable click.

Soft *systolic murmurs* are heard in many newborn infants. They are usually of no significance and disappear after a few weeks but may, if they persist, indicate a congenital abnormality of the heart.

Examine the *hands* for abnormalities such as extra digits and for the single transverse palmar crease associated with Down's syndrome. Look for deformities of the *feet*. Talipes equino-varus is the common type of 'club foot' in which the foot is plantar flexed and rotated inwards.

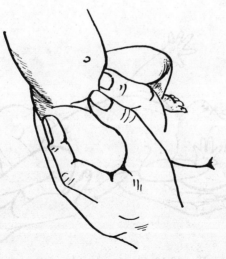

Fig. 12.12 Examination of the hips in the newborn.

Gently feel the *abdomen* for abnormal masses such as an enlarged kidney or bladder. The umbilical cord begins to shrivel up soon after birth and normally drops off at about the seventh day to leave a moist slightly infected stump, but redness and oedema of the skin around the stump indicate more serious infection.

In the neurological examination note the muscle tone and observe the posture and movement of the limbs. Any marked difference between the two sides is abnormal. The normal position of the limbs is in flexion. Look for weakness or paralysis in the face and in the arms suggesting injury to the facial nerve or brachial plexus. Flaccid paralysis in both legs is usually due to spina bifida with myelomeningocoele.

Primitive reflexes

Primitive reflexes are present in the normal newborn infant and disappear between three and six months of age. They are responses to specific stimuli and depend to some extent on the baby's state of wakefulness. The absence of one or more of these reflexes in the newborn period may indicate some abnormality of the brain or perhaps a local abnormality in the affected limb or neuromuscular pathway.

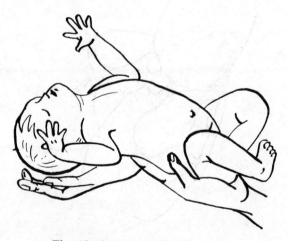

Fig. 12.13 Eliciting the Moro reflex.

The most useful of the primitive reflexes is the *Moro reflex*. This is correctly called the 'startle' reflex and should be elicited with care and gentle handling. The baby's body is supported with one arm and his hand and head with the other hand. The hand holding the head is suddenly lowered a few centimetres allowing the baby's head to drop back (Fig. 12.13). In a positive response the baby abducts and extends his arms and finally flexes them. A diminished or absent response suggests some cerebral abnormality. A clearly unilateral response suggests some local abnormality such as a fracture or brachial plexus injury in the arm on the side which does not respond.

Other primitive reflexes are:

Rooting reflex.   In this reflex the baby turns his head towards the stimulus of a touch on the side of the face, searching for the nipple.

Palmar grasp reflex.   A finger is placed across the palmar surface of the baby's fingers which flex and grip the examiner's.

Stepping reflex.   The baby is held upright with his feet resting on a firm surface. As one foot presses down on the surface the other leg flexes at the hip and knee in a stepping movement. As this response is alternated from one leg to the other the baby makes a walking movement.

13

The blood

The investigation of a patient with a blood disorder includes a history and clinical examination as well as the examination of the blood in the laboratory

CLINICAL EXAMINATION

Symptoms and signs in blood disease are due to:

1. Anaemia (lack of haemoglobin) and polycythaemia (excess haemoglobin)
2. leukopenia, leukocytosis and functional disorders of white cells
3. Failure of haemostasis

It is particularly important to take a careful past history, family history and drug history as many blood disorders are chronic, inherited or drug-induced. Details of history taking will be found in the various sections of this chapter. Physical examination is often concentrated on the lympho-reticular system (i.e. lymph nodes, liver and spleen) and the skin gives valuable information on anaemia, infection and bleeding tendencies. A full physical examination cannot be neglected as many blood disorders have general effects and many illnesses in the field of general medicine affect the blood.

The lymph nodes

Figure 13.1 shows the distribution of the principal lymph node groups which may be felt. These areas should be examined and if lymph nodes are found the following points should be considered.

1. How many nodes are palpable?
2. What is their approximate diameter in centimetres?
3. What is their consistency?
4. Are they discrete or confluent?
5. Are they mobile or fixed?
6. Is the skin in the vicinity of the nodes abnormal?

The liver and spleen

Blood disorders often cause very marked enlargement of the liver and spleen. The examination should begin in the iliac fossae to

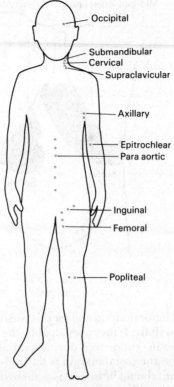

Fig. 13.1 The lymph nodes: clinical examination.

avoid missing the edge of an organ which has reached the level of the pelvic inlet. The liver is often difficult to feel even when enlarged and useful information can be gained by percussion. The spleen is difficult to feel when only slightly enlarged and it may be useful to instruct the patient to lie slightly on his right side. The physician then places his left hand over the left lower lateral rib cage of the patient and supports it. With the physician's right hand at the costal margin the patient should be asked to relax and breathe deeply through the mouth. This manoeuvre can make the spleen more prominent. Whilst the spleen usually enlarges in the direction of the right iliac fossa, it can sometimes be felt in a

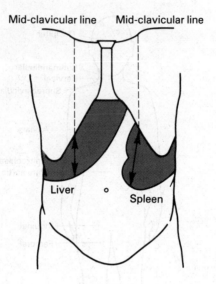

Fig. 13.2 The liver and spleen: clinial examination. CM = costal margin

vertical posterior position and for this reason the left loin should be palpated carefully. If they are palpable, the liver and spleen should be measured in centimetres, during natural expiration. A suitable landmark on the costal margin is the mid-clavicular line and the measurement should be from this point to the furthest extent of the organ (see Fig. 13.2).

The skin

The skin surface itself may be infected or ulcerated and various forms of haemorrhage into the skin may occur. Haemorrhages are classified as follows:

1. *Purpura and petechial haemorrhages*: tiny pinpoint haemorrhages into the skin which do not blanch on compression with a glass slide
2. *Ecchymoses*: haemorrhages which are larger than petechiae and with more obvious confluence
3. *Bruises*

Telangiectasia are small dilated blood vessels which may be visible on the skin surface, particularly on the lips. They blanch on compression and are sometimes a source of severe haemorrhage when the nose, gastrointestinal tract or bladder are affected.

Skin infiltration occurs in some malignant conditions of the blood, e.g. Hodgkin's disease.

The conjunctiva should be inspected for pallor or jaundice and the mouth may show evidence of haemorrhage, ulceration or infection. The tongue may be smooth or red and cracking may be noted at the corners of the mouth (angular cheilosis).

The fundus oculi

Fundal haemorrhages are often visible in disorders of haemostasis, especially thrombocytopenia. When blood viscosity is increased (e.g. in macroglobulinaemia or chronic granulocytic leukaemia with a high white cell count) there may be engorgement of retinal vessels with papilloedema and retinal haemorrhage.

LABORATORY EXAMINATION

Sampling

Blood should be collected by venepuncture, usually from the antecubital fossa. Venous occlusion by a cuff is permissible in most haematological investigations but should not be severe or prolonged. A medium-sized needle should be used; undue suction should not be applied to the syringe as this may cause haemolysis. The patient should be resting comfortably during venepuncture and the procedure should be explained clearly before starting.

The treatment of many blood disorders is by the intravenous route and every effort should be made to avoid laceration of veins or haemorrhage around the vein punctured. At the end of the procedure the arm can be held up in the air while the venepuncture site is pressed.

Blood clots when removed from the body and this occurs more rapidly in glass than in plastic tubes. If clotted blood is required, e.g. for blood grouping, it should be taken into a new plain glass tube and allowed to stand at room temperature for 10 minutes before separation of clot from serum. Most other samples are taken into plastic tubes to which some anticoagulant has been added. Anticoagulants commonly used include:

1. *Sequestrene (EDTA)*, which binds calcium by chelation and is used for routine blood counts.
2. *Citrate*, which also removes calcium and is used in coagulation work.
3. *Heparin*, which inhibits many parts of the coagulation mechanism and is useful for chemical estimations, e.g. plasma iron.

The peripheral blood film

If blood is required only for the making of a stained film then the patient's finger may be pricked with a lance and the blood spread directly onto a slide. Unfortunately this causes platelet clumping and films are best made from freshly collected blood placed in a sequestrene tube, spread expertly and correctly stained with a Romanowsky method.

The high power of the microscope is generally used to examine blood films except where the presence of large blood parasites (e.g. microfilaria) is suspected. Each element of the peripheral blood should be examined systematically i.e.

red cells	size, shape, colour, presence of nucleated cells, rouleaux
white cells	distribution of various types, maturity, morphology
platelets	numbers (normal, reduced or increased), morphology

A more detailed account of the peripheral blood will be found in the various sections.

The bone marrow

In the adult, blood production is confined to the skull, spine, pelvis, and upper ends of the long bones. It is often necessary to examine the bone marrow in disorders of the blood and this can be done either by aspiration with a syringe and a specially designed needle or by removing a core of bone marrow tissue (trephine biopsy). Aspirates may be taken from the manubrium or body of the sternum or from the anterior or posterior iliac crest, but trephine samples must be obtained from the iliac crest.

Bone marrow aspirates can be spread on slides and stained in the same way as peripheral blood, or they may be examined histologically after formalin fixation. Trephine samples are fixed in formalin and decalcified before examination.

Examination.   The principles of examination of bone marrow aspirates are the same as those for the peripheral blood but the slide must be examined under the low power of the microscope to assess cellularity in the fragments at the ends of the trails and to assess megakaryocyte numbers. Erythropoiesis, granulopoiesis, lymphocytes and plasma cells are examined under the high power of the microscope and a search is made for any evidence of infiltration by cells not usually found in the bone marrow (e.g. carcinoma cells). It is important to stain the aspirate by Perls' ferrocyanide method to assess iron (haemosiderin) in fragments and erythroblasts.

Bone marrow appearances are considered in more detail in the various sections as are the more complex investigations associated with particular disorders. Photomicrographs of normoblastic and megaloblastic marrow are shown in Plate VIII.

ANAEMIA

Common symptoms of anaemia are usually the result of deficient oxygen supply to the tissues. They include:

Dyspnoea appears at first only on exertion, but with progressive anaemia the cardiac function becomes affected and shortness of breath occurs also at rest.

Ankle oedema also occurs late in anaemia and is associated with cardiac dysfunction.

Palpitations occur when anaemia is severe and the cardiovascular dynamics are affected.

Lassitude is variable, but tends to become more pronounced as the haemoglobin level falls.

Anaemia will also accentuate features of vascular insufficiency thus emphasizing *angina, claudication* and *cerebral ischaemic symptoms*.

Clinical evidence of anaemia can only be assessed by examination of the mucous membranes of the mouth, the conjunctivae, nails and skin creases. Due to variation in thickness and depth of pigmentation, the skin colour is an unsuitable clinical index of anaemia.

Examination of the peripheral blood

Sampling.   The initial screening for anaemia is best carried out on a small (4·5 ml) sample of venous blood taken into a container

Table 13.1.   NORMAL RED CELL VALUES

	Men	Women
Red cell count $\times 10^{12}$/litre	4·4–6·1	4·2–5·4
Haemoglobin g/dl	13·0–18·0	11·5–16·5
Haematocrit	0·40–0·54	0·37–0·47
Mean corpuscular volume fl	75–99	75–99
Mean corpuscular haemoglobin pg	27–31	27–31
Mean corpuscular haemoglobin concentration g/dl	32–36	32–36

Table 13.2.   TYPICAL RED CELL VALUES IN ANAEMIA

	Iron deficiency	Macrocytic anaemia
Red blood cell $\times 10^{12}$/litre	4·9	2·7
Haemoglobin g/dl	10·4	10·4
Haematocrit	0·35	0·32
Mean corpuscular volume fl	72	119
Mean corpuscular haemoglobin pg	21	38
Mean corpuscular haemoglobin concentration g/dl	29	32

In these two examples there is a similar degree of anaemia (haemoglobin 10·4 g/dl). Note the differences in size (MCV) and haemoglobinization (MCHC) of the red cells in the two types of anaemia. The MCH is increased in the macrocytic anaemia because the red cells are *larger* than normal.

In iron deficiency, on the other hand, the MCH is reduced because the red cells are smaller than usual, and also because they are poorly haemoglobinized. Generally, in iron deficiency anaemia the red cell count is well maintained, but in macrocytic anaemia the red cell count is lower.

prepared with dipotassium ethylene diamine tetra-acetic acid (EDTA: sequestrene). A sample of this size is necessary for the requirements of the automatic counting machines which are much more accurate than the older capillary methods; furthermore, additional tests can be carried out on the same specimen should preliminary tests indicate that they are necessary.

Red cell indices. Estimations of red cell indices (Table 13.1) provide invaluable information for the basic differentiation of the type of anaemia. Accurate estimation of the *haemoglobin* and the *haematocrit* (or *packed cell volume*) are the basic values indicating the degree of anaemia. A simple calculation relating these two estimations produces the *mean corpuscular haemoglobin concentration (MCHC)*; this is a useful index of the average haemoglobin concentration of the red cells. The accuracy of the *total red cell count* is considerably greater when an automatic electronic (particle) counter is used because a very large number of cells can be enumerated in a short time. A reliable red cell count enables the computation of other useful indices such as the *mean corpuscular haemoglobin (MCH)* and the *mean corpuscular volume (MCV)* which can be derived by relating the red cell count to the haemoglobin and PCV values respectively. The MCH indicates the average weight of haemoglobin per red cell and the MCV provides an estimate of the mean cell size. In some machines the MCV is obtained automatically by sizing the individual cells.

Confirmatory information on the size and haemoglobin content of the red cells can be obtained in the course of examining a blood film.

The blood film. Morphological abnormalities of individual red cells often provide clues to the nature of the anaemia.

Anisocytosis, or variation in cell size, is an observation almost valueless in small degree; in marked degree it is much more important to know the types of cell involved, such as microspherocytes or macrocytes.

Macrocytosis may be due to the presence of large *polychromatic* (grey-blue staining) immature red cells (Plate VIII) produced by increased erythropoietic stimulation, or from megaloblastic red cell precursors.

Microcytosis is usually associated with iron deficiency but also occurs in sickle cell anaemia (Plate VIII).

Normocytic red cells are found in acute blood loss and bone marrow failure.

Poikilocytosis or variation in cell shape is found with significant ineffective erythropoiesis as in megaloblastic anaemia, myelofibrosis or when the cells are damaged in their circulation.

Abnormally pale-staining red cells (*hypochromasia*) usually indicate that they are deficient in haemoglobin content (Plate VIII).

Bone marrow examination.   Frequently it is necessary to study an aspirate of marrow tissue to identify the underlying disorder more exactly.

IRON DEFICIENCY

Clinically the patient with iron deficiency shows symptoms and signs of anaemia. More specific evidence in long-standing iron lack is indicated by *glossitis* with atrophy of papillae and *angular stomatitis (cheilosis)*. These may be associated with *dysphagia* to form the *Plummer-Vinson* or *Paterson-Kelly* syndrome. The nails may be brittle and spoon-shaped (koilonychia) (Plate I).

The history may reveal evidence of dietary lack or a cause of chronic blood loss such as menorrhagia, gastrointestinal symptoms of neoplasm, peptic ulcer, hookworm or haemorrhoids. The diagnosis of iron deficiency is not complete without an indication of its cause.

Red cell indices.   Table 13.2 shows evidence of reduced haemoglobin content (low MCH and MCHC) and reduction in mean cell size (low MCV). The hypochromic microcytic state of the red cells is confirmed on examination of the *blood film* in which the *central* pallor of the cells is considerably enlarged.

Estimation of plasma iron is essential to confirm the deficiency; the plasma iron binding capacity is typically increased.

Hypochromic anaemia without iron deficiency is a feature of 'anaemia of chronic disorders', thalassaemia syndromes, sideroblastic anaemias and occasionally renal failure.

Bone marrow aspiration.   Though not usually necessary, bone marrow aspirates show erythroblasts in increased numbers in the later stages of maturation, with deficient haemoglobin formation. Staining the film to determine its iron content reveals a deficiency of storage iron (haemosiderin).

DEFICIENCY OF VITAMIN B₁₂ AND FOLIC ACID

In addition to the symptoms and signs of anaemia, the history may reveal a primary causation such as dietary deficiency or total or partial gastrectomy. Pregnancy may also cause folate deficiency. Other important clinically related conditions include pernicious anaemia and malabsorption syndrome.

Deficiency of vitamin B_{12} and of folate can be confirmed by serum assays of these vitamins; malabsorption of vitamin B_{12} is best demonstrated by the radioactive B_{12} urinary excretion (Schilling) test.

Pernicious anaemia (Plate VIII) is the most common cause of vitamin B_{12} deficiency in the United Kingdom. It is rare in Africa and Asia. It presents uncommonly before the age of 30. A sore tongue is a usual symptom and the features of subacute combined degeneration of the nervous system may precede or succeed the symptoms of anaemia. Indigestion and diarrhoea may occur.

In addition to the anaemia, mild jaundice is common and the tongue becomes reddened, smooth and shiny. The spleen is often moderately enlarged.

Additional and more specific tests for pernicious anaemia include *gastric analysis* following pentagastrin stimulation to demonstrate achlorhydria. This is not usually done when the other tests are available.

Auto-antibody studies in the serum are positive for parietal cell antibodies in 95% of cases and for *intrinsic factor antibodies* in 60%.

Malabsorption syndrome produces folic acid deficiency and is found in association with tropical sprue, adult coeliac disease and other small bowel pathology such as blind loops, fistulae, ileitis and jejunal diverticulosis. Sprue and coeliac disease may be accompanied by steatorrhoea and features due to lack of absorption of other important dietary components such as protein and calcium.

Red cell indices.   The total red cell count is reduced in number but each cell is well haemoglobinized (normal MCH and MCHC) and larger than normal (high MCV). In the *blood film* the macrocytes are typically oval in outline and a number of 'tear-drop' poikilocytes are seen. They are normochromic unless there is a complicating iron deficiency also. The polymorph leucocytes tend to be reduced in number and have hypersegmented nuclei.

Bone marrow films.   Bone marrow films show marked increase in cellularity due to proliferative (but ineffective) erythropoiesis with defective maturation of the cell nuclei resulting in the formation of megaloblastic red cell precursors and giant metamyelocytes. Iron stores are increased due to the excessive breakdown of the abnormal red cell series.

HAEMOLYTIC ANAEMIAS

Anaemia due to premature destruction of the cells may be congenital or acquired. The congenital forms have a history of anaemia and usually hyperbilirubinaemia dating from early life often accompanied by a family history. They are usually due to intrinsic abnormalities of the red cell membrane (e.g. congenital spherocytosis), metabolism (e.g. enzyme deficiencies) or haemoglobin structure. Acquired haemolysis is usually of recent onset and arises as the result of the cells being exposed to the destructive effects of, for example, antibodies and poisons. A rare form of acquired red cell membrane abnormality is *paroxysmal nocturnal haemoglobinuria.*

Clinically the patient presents with a variable degree of anaemia and jaundice, though in mild cases the latter may be absent. On examination the spleen is usually palpable in established cases. In severe long-standing haemolysis of congenital origin the increased red cell production tends to produce stunted growth with distortion of the bones of the skull due to the marrow hyperplasia. Typically, this results in mongoloid facies and radiological thickening of the diploe. There is a tendency for skin ulceration to occur particularly on the lower legs.

The laboratory findings in addition to a degree of anaemia are:
1. Abnormal red cell morphology, e.g. spherocytes
2. Reticulocytosis
3. Erythroid hyperplasia of the bone marrow
4. Increased indirect plasma bilirubin
5. Increased urobilinogen
6. Shortened survival of isotope-labelled red cells
7. Typically, the urine contains no bilirubin

Intravascular haemolysis

In many cases of acquired haemolysis, the damaged red cells are removed by the reticulo-endothelial tissues, particularly the spleen. When red cell destruction is acute they are broken down in the circulation. This is the intravascular haemolysis which results in loss of serum *haptoglobins*, the presence of *methaemalbumin* in the serum, *haemosiderinuria* and *haemoglobinuria*.

The saline osmotic fragility test

The saline osmotic fragility test essentially measures the ratio of thickness to volume in the red cell. Spherocytes are therefore more fragile, and *leptocytes* (e.g. target cells) less fragile than normal. The degree of increased fragility of a red cell sample is entirely proportional to its spherocyte population.

Red cell enzymes deficiencies

A breakdown in the mechanism of red cell carbohydrate metabolism may occur either in the pentose phosphate pathway, when deficiency of glucose-6-phosphate dehydrogenase (G6PD) is the more common defect, or in the Emden-Meyerhof glycolytic pathway which is particularly affected by a lack of pyruvate kinase. These enzymes can be quantitated by fairly simple methods. G6PD deficiency may be recognized by a simple qualitative dye screening test.

Each of these important inherited enzyme deficiencies may be associated with forms of non-spherocytic congenital haemolytic anaemia. Severe G6PD deficiency occurs particularly in Mediterranean peoples. An additional factor in some of these individuals, which may produce severe haemolysis, is an associated sensitivity to the fava bean or its plant pollen. A less severe variety of G6PD deficiency occurs in some 10% of African males and less frequently in African females, the character being sex linked. Such deficient individuals show no adverse effects except after treatment with certain drugs such as primaquine.

Family studies should always be carried out.

Abnormal haemoglobin formation

Abnormal haemoglobin may arise as a result of substitution of abnormal variants of haemoglobin for the normal adult (A) type, or it may occur when normal adult haemoglobin formation is inhibited as in the *thalassaemia* syndromes.

A prominent example of a substituted abnormal variant is haemoglobin S which produces *sickle cell disease* (Plate IX). If sickle cell haemoglobin is deoxygenated, it becomes insoluble and crystallizes out in the red cell. Such red cells take on a characteristic sickle shape and may obstruct the blood flow in nutrient vessels and cause infarction. When sickle formation is not obvious as is likely to be the case in the heterozygous form, sickling may be provoked *in vitro* by incubating a wet preparation of the erythrocytes under conditions of reduced oxygen tension. Alternatively the haemoglobin S component can be detected by a simple tube test which depends upon the fact that sickle haemoglobin is less soluble than the normal form. Sickle cell disease is common in African and New World negroes. Other qualitatively abnormal haemoglobins of note are C (in West African and New World negroes), D punjab (in northern Indians) and E (in south east Asians). These abnormal components can be identified separately in the haemolysate by employing various electrophoretic techniques.

Of the *thalassaemias*, the common variety is β-thalassaemia in which the production of β-polypeptide chains of the globin is lacking. It is distinguished by an increase in the minor normal haemoglobin components A2 and F. In α-thalassaemia, where α chains are deficient, there is no increase in A2 or F but the formation of haemoglobin Barts ($\gamma4$) and haemoglobin H ($\beta4$) may occur. These haemoglobin variants can be individually identified by electrophoretic techniques and haemoglobin F can be estimated by a method which employs its relatively increased resistance to denaturation by alkali.

The overall picture of thalassaemia is that of hypochromia due to the genetically determined deficiency of haemoglobin A production. The abnormally thin red cells that are produced frequently appear as *target cells*. The *leptocyte* has an increased resistance to more dilute solutions of saline compared with normal cells when the osmotic fragility test is applied. The level of iron in the plasma is high in these conditions and the iron-binding capacity is greater than normal. In the marrow there are abundant iron stores and the metabolic defect in haemoglobin synthesis results in the presence of iron granules in the developing red cells.

Acquired haemolytic anaemia may be due to red cell damage by autoantibodies or toxic chemicals, poisons and therapeutic agents or by red cell trauma.

The direct antiglobulin (Coombs) test. Red cells which have been sensitized by antibodies are coated with immunoglobulin (IgG, IgA or IgM) and sometimes components of complement also. An anti-human globulin (Coombs) serum, obtained by deliberately immunizing an animal (e.g rabbit) to human globulin, will agglutinate cells sensitized in this way and so demonstrate the presence of the antibody. The affected cells in *haemolytic disease of the newborn* due to Rhesus fetal-maternal incompatibility can be detected by the same technique.

POLYCYTHAEMIA

If the red cell count is in excess of normal, polycythaemia is present. This is usually associated with increases in the haemoglobin level and PCV. The condition may be due to a primary bone marrow disorder, for example polycythaemia rubra vera, or may be secondary, for example in congenital heart disease, chronic lung disease, and some renal conditions.

Clinically, polycythaemia causes headache, plethora and tinnitus. Patients with the primary condition often complain of pruritus and on examination the spleen is usually palpable.

In polycythaemia rubra vera the neutrophil and platelet counts are typically increased and the neutrophil alkaline phosphatase and plasma uric acid levels are elevated. The red cell mass is increased in all forms of polycythaemia except when the plasma volume is reduced, e.g. dehydration.

BLOOD TRANSFUSION

Collection of donor blood

In the United Kingdom a highly organized blood collection service is available on a nation-wide basis. Donors are selected from healthy adults of either sex between the ages of 18 and 65, except for pregnant and lactating women. Usually about 500 ml of blood is taken into a special plastic bag containing 75 ml of a citrate anticoagulant. Donors are safeguarded by a routine haemoglobin estimation prior to donation using a simple finger prick method based on the specific gravity of a drop of blood in copper sulphate solution. Males are accepted if their haemoglobin equivalent is over 13·5 g/dl; for females the minimum level is 12·5 g/dl. Usually donors give only two donations in a year. Care must be taken to avoid air embolism during donation.

Processing of donor blood

In order to protect the recipient, measures must be taken to avoid the possibility of *transmitting disease* in the transfused blood (p. 450). An attempt to avoid *hepatitis* is made by rejecting donors with a history of jaundice and testing all donor samples for hepatitis associated antigen (HAA) and antibody. The serum of all donors is also tested for *syphilis*. The ABO and Rh(D) blood groups are determined routinely before transfusion. If the donor is group O, the serum should be tested for immune anti-A and anti-B. When these antibodies are present the blood should be reserved for group O recipients only. *Storage* of whole donor blood in acid-citrate dextrose (ACD) or citrate-phosphate-dextrose (CPD) must be maintained at a constant temperature of 4°C. Optimally this should be for a maximum period of three weeks.

Blood components

It is now possible to separate individual components of whole donor blood and make them available for specific therapeutic requirements. Transfusion thus becomes both more economical and more specifically effective. Such components include packed red cells, platelets, leucocytes (occasionally), whole plasma (fresh frozen at −20°C) and factor VIII (as cryoprecipitate at −20°C). Dried preparations of whole plasma, fibrinogen and factor VIII and IX concentrates are also available.

Compatibility testing of blood for transfusion

When a patient requires a transfusion, blood of the same ABO and Rh(D) group must be selected. The red cells of each donor sample must be tested with the recipient's serum by several methods at different temperatures. Agglutination by complete cold antibodies in saline is tested for at room temperature and at 37°C. Tests for incomplete warm antibodies should be done in bovine albumin at 37°C and by the indirect antiglobulin (Coombs) test using 'broad spectrum' antiglobulin serum that will detect both IgG antibody and complement. Treatment of the donor red cells with proteolytic enzymes may also be used as a technique for discovering potentially incompatible antibodies in the recipient's serum.

Indications for blood transfusion

It is important to confine blood transfusion to clinical conditions in which there is a clear indication; there are very real hazards which may occur as a direct consequence.

Acute blood loss must be rectified by giving whole blood sufficient to restore blood volume. *Trauma* may additionally involve excessive loss of plasma which may require proportionately more plasma to restore equilibrium. *Burns*, when extensive, need almost exclusively plasma replacement to rectify the marked haemoconcentration following severe plasma loss.

Most *chronic anaemias* of nutritional type can be corrected by giving the appropriate replacement therapy such as iron, folic acid or vitamin B12. Transfusion of packed red cells may be necessary if rapid restoration is required in iron deficiency of pregnancy or if anaemia is severe in B12 or folate deficiency. Chronic *bone marrow failure* due to aplasia, fibrosis or leukaemic infiltration requires correction at intervals with donor red cells.

Transfusion of *platelet concentrate* is indicated when spontaneous bleeding occurs due specifically to thrombocytopenia.

In cases of leucopenia with severe infection, *granulocyte transfusion* may be accomplished by separating neutrophils from the fresh blood of normal donors. Patients with chronic granulocytic leukaemia have also been used as a source of cells.

Complications of blood transfusion

Incompatibility. Incompatibility is the most serious hazard associated with blood transfusion. Acute haemolysis arises from ABO blood group incompatibility. Massive red cell agglutination and destruction is followed by intense haemoglobinaemia, jaundice and acute renal failure due to tubular necrosis. The renal lesion is partly due to circulatory shock and hypotension and partly to the presence of haemoglobin casts and red cell debris. Careful documentation and sample labelling are required to avoid this potentially fatal consequence.

Pyrogen reaction.   The pyrogen reaction is probably due to the presence of antibodies to transfused leucocytes and platelets in the patient.

Allergic reactions.   Urticaria and asthma may occur during transfusion if the donor blood contains material to which the patient is sensitive.

Toxic effects   due to excess of citrate may occur following multiple transfusion and symptoms of hypocalcaemia develop.

Air embolism   is much less likely to occur with the use of plastic bags which collapse down as they empty of blood.

Circulatory overload   is more likely to occur in elderly patients with chronic anaemia. The use of packed cells for transfusion and potent diuretics help to prevent its occurrence.

Iron overload   occurs in patients who have been sustained over a long time with numerous blood transfusions.

Thrombophlebitis   tends to occur when the same infusion needle remains in the same site for over 12 hours.

Transmission of disease.   *Malaria* parasites survive for about three weeks at 4°C and can easily be transmitted. In non-malarious countries, potentially infected donors are rejected. In malarious areas the simultaneous administration of anti-malarials may be necessary.

Hepatitis due to hepatitis-associated antigen (HAA) should be avoided by screening the serum of all donors. Some anicteric cases have sera positive for the antigen and are capable of giving the recipient hepatitis. Furthermore hepatitis may result even when no HAA has been identified in the donor sample

Syphilis is due to treponema pallidum which may survive for six days at 4°C. All donors in the UK are screened serologically.

Brucellosis and *cytomegalovirus* may also be transmitted.

Faulty storage. Blood stored at freezing temperatures or over-heated prior to transfusion may result in massive haemolysis of donor red cells with dangerous consequences if transfused into a patient. Grossly infected blood may result from storage at temperatures above 4°C.

DISORDERS OF WHITE CELLS

The clinical effects of white cell disorders arise from lack of white cells, disturbances in white cell function and the effects of white cell proliferation. When taking a history the following points should be considered.

Has the patient noticed a reduced resistance to infection, e.g. frequent colds or influenza, sore throats, chest infections, earache, boils, pustules, dysuria and fever or sweats?

Does the patient complain of mouth ulceration, skin rash or irritation (pruritus)? Has the patient noticed any enlargement of lymph nodes or the sensation of dragging or pain in the left hypochondrium which can arise from an enlarged spleen?

In practice it is remarkable how few symptoms may arise from very enlarged lymph nodes, liver and spleen. One may see a patient whose spleen is enormous presenting with an entirely different complaint.

Symptoms may be related to invasion and displacement of normal tissues by tumour. Thus patients with acute leukaemia also suffer from symptoms of anaemia and thrombocytopenia and may develop bone pain. When the meninges are invaded symptoms of headache and neck stiffness may be prominent and deposits may damage the spinal cord causing paraplegia. If lymph nodes in the mediastinum become sufficiently large as a result of lymphoma they may cause mediastinal obstruction with venous engorgement of the head and respiratory embarrassment, whilst in the abdomen large nodes may cause lymphatic and/or venous obstruction in the lower limbs. Bone pain is also a prominent symptom of the plasma cell tumour myelomatosis in which pathological fractures also occur.

A variety of symptoms may be caused by the systemic effects of white cell tumours. These include fever without evidence of infection, weight loss, pruritus, polyneuropathy, myopathy and renal failure from a variety of causes. In myelomatosis an abnormal globulin may circulate in the blood and contribute to renal failure and may cause visual and circulatory disturbances. Autoimmune haemolytic anaemia may occur in some lymphomas.

When the white cell count is very high i.e. greater than 300×10^9/litre this alone may cause symptoms due to failure of the peripheral circulation. Thus in chronic granulocytic leukaemia patients may present with priapism, visual loss or dyspnoea.

Physical examination is mainly concentrated on the mouth, skin and lymphoreticular system; neutropenic mouth ulceration may be very severe. The lymph nodes are usually enlarged in the lymphoid malignancies but many viral illnesses (e.g. glandular fever) may cause lymphadenopathy. The liver and spleen are also often enlarged in lymphoid diseases.

In the *laboratory*, investigation centres on the *peripheral blood* and *bone marrow*.

The peripheral blood

The white cell count ranges from $4 \cdot 5 - 11 \times 10^9$/litre in the normal adult. With modern apparatus the white cell count is usually measured automatically at the same time as the haemoglobin and other red cell values. The differential white cell count is usually calculated by examination of the stained film and in health a typical result would be:

Neutrophils	60%
Lymphocytes	30%
Monocytes	6%
Eosinophils	3%
Basophils	1%

Variations of normality are very wide and values are different for infants and young children. The actual process of differential counting using the microscope is very inaccurate so that one should not put too much emphasis on individual results. Trends in serial counts are easily seen by charting figures. Automatic differential counters are now being developed and these are potentially much more accurate than manual methods and will allow valid calculation of absolute white cell numbers which are derived from the total white cell count and the differential count.

An abnormality in the number and/or distribution of white cells does not necessarily imply a white cell disorder as almost any illness may alter the total or differential white cell counts. The typical response to bacterial infection or any stress is a neutrophil leukocytosis, though in children a lymphocytosis often occurs, especially in whooping cough. Sometimes the reaction may be so marked as to mimic a leukaemic process, and is termed a leukaemoid reaction. Glandular fever is an infectious illness which causes a nonspecific lymphocytosis in which the lymphocytes are morphologically abnormal and in some respects resemble leukaemic cells, but the illness is self-limiting (Plate IX).

The white cell count is also increased in most types of leukaemia due to the presence of abnormal white cells in the peripheral blood. In acute leukaemia these will be lymphoblasts (Plate X) or myeloblasts (see below). In chronic lymphocytic leukaemia mature lymphocytes (Plate X) form the majority of the white cells and in chronic granulocytic (myeloid) leukaemia a spectrum of maturing granulocytes is found (Plate X).

The white cell count may be reduced due to:

1. Aplasia—idiopathic or due to drugs, chemicals or irradiation
2. Infiltration, e.g. myelofibrosis
3. Vitamin B12 or folic acid deficiency
4. Sequestration and/or destruction due to an enlarged spleen, e.g. Felty's syndrome
5. Overwhelming infection
6. Inherited conditions

Inherited defects may also lead to disorders of neutrophil function as in the sex-linked chronic granulomatous disease of childhood. Both inherited and acquired disorders of lymphocytes are described but the acquired defects are more common and are often found in patients with Hodgkin's disease, lymphoma or myeloma.

Apart from white cell numbers and distribution, morphology is also studied.

The lymphoid series. Many morphological alterations are nonspecific, as discussed above, but malignant lymphoid cells are often larger than normal and contain a prominent nucleolus (lymphoblasts). Morphological abnormalities may also be seen in the more 'mature' lymphocytic and plasmacytic malignancies.

The myeloid series.   More primitive white cells may appear in the peripheral blood in various forms of myeloid leukaemia and also in infection (see above). The most primitive myeloid cells (myeloblasts) are large cells with more plentiful cytoplasm than lymphoblasts and the nuclei often contain multiple nucleoli. In the cytoplasm, rod-like structures (Auer rods) may sometimes be seen. Abnormal myeloid cells often resemble monocytes morphologically. Some forms of myeloid leukaemia are specifically monocytic (Plate X).

The bone marrow

It is difficult to give precise indications for examination of the bone marrow and details of interpretation are outside the scope of this chapter. However, bone marrow aspiration is indicated in the investigation of disorders associated with diffuse marrow infiltration, e.g. leukaemias and myelomatosis (Plate IX), whilst a combination of aspiration and trephine biopsy is to be preferred in those conditions associated with patchy marrow involvement, e.g. lymphomas. A bone marrow trephine may be necessary to confirm the diagnosis of aplastic anaemia. In myelofibrosis the 'solidification' of the marrow makes aspiration impossible and a trephine sample must be obtained. It is important to note that bone marrow infiltration in acute leukaemia does not always spill over into the peripheral blood though there is usually a clue to be found in the associated pancytopenia. This is known by the rather unsatisfactory term of 'sub-leukaemic leukaemia'.

A number of other investigations may be useful in the diagnosis of white cell disorders including special white cell stains, chromosome analysis and lymphocyte typing. An example of a white cell staining technique is the neutrophil alkaline phosphatase test. Investigations available in the other branches of pathology are also of great importance, e.g. chest radiography, lymphangiography and tests of hepatic function and protein chemistry. These cannot be considered here but close cooperation between different disciplines is essential.

HAEMOSTASIS

The haemostatic mechanism involves the following:
1. The properties of the vessel wall
2. The platelets
3. The coagulation mechanism
4. The fibrinolytic mechanism

These mechanisms are closely interrelated and are separated conventionally only for ease of description.

The majority of haemostatic defects result in a tendency to bleed excessively. Hypercoagulable states are comparatively rare and are outside the scope of this chapter. Different defects produce different clinical syndromes and in defects of haemostasis the history is often more important than the physical examination.

First it is important to establish whether excessive bleeding has taken place or not. This may be very difficult as 'a little blood goes a long way'. A history often has to be taken from the anxious mother of a child who has bled after dental extraction or tonsillectomy and it is useful to have some objective evidence of excessive haemorrhage from another source, e.g. the need for blood transfusion recorded in the hospital notes.

The history should include the following questions:

Does spontaneous bleeding occur (e.g. epistaxis, joint or muscle haemorrhage)? Is haemorrhage excessive after trivial trauma (e.g. easy bruising or haematoma formation during every-day life or gentle sports)? Is haemorrhage excessive only after severe trauma? E.g. has there been severe haemorrhage after tonsillectomy, dental extraction or appendicectomy? If so has this happened on more than one occasion?

Has there been any blood in the vomit (haematemesis), altered blood in the stools (melaena) or blood in the urine (haematuria)? Has the patient noticed any small red blood spots (purpura) on the skin or in the mouth? Do the gums bleed? In women, has menstruation been excessive? Does the patient enjoy good general health? Follow up any specific points.

Can the patient remember any previous incident involving excessive haemorrhage at any time? Is there a family history of excessive haemorrhage and if so what is the pattern of inheritance?

What drugs is the patient taking and what drugs have been taken in the recent past? Aspirin is the most common drug to consider because of its various effects on the haemostatic mechanism and because it is often included in proprietary preparations which the patient may not regard as 'drugs'. It is also important to make sure that the patient is not taking oral anticoagulants.

What is the patient's occupation? Does he come into contact with any dangerous chemicals? These questions are obviously important in the analysis of the cause of any defect. If a defect is found it may influence the choice of occupation for the patient in the future, e.g. a patient with haemophilia makes a poor security guard.

Physical examination will demonstrate whether or not there is any damage from previous excessive haemorrhage: large untidy scars may be due to previous wound haematomata and recurrent haemarthroses may cause degenerative joint disease. The skin, mucous membranes and fundi should be examined for purpura, petechial haemorrhages and bruises. Examination of the lymph nodes, liver and spleen may reveal a white cell abnormality.

Having discussed the clinical aspects of haemostasis it is worth discussing interpretation briefly. Haemorrhage due to vessel wall and platelet defects tends to be from the mucous membranes and into the skin. In patients with hereditary telangiectasia, bleeding occurs from the nose, mouth and gastrointestinal tract and also sometimes from the urinary tract. Patients with reduced numbers of platelets (thrombocytopenia) also suffer from nose bleeds and purpura, and bleed excessively at surgery. The degree of haemostatic defect depends on the number of circulating platelets (see below). In patients with a coagulation defect primary haemostasis, which relies on platelet function, may be normal but haemorrhage occurs after surgery often after a short delay. In severe coagulation defects spontaneous haemorrhage may occur especially into joints and muscles but intra-abdominal and intracranial haemorrhage are also well described. In von Willebrand's disease both platelet function and the coagulation mechanism are abnormal and there is a mixed clinical picture though the platelet functional defect predominates.

Laboratory tests can only be undertaken after a full clinical assessment. There is little place in modern haematology for bedside tests such as the Hess capillary fragility test, but the Lee and White clotting time may be useful in the bedside control of heparin treatment. The bleeding time test is still frequently performed.

The bleeding time

The bleeding time test is an in vivo test of platelet function. It involves making a small wound and measuring the time taken for bleeding to cease. The two methods commonly used are Ivy's method and Duke's method.

Ivy's method. A cuff is placed round the upper arm and is inflated to 40 mmHg. The forearm is cleaned and three cuts or puncture marks are made with a standard lance taking care to avoid damaging veins. Every 15 seconds the blood is gently removed with a filter paper, without pressing on the arm, until bleeding ceases. This usually takes less than six minutes but varies with the method used. The average of the three readings is taken ignoring wounds that fail to bleed and wounds that have obviously damaged veins. As can be seen, this test is not easy to reproduce or standardize. It should be avoided when a patient is known to be thrombocytopenic as it then serves no useful purpose and may cause severe bleeding into the forearm.

Duke's method. The ear lobe is stabbed by a standard lance and the blood removed as for the Ivy method. This technique is even more difficult to standardize than the Ivy method but it may be less traumatic especially in young children.

Laboratory tests of haemostasis

A peripheral film should always be examined and particular attention paid to platelet numbers and morphology.

The standard tests are the platelet count and the tests which measure the various parts of the coagulation mechanism (Fig. 13.3). Other tests are useful in special circumstances.

Platelet count. The normal range of platelet count is 150–400 $\times$ 10^9/litre. Platelet numbers can be estimated roughly from the peripheral film and this examination is usually enough for emergencies. Platelets can also be counted visually but automatic machines are usually used. These rely on interruption of an electric field or a light path and details of these methods are outside the scope of this chapter.

The platelet count is reduced in bone marrow failure from any cause and in conditions where peripheral destruction of platelets

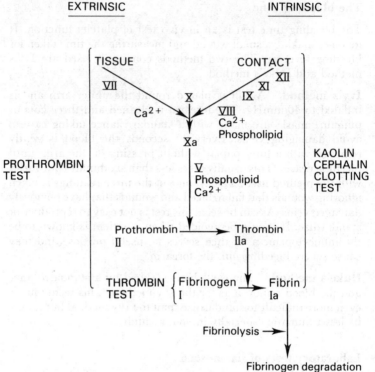

Fig. 13.3 The coagulation and fibrinolytic mechanisms.

takes place for immunological reasons (e.g. idiopathic thrombocytopenic purpura) or because of trapping and/or destruction by an enlarged spleen (e.g. myelofibrosis). Thrombocytopenia also takes place after massive blood transfusion as stored blood does not contain viable platelets. When the platelet count is above 100×10^9/litre no clinical symptoms arise; between 50 and 100×10^9/litre bleeding may occur after major surgery or trauma and between 20 and 50×10^9/litre after minor trauma. Below 20 and 10^9/litre spontaneous haemorrhage may occur and purpura is very likely. At very low platelet counts there is a risk of fatal cerebral haemorrhage.

The platelet count is increased in many myeloproliferative diseases and thrombocytosis may occur in Hodgkin's disease or after chronic haemorrhage. Sometimes thrombosis or bleeding may occur as a result.

Many qualitative platelet defects are described. Apart from the effects of aspirin ingestion most of these are very rare and their investigation requires sophisticated tests of platelet function such as platelet adhesion and aggregation which cannot be described here.

The prothrombin test and ratio (PTR). The PTR is the most commonly performed coagulation test and measures the extrinsic coagulation pathway (Factors VII, X, V, II and I) (Fig. 13.3). Citrate is used as an anticoagulant in a volume of one part citrate to nine parts blood. Platelet-poor plasma is obtained by centrifugation and is added to an equal volume of human brain extract at $37°C$ (tissue thromboplastin). After recalcification with 0.025 M calcium chloride a clot forms in approximately 13 seconds using normal plasma. The test is performed in duplicate and the result is compared with that obtained from a pooled normal control. The result is expressed as a ratio of the control sample, i.e. if the test sample takes 26 seconds to clot the ratio is 2.0. Human brain thromboplastin is now standardized in the United Kingdom so that prothrombin ratios should be comparable in different parts of the country.

Situations in which the PTR is abnormal include:

1. The use of oral anticoagulants (therapeutic ratio 2:3 and heparin)
2. Hepatic failure
3. Haemorrhagic disease of the newborn
4. Intravascular coagulation

In practice the test is usually performed to control the dose of oral anticoagulants (e.g. warfarin). These vitamin K antagonists inhibit the formation of factors II, VII, IX and X. The prothrombin ratio is chosen mainly because it is easy and rapid to perform.

A commercial test (Thrombotest) is also available for the control of oral anticoagulants and works on the same basic principle as the prothrombin test. It can be performed on plasma or capillary blood but is not as popular as the prothrombin test.

The Kaolin Cephalin Clotting Test (KCCT). The KCCT, also known as the partial thromboplastin test (PTT), also uses citrated platelet-poor plasma and measures the intrinsic coagulation pathway (Factors XII, XI, IX, VIII, X, V, II, I) (Fig. 13.3). Plasma is added to a mixture of kaolin (surface contact) and cephalin (phospholipid) and is incubated for two minutes at 37°C. After calcification with 0·025 M calcium chloride a clot forms in approximately 40 seconds. The result is not usually expressed as a ratio and the test is more difficult to standardize than the PTR.

Situations in which the KCCT is abnormal include:

1. Haemophilia (Factor VIII or IX deficiency)
2. Von Willebrand's disease (Factor VIII deficiency with associated Factor VIII related platelet defect)
3. Contact factor deficiency (Factor XII or XI deficiency)
4. Anticoagulant therapy
5. Hepatic failure
6. Intravascular coagulation

Factor VIII and IX deficiency (haemophilia) make up over 90% of inherited coagulation defects and the test is used as a screening test for these conditions. It has also been used for the laboratory control of heparin treatment (see below).

Thrombin Test (TT). An equal volume of thrombin (or a calcium and thrombin mixture) is added to citrated platelet-poor plasma. A clot forms in about 10 seconds. Only the final reaction of fibrin formation from fibrinogen is measured (see Fig. 13.3). The test is abnormal in the presence of hypofibrinogenaemia, dysfibrinogenaemia, heparin or fibrinogen degradation products (FDPs). It is used to monitor heparin therapy and is preferable to the KCCT for this purpose as the clot takes a shorter time to form. It is also used in the diagnosis of intravascular coagulation.

PARASITES IN THE BLOOD

In fresh blood viewed under a coverslip, some parasites, such as microfilariae and trypanosomes, may be seen alive and moving; others may be seen in thick or thin, fixed and stained films. The important parasites of the blood are those of malaria, microfilariae of several varieties, trypanosomes, Leishman–Donovan bodies and the spirochaetes of relapsing fever.

Malaria

For the diagnosis of malaria, thick films should be used for the detection of parasites and thin films for their identification. Films should preferably be taken when the patient's temperature is raised. Thick films should be examined systematically for 10–15 minutes before concluding that no parasites are present. The recognition of parasites in thick films requires practice. White cells, platelets, bacteria, the remains of reticulocytes and miscellaneous dirt can be mistaken for parasites. Parasites have definite morphological and staining properties and objects which do not show these are not parasites.

For details of the identification of the different types of parasites in thin films, larger works must be consulted. The main distinguishing points are as follows (Plate XI).

In infection with *Plasmodium falciparum*, which produces malignant tertian malaria, schizogony generally takes place in the tissues, so that except in rare cases in moribund patients, only ring forms and a few crescent-shaped gametocytes are seen in the peripheral red blood cells. Ring forms of any species consist of a rim of cytoplasm which stains blue and a small nucleus or chromatin dot which stains red. The rings of *Plasmodium falciparum* are usually, though not invariably, small and delicate, and the red cells are not enlarged. More than one ring may appear in a single red cell and some rings may have two chromatin dots. Marginal forms or *formes appliquées* with the parasite lying along the edge of the cell may be seen. A few crescent-shaped gametocytes, which are easily recognized (Plate XI), may have been seen in films from untreated patients, but if absent at this time they may appear some 7–10 days after the beginning of treatment.

In the remaining three species, schizogony takes place in the peripheral blood, so that ring forms, large trophozoites and schizonts will be present together in films.

In infections with *Plasmodium vivax*, which produces benign tertian malaria, the rings are large and stout and often measure one-third of the diameter of the red cell. The red cells may be enlarged, and if properly stained may show well marked

Schüffner's dots (Plate XI). Large irregular trophozoites containing brown pigment, and mature schizonts with 12–24 merozoites, may be seen (Plate XI).

In infections with *Plasmodium malariae*, which produces quartan malaria, the ring forms are also large and stout, but the larger trophozoites are more compact and dense-looking and frequently take a characteristic band form (Plate XI). Mature schizonts contain some 8 merozoites arranged in a rosette form around a mass of golden yellow pigment. Further, Schüffner's dots are not seen and the red cells are not enlarged.

In infection with *Plasmodium ovale*, which is much the rarest of the four species, the parasites have some of the characteristics of *Plasmodium vivax* (e.g. large and prominent Schüffner's dots) and others of *Plasmodium malariae* (e.g. compact large trophozoites and occasional band forms). The most characteristic feature is the distortion in shape of the red cells, which become oval or fimbriated, and the schizonts only contain 8–10 merozoites (Plate XI).

In some cases, mixed infections may be present.

Trypanosomiasis

In the diagnosis of trypanosomiasis, examination of the blood is generally less efficient than the examination of fluid obtained by gland puncture. An enlarged gland, usually in the posterior triangle of the neck, is held firmly between the thumb and fingers of the left hand, while a moderate sized hypodermic needle is plunged through the skin and into the substance of the gland. A small amount of gland fluid passes into the needle and suction is neither necessary nor desirable. The needle is withdrawn and its contents blown out on to clean glass slides. The fluid should be examined fresh and unstained as described for fresh blood films; thin films should be stained with Leishman's stain.

Trypanosomes (Plate XI) may also be found in thick or thin blood films and, in advanced cases, in films made from the deposit of centrifuged cerebrospinal fluid. (For methods of concentrating trypanosomes in the blood, larger works must be consulted.)

The important trypanosomes of man are *Trypanosoma gambiense* and *T. rhodesiense*, which cause African sleeping sickness, and, as seen in human blood, are usually morphologically indistinguishable; and *Trypanosoma cruzei*, which causes Brazilian trypanosomiasis (Chagas's disease). The latter exists chiefly in a non-flagellated form in the organs and muscles and only occasionally appears in the blood as a flagellate trypanosome (Plate XI).

In a suspected case of trypanosomiasis, several specimens of gland fluid and of blood should be examined, both fresh and unstained, and in stained films. Trypanosomes may be seen 'lashing' their way amongst the cells and are often first detected by the commotion they produce in the latter. This movement must not be confused with that produced by the organisms of relapsing fever (*Borrelia recurrentis*) (Plate XI).

In stained films, typical trypanosomes are seen as elongated fusiform structures some 14–30 μm long and 1–3 μm broad with a longitudinal undulating membrane and a terminal flagellum projecting from the anterior end (Plate XI). There is a centrally placed nucleus, and at the posterior end a smaller black-staining kinetoplast. The shorter forms are more stumpy and may have little or no free flagellum.

Kala-azar

In the diagnosis of *kala-azar*, Leishman–Donovan bodies may be looked for in the blood or in material obtained by sternal, gland, spleen or liver puncture. Of these, examination of marrow obtained by sternal puncture (p. 438) is probably the simplest and safest method, but in occasional cases the parasites may be found by the examination of stained blood films, when they are seen in the cytoplasm of large mononuclear cells. When direct microscopic examination fails, culture methods (for which larger works must be consulted) are frequently successful.

The bodies may be seen in thick or thin stained blood films which should be searched systematically. The parasites are seen as round or oval bodies from 2 to 5 μm in diameter, containing a large round or oval solid-looking nucleus and a smaller more deeply stained and usually rod-shaped kinetoplast. In Leishman-stained films the cytoplasm is blue and the nucleus and kinetoplast are red (Plate XI). Giemsa staining is preferable.

While the term Leishman–Donovan bodies strictly applies to the Indian form of kala-azar, exactly similar *Leishmania* may be found in the blood or tissues in cases of Mediterranean kala-azar, from fluid obtained by puncture at the margin of the lesion in the various forms of cutaneous leishmaniasis or 'tropical sore', and from the mucous membranes of the mouth, nose or throat in espundia or South American leishmaniasis.

Microfilariae

Adult filarial worms or microfilariae are parasites of the lymphatic system or connective tissues. Their presence is diagnosed by the finding of their larvae or microfilariae in the blood stream. Three main varieties of microfilariae are found in the blood of man. These are:

1. *Filaria bancrofti* (*Wuchereria bancrofti*) which is found in the blood stream in any numbers only at night and which causes filariasis, characterized by irregular fever, lymphangitis and various forms of elephantiasis.

2. *Filaria loa-loa*, which is found in the blood stream only by day, and which causes loaisis, characterized by transient red painful swellings known as calabar swellings.

3. *Filaria perstans*, which is non-periodic, appearing equally by day and night, and has no recognized pathogenic effects.

If filariasis is suspected, blood should be examined say at 8 a.m., noon and 4 p.m., and again at 8 p.m., midnight and 4 a.m. Fresh unstained films should be used for the detection of the filariae, and stained ones, thick if the larvae are scanty and thin if they are plentiful, for their identification.

In fresh unstained films microfilariae are easily seen as actively moving linear objects. In stained films they are seen as wormlike objects with a round head and a pointed tail, from 5 to 8 μm broad (i.e. about the diameter of a red cell) and from 100 to 300 μm long (Plate XI). The main differentiating features of the three species, apart from their periodicity, are as follows. *Filaria bancrofti* and *F. loa-loa* have a delicate sheath, which can be seen where it projects beyond the rounded head and pointed tail of the larva, whereas *F. perstans* is unsheathed. All larvae have a central column of nuclei extending from the head more or less to the tail. In *F. loa-loa* and *F. perstans* the nuclei extend to the extreme tip of the tail, whereas in *F. bancrofti* the column ends short of the tip.

Microfilariae do not stain well by Leishman's stain. Thick films should be dehaemoglobinized and stained by Giemsa.

Microfilariae are readily recognized by the intense staining of their nuclei, and the sheath, if present, is easily seen.

Relapsing fever

The *Borrelia recurrentis* of relapsing fever should be sought in fresh unstained films of blood and in thin films stained by Leishman's method under the oil-immersion. Fresh unstained films should be examined with the light well cut down. Agitation of the red cells usually calls attention to the presence of parasites, which may otherwise be difficult to detect.

In thin stained films the spirochaete is seen as a linear object with tapering ends, 0.4 μm in breadth and $10-30$ μm in length. The spiral shape which it possesses in life is lost and the body lies in irregular curves. In searching for the oganism, it is important to direct the eyes deliberately to the spaces between the red cells rather than to the red cells, or the parasite may be missed.

14

Using the laboratory

What investigation to request
What information to send
Collection of specimens
Making the best use of results

Cooperation with laboratories requires mutual understanding between clinicians and laboratory workers. Pathology now embraces a series of specialized subjects and clinicians cannot be expected to be familiar with the detailed performance of all tests that they request. However they should know the following:

1. What *investigation* to request in given circumstances.
2. The discomfort and possible risk to the patient of an investigation.
3. What *information* the pathologist requires about the patient.
4. What *specimens* are required and how they should be obtained and transmitted to the laboratory.
5. The approximate cost in time and money of an investigation.
6. The possible risk of a specimen to the laboratory worker (infected material or Australia antigen-positive sera).
7. How to make the *best use* of the results received from the laboratory. In the case of complicated investigations, the clinician and the pathologist should agree a programme of investigation and discuss the results.

WHAT INVESTIGATION TO REQUEST

The result of any laboratory investigation is only one part of the information required to make a diagnosis. It may have as much or as little significance as any other physical finding. The plan of investigation has to be decided from the facts elicited by history taking and physical examination. However the widespread use of automation in haematology and biochemistry means that tests are often performed in a 'package'. It is necessary to know what is offered in each package and to choose the appropriate one, rather than the single test. The availability of these routines should not lead to the abandonment of the eclectic approach that adds to the patient's comfort, the speed of diagnosis and the continued education of the doctor.

Certain investigations are often necessary to monitor the natural history of a disease and its treatment. For example the white blood cell count has to be followed serially in cases of leukaemia and the sedimentation rate in rheumatoid arthritis. There should therefore be a planned series of repeat tests, as is often necessary when following the resolution of a metabolic disorder. Tests should not be repeated without good reason and, if repeated, the interval between them should be logically decided.

WHAT INFORMATION TO SEND

A source of serious error can be failure to identify correctly the source of a specimen from a given patient. Therefore laboratories design their request forms with care and it is essential that all details required are filled in, accurately and legibly. Usually it is necessary to record the patient's surname and first name, address (or ward and bed number), the hospital serial number and the sex and date of birth of the patient. These details are all the more necessary in parts of the world where many family names are very similar.

Requests must also indicate the exact nature of the material sent, its source and the precise nature of the investigations required. The date on which the specimen is collected must be recorded. For many biochemical tests it is necessary to record the exact time at which the specimen is collected.

It is desirable that the patient's tentative diagnosis should be recorded together with any relevant clinical comment. A note of current antibiotic therapy is necessary with all requests for bacteriologial examinations. Any therapy that might influence biochemical investigations should be recorded.

COLLECTION OF SPECIMENS

It is essential that specimens reach the laboratory fresh and in the correct kind of containers. Specimens are best taken by hand to the laboratory as soon as they are obtained, but they can, if necessary, be sent by post (letter post only), provided they are suitably packed and labelled 'Fragile, With Care' and 'Pathological Specimen'. Such specimens must be placed in a sealed inner container and then packed in a wooden or metal box containing sufficient absorbent material to soak up all the liquid contents if the inner container is broken. Local and international regulations about the transmission of pathological material must be strictly adhered to.

Suitable containers are best obtained from the laboratory that is going to make the investigations. All containers must be perfectly clean and preferably sterile. This is of course essential for bacteriological specimens. Containers for blood should be completely dry. All containers must have properly fitting lids or caps. It is usually essential that the correct container should be used for each particular investigation (e.g. particular anticoagulants are necessary for particular chemical or other tests on blood). It is also desirable that the amount of material specified for a particular container should be placed in that container, and in any case no more than the amount specified.

All syringes and needles must be sterile and should either be of the disposable type or be dry-sterilized in a laboratory.

Venepuncture

A piece of rubber tubing is used as a tourniquet and applied round the upper arm over the middle of the biceps, so as to impede the venous but not the arterial flow. The skin at the bend of the elbow is 'painted' with 0·5% chlorhexidine in 70% alcohol or simply 70% spirit (iodine is expensive and can give rise to severe skin reactions). The skin is rendered tense by the operator's left hand; the syringe with the needle attached is held in the right hand and almost parallel with the patient's arm; the patient is asked to 'make a fist' and then the needle with the bevel upwards is inserted into a prominent vein—the median basilic is usually convenient—and the needle is pointed in the direction of the blood flow. The required amount of blood is then drawn up into the syringe and the tourniquet is removed before the needle is withdrawn, as otherwise a haematoma may form. For some purposes it is necessary to remove the tourniquet as soon as the needle enters the vein, so that free-flowing blood is withdrawn. As soon as the needle is withdrawn a swab is placed on the puncture site and the patient is instructed to hold his forearm firmly flexed against his arm for a minute or so. Occasionally a vein in the forearm or wrist may prove more convenient than one at the elbow, but the procedure is then usually more painful. A vein which can be *felt* is generally easier to enter than one which can only be *seen*.

Blood obtained by venepuncture should be placed immediately in a container suitable for the purpose for which it is to be used. The needle should first be removed from the syringe, since forcing the blood through the needle may cause haemolysis. Appropriate containers for particular investigations should be obtained from the laboratory, since, when unclotted blood is required, different anticoagulants are needed for particular purposes.

Heparin and sequestrene (EDTA) are the most generally useful anticoagulants. Sequestrene can be used for most haematological investigations and heparin for most simple chemical tests, with the exception of blood glucose for which bottles containing sodium fluoride are necessary.

For blood groups and serological investigations blood should be taken into a dry sterile bottle or tube. If the specimen has to be sent to the laboratory by post, it is best to wait till the blood has clotted. Some serum should then be removed with a sterile needle and syringe, and this serum should be sent separately, together with the blood clot.

Lumbar puncture.   See p. 333.

MAKING THE BEST USE OF RESULTS

It is merely stating the obvious to say that the interpretation of any laboratory test will depend on the relevance of the test to the presumptive diagnosis and the interpreter's knowledge of pathology, biochemistry and physiology. The task of a clinical laboratory is to put these disciplines to work in the solution of a diagnostic problem.

All tests are subject to errors of performance. Fortunately these are rare but the clinician will help the pathologist if he tells him of any 'rogue' result that does not accord with other data. All results will depend on the precision of the method used and the variability of the quality measured amongst a healthy population.

In non-quantitative tests, as in cytology, there may be false positives and false negatives. The laboratory should be able to say with what frequency these may occur. For instance, in cases of bronchial carcinoma, malignant cells are often to be detected in the sputum; however, in a very small proportion of examinations, apparently malignant cells in the sputum will be reported when there is no bronchial carcinoma. The clinician can give some weight to such finding by considering the patient. If the patient is a middle-aged man who smoked heavily, the report of malignant cells would be likely to be a true positive as bronchial carcinoma is prevalent in such patients. Conversely, if the patient is a non-smoking girl the positive sputum report would be likely to be false.

For quantitative tests, as in biochemistry and much of haematology, the precision of a test can be determined statistically and its performance monitored within the laboratory and by co-operation with other laboratories.

Precision is the measure of the repeatability of a determination. If the method is very precise the spread of results around the 'true' value will be small and vice versa. The precision of measurement has to be linked to the variations of the 'true' value as found in a population of, say, 1000 healthy people. The results of the measurement performed on this group of normals can be plotted as a Gaussian curve on either side of the mean value. It is conventional to express this normal range as the mean value of plus/minus two standard deviations. Within this range will fall 95% of all normal results. However it has to be remembered that one in 20 of normal results will fall just outside the normal range. Therefore a value just outside the range of normal does not necessarily indicate abnormality. It should also be remembered that normal ranges have to be established for the sex and age of the groups studied and also for the method as performed in each laboratory.

Appendix

Centigrade and Fahrenheit scales
SI units
Some approximate conversion tables

CENTIGRADE AND FAHRENHEIT SCALES

The Centigrade (Celsius) scale is preferred.
The following table shows the relationship of the Centigrade and Fahrenheit scales, as far as is likely to be required in clinical work.

Centigrade	Fahrenheit	Centigrade	Fahrenheit
110	230	36·5	97·7
100	212	36	96·8
95	203	35·5	95·9
90	194	35	95
85	185	34	93·2
80	176	33	91·4
75	167	32	89·6
70	158	31	87·8
65	149	30	86
60	140	25	77
55	131	20	68
50	122	15	59
45	113	10	50
44	111·2	5	41
43	109·4	0	32
42	107·6	⁻5	23
41	105·8	⁻10	14
40·5	104·9	⁻15	5
40	104	⁻20	⁻4
39·5	103·1		
39	102·2	0·54	1
38·5	101·3	1	1·8
38	100·4	2	3·6
37·5	99·5	2·5	4·5
37	98·6		

To convert Fahrenheit to Centigrade:

$$X°F - 32 \times \frac{5}{9} = Y°C$$

To convert Centigrade to Fahrenheit:

$$X°C \times \frac{9}{5} + 32 = Y°F$$

SI UNITS

In this book the Système International d'Unités has been used as far as possible. This system aims to derive all measurements from seven basic units and to express all measurements as decimal fractions or multiples of these. Of the seven basic units the four which appear in this book are:

Physical quantity	Name of SI unit	Symbol
length	metre	m
mass	kilogram	kg
time	second	s
amount of substance	mole	mol

and the prefixes indicating the decimal fractions and multiples are:

Fraction	Prefix	Symbol
10^{-1}	deci-	d
10^{-2}	centi-	c
10^{-3}	milli-	m
10^{-6}	micro-	μ
10^{-9}	nano-	n
10^{-12}	pico-	p
10^{-15}	femto-	f

Multiple	Prefix	Symbol
10	deca-	da
10^2	hecto-	h
10^3	kilo-	k
10^6	mega	M

The litre ($1 = dm^3$) is also recognized as the unit of volume.

It follows that when SI is adopted certain familiar terms will no longer be used, as is the case with measures of volume. A cubic centimetre (cc, cm^3) is replaced by the millilitre (ml) and the cubic millimetre (cmm, mm^3) by the microlitre (μl). In linear measure the micron (μ) should no longer be used; the correct unit is the micrometre (μm). Blood, intrauterine and intra-ocular pressures are measured in millimetres of mercury (mmHg) and intrathecal pressures in centimetres of CSF (cm CSF). It is recommended that the medical calorie or kilocalorie should now be converted to the joule (1 kCal = 4186·8 J).

Further information on SI units may be obtained from *The Use of SI Units*, Publication PD 5686 of the British Standards Insitution, and useful information on the SI units commonly used in medicine and biology is available in *Units, Symbols and Abbreviations: A Guide for Biological and Medical Editors and Authors*, published by the Royal Society of Medicine.

SOME APPROXIMATE CONVERSION TABLES

1 fluid ounce (fl oz)	= 28 ml
1 gallon UK (gal)	= 4·5 litres
1 grain (do not abbreviate)	= 65 mg
1 inch (in)	= 25·4 mm
1 foot (ft)	= 0·3 m
1 ounce (oz)	= 28 g
1 pound (lb)	= 0·45 kg
1 calorie (cal)	= 4·2 J
1 kilocalorie (medical calorie)	= 4·2 kJ

Index

Note: Page numbers of figures and tables are in *italic* type.